Child, Adolescent and Family Refugee Mental Health

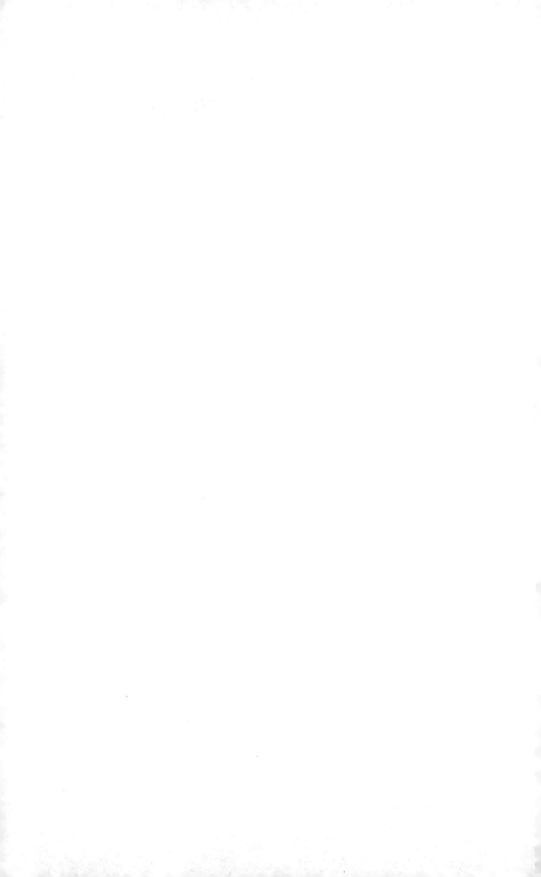

CPSIA information can be obtained
at www.ICGtesting.com
Printed in the USA
LVHW081409170620
658353LV00008B/1034

9 783030 452773

Suzan J. Song • Peter Ventevogel
Editors

Child, Adolescent and Family Refugee Mental Health

A Global Perspective

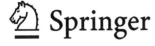

Editors
Suzan J. Song
Department of Psychiatry
George Washington University
Washington, DC
USA

Peter Ventevogel
Public Health Section (Division
of Resilience and Solutions)
United Nations High Commissioner
for Refugees
Genève
Geneve
Switzerland

ISBN 978-3-030-45277-3   ISBN 978-3-030-45278-0   (eBook)
https://doi.org/10.1007/978-3-030-45278-0

This Springer imprint is published by the registered company Springer Nature Switzerland AG
The registered company address is: Gewerbestrasse 11, 6330 Cham, Switzerland

Foreword

Meeting the mental health needs of child and adolescent refugees poses major problems for all communities. Most mental health workers are well trained in helping individual families and children, but few are experienced in meeting the very complex needs of refugees. For a start, the sheer numbers are currently overwhelming. With many low- and middle-income countries having few qualified mental health personnel, how can they be expected to meet the acute and chronic needs of forced migrants? Faced with such challenges, people usually fall back on adapting and applying their existing skills and knowledge which may not always be appropriate. This welcome text in turn challenges many assumptions and points the way to applying better understanding based on contemporary models of child and family development.

Historically, it has to be conceded that many mental health workers responded to the perceived needs of refugees focusing on mainly individual therapeutic interventions. However, it soon became clear that these were insufficient in themselves and may even have been harmful. Cultural differences in understanding of mental health and widely differing contexts of family life rightly posed challenges. Focusing on stress reactions was seen as ignoring strengths and resilience. Outsiders rushing in to help without understanding the background of survivors and without knowing the supports and barriers within communities were inevitably less effective than they might have been.

This book provides helpful lessons from a wide range of academic and applied perspectives. Considerations of culture and the need to see the child in the context of family and community provide suggestions for improving the assessment of needs. Good, sensitive interviewing techniques—both with parents and children—form the basis of most assessments. Healthy skepticism is aired about questionnaires but screening remains a necessity. Similarly, while warning against an exclusive individual therapeutic approach, the particular needs of children with developmental disabilities, substance abuse, depression, grief and, yes, even PTSD are discussed. Throughout there are clinical examples that bring the issues to life.

One overriding problem is the great lack of acceptable evidence for the approaches recommended. At the wider community level, psychosocial interventions that claim they are not "clinical" offer help at what seems to be an acceptable level. But where is the evidence that safe child spaces or even psychological first aid are really effective in helping refugee children adjust to their reactions to being uprooted? Difficult as it is, there is a moral as well as scientific imperative to evaluate all efforts to help.

While the main approaches discussed rightly argue that children should be supported along with and within their families, a high percentage of child refugees arrive at a hopefully safe and welcoming country but alone. The additional issues that unaccompanied minors pose to authorities require even greater planning. This, and evaluation, will feature in the next edition of this book, provided the mental health community takes heed of the lessons given here.

London, United Kingdom   William Yule

Contents

Contributors

Abdirahman Abdi Shanbaro Community Association, Chelsea Collaborative, Chelsea, MA, USA

Julia Bala, PhD ARQ National Psychotrauma Centre, Diemen, The Netherlands

Cyril Bennouna, MPH Political Science, Brown University, Providence, RI, USA

Lidewyde H. Berckmoes, PhD African Studies Centre, Leiden University, Leiden, The Netherlands

Jenna M. Berent, MPH Research Program on Children and Adversity, Boston College School of Social Work, Chestnut Hill, MA, USA

Theresa S. Betancourt, ScD, MA Research Program on Children and Adversity, Boston College School of Social Work, Chestnut Hill, MA, USA

Vanessa Cavallera, MD, MPH Independent Consultant, Milan, Italy

Neerja Chowdhary, MD Department of Mental Health and Substance Abuse, World Health Organization, Geneva, Switzerland

Matty R. Crone, PhD Department of Public Health & Primary Care, Leiden University Medical Center (LUMC), Leiden, The Netherlands

Anne-Sophie Dybdal, MSc Save The Children Denmark, Frederiksberg, Denmark

Rochelle L. Frounfelker, ScD, MPH, MSSW Division of Social and Transcultural Psychiatry, Department of Psychiatry, McGill University, Montreal, QC, Canada

Melanie M. Gagnon, PhD CIUSSS West-Central Montreal, Montreal, QC, Canada

Bhuwan Gautam, MPA Bhutanese Society of Western Massachusetts, Inc., Springfield, MA, USA

M. Claire Greene, PhD, MPH Department of Psychiatry, Columbia University/ New York State Psychiatric Institute, New York, NY, USA

Johns Hopkins Bloomberg School of Public Health, Baltimore, MD, USA

Zeinab Hijazi, MsC, PsyD Mental Health and Psychosocial Support Specialist, Child Protection in Emergencies, Programme Division, New York, NY, USA

Lynne Jones, OBE, FRC Psych., PhD FXB Center for Health and Human Rights, Harvard University, Cambridge, MA, USA

Joop T. V. M. de Jong, MD, PhD Cultural Psychiatry and Global Mental Health, Amsterdam UMC, Amsterdam, The Netherlands

Boston University School of Medicine, Boston, MA, USA

Jeremy C. Kane, PhD, MPH Johns Hopkins Bloomberg School of Public Health, Baltimore, MD, USA

Department of Epidemiology, Columbia University, New York, NY, USA

Nancy H. Liu, PhD Department of Psychology, University of California, Berkeley, Berkeley, CA, USA

Tej Mishra, MPH Research Program on Children and Adversity, Boston College School of Social Work, Chestnut Hill, MA, USA

Trudy Mooren, PhD ARQ Centrum'45, Diemen, The Netherlands

Kerim Munir, MD, MPH, DSc Boston Children's Hospital, Harvard Medical School, Boston, MA, USA

Ramzi Nasir, MD, MPH Consultant in Developmental Behavioral Pediatrics, London, UK

Julia Oakley, LCSW Northern Virginia Family Services, Program for Survivors of Severe Torture and Trauma, Arlington, VA, USA

Yoke Rabaia, PhD Institute of Community and Public Health, Birzeit University, Birzeit, Palestine

Ria Reis, PhD Department of Public Health & Primary Care, Leiden University Medical Center (LUMC), Leiden, The Netherlands

Department of Anthropology, University of Amsterdam, Amsterdam, The Netherlands

Amsterdam Institute for Global Health and Development (AIGHD), Amsterdam, The Netherlands

The Children's Institute, School of Child and Adolescent Health, University of Cape Town, Cape Town, South Africa

Cécile Rousseau, MD Division of Social and Cultural Psychiatry, McGill University, Montreal, QC, Canada

Leslie Snider, MD, MPH The MHPSS Collaborative, Save the Children, Copenhagen, Denmark

Suzan J. Song, MD, MPH, PhD Department of Psychiatry, George Washington University, Washington, DC, USA

Lindsay Stark, DrPH Brown School, Washington University in St. Louis, St. Louis, MO, USA

Peter Ventevogel, MD, PhD Public Health Section (Division of Resilience and Solutions), United Nations High Commissioner for Refugees, Geneva, Switzerland

An Verelst, PhD Department of Social Work and Social Pedalogy, Ghent University, Gent, Belgium

Sophie Vindevogel, PhD Department of Social Educational Carework, University of Applied Sciences and Arts Ghent, Gent, Belgium

Michael G. Wessells, PhD Program on Forced Migration and Health, Columbia University, New York, NY, USA

About the Authors

Abdirahman Abdi is a Somali Bantu community leader and partner with the "Refugee Behavioral Health Program" at the Research Program on Children and Adversity at Boston College School of Social Work, Chestnut Hill, Massachusetts, USA.

Julia Bala, PhD is a clinical psychologist, psychotherapist, and independent consultant, a former staff member of ARQ Centrum45 in the Netherlands. Her main fields of interest include the intergenerational consequences of trauma, preventive multi-family interventions, and strengthening family resilience.

Cyril Bennouna, MPH is a Fellow at the Center for Human Rights and Humanitarian Studies and a PhD student in comparative politics and international relations at Brown University. His research focuses on the politics of forced migration and efforts to reduce violence against civilians during armed conflict.

Lidewyde H. Berckmoes, PhD is assistant professor at the African Studies Centre at Leiden University in the Netherlands. Having a background in anthropology, her research focus is on the long-term effects of conflict and violence on children and youth in war-affected and refugee contexts. She has extensive research experience in the Great Lakes region, particularly Burundi.

Jenna M. Berent, MPH is a program manager for the "Refugee Behavioral Health Program" at the Research Program on Children and Adversity at Boston College School of Social Work, Chestnut Hill, Massachusetts, USA.

Theresa S. Betancourt, ScD, MA is the inaugural Salem Professor in Global Practice at the Boston College School of Social Work and Director of the Research Program on Children and Adversity, Chestnut Hill, Massachusetts, USA.

Vanessa Cavallera, MD, MPH is child neurologist and psychiatrist with a Master's Degree in Public Health. She has been working for the World Health Organization and other UN agencies and NGOs focusing on early childhood development and child and adolescent mental health in developing and humanitarian contexts.

Neerja Chowdhary, MD Technical Officer in the Department of Mental Health and Substance Use, World Health Organization, Geneva.

A psychiatrist by training, she works as part of WHO's brain health team, supporting implementation of the global action plan on the public health response to dementia 2017–2025. Her other areas of work include provision of technical assistance for WHO's mental health Gap Action Programme (mhGAP) including development of training and guidance documents and providing technical support to country implementation. She is one of the co-authors of the WHO guidelines for the management of physical health conditions in people with severe mental disorders.

Mathilde R. Crone, PhD is a health scientist and has extensive research experience in the field of public health, in particular child health. She has particular expertise in exploring the determinants of (un)healthy behavior and chronic physical and mental health conditions of children/adults, evaluation studies of (preventive) care programs, and implementation studies. https://www.researchgate.net/profile/Matty_Crone/publications

Anne-Sophie Dybdal, MSc is a Licensed Clinical Child Psychologist from University of Copenhagen. She has 28 years of experience working with children and families with a focus on child development, resilience and well-being. Anne-Sophie Dybdal has worked in the humanitarian sector since 2000 and from 2006 as senior child protection and MHPSS advisor for Save The Children Denmark. For the last 5 years she has been involved in implementation of the Save The Children Youth Resilience Programme, currently running in 10 countries globally, including in refugee camps and extremely vulnerable communities.

Rochelle L. Frounfelker, ScD, MPH, MSSW is a social epidemiologist and postdoctoral fellow in the Division of Social and Transcultural Psychiatry, Department of Psychiatry, McGill University, Montreal, Canada.

Melanie M. Gagnon, PhD is a clinical psychologist. She is also responsible for coordinating the Center of Expertise for the Wellbeing and Physical Health of Refugees and Asylum Seekers at the Centre-Ouest-de-l'Île-de-Montréal CIUSSS. She is involved in the field of research and is a researcher-practitioner at the Sherpa Research Center, University Institute for Ethnocultural Communities.

Bhuwan Gautam, MPA is a Bhutanese community leader and co-investigator in the "Refugee Behavioral Health Program" at the Research Program on Children and Adversity at Boston College School of Social Work, Chestnut Hill, Massachusetts, USA.

M. Claire Greene, PhD, MPH is a psychiatric epidemiologist in the Department of Psychiatry at Columbia University. Her research focuses on the implementation and evaluation of interventions to address alcohol and other drug use, mental health, and psychosocial problems in humanitarian settings.

Zeinab Hijazi, MsC, PsyD is a Global Mental Health and Psychosocial Support Specialist, UNICEF, New York Headquarters.

Zeinab has 14 years of experience supporting MHPSS programs globally, and was in an advisory role with International Medical Corps providing guidance and oversight in the development, monitoring, evaluation, and running of culturally appropriate MHPSS activities in Lebanon, Jordan, Syria, Turkey, Palestine, Iraq, Tunisia, Libya, and Yemen.

At present, Zeinab is the MHPSS specialist and technical lead at UNICEF, and provides program guidance and technical support to enhance UNICEF's approach to the provision of mental health and psychosocial support for children and families in humanitarian settings. This includes supporting UNICEF country teams in designing and implementing locally relevant, comprehensive, and sustainable MHPSS strategies that (1) promote safe, nurturing environments for the recovery, psychosocial well-being, and protection of children; and (2) engage children, care-givers and families, community systems, and service providers at all levels of the social-ecological framework.

Lynne Jones, OBE, FRC Psych., PhD is a child psychiatrist, relief worker, and writer. She has spent much of the last 25 years establishing and running mental health programs in areas of conflict or natural disaster including the Balkans, East and West Africa, South East Asia, the Middle East, Haiti, and Central America. Most recently she has worked in the migrant crisis in Europe and Central America. She is a course director for the annual course on Mental Health in Complex Emergencies, run by the Institute of International Humanitarian Affairs at Fordham University, in collaboration with UNHCR. Her most recent book is *Outside the Asylum: A Memoir of War, Disaster and Humanitarian Psychiatry* (Orion 2017). Jones has an MA in human sciences from the University of Oxford. She qualified in medicine before specializing in psychiatry and has a PhD in social psychology and political science. In 2001, she was made an Officer of the British Empire for her work in child psychiatry in conflict-affected areas of Central Europe. She regularly consults for UNICEF and WHO. She is an honorary consultant at the Maudsley Hospital, London, and with Cornwall Partnership NHS Foundation Trust. She is a visiting scientist at the François-Xavier Bagnoud Centre for Health and Human Rights, Harvard University.

Joop T. V. M. de Jong, MD, PhD is Emeritus Professor of Cultural Psychiatry and Global Mental Health at UMC Amsterdam, Adjunct Professor of Psychiatry at Boston University School of Medicine, and Emeritus Visiting Professor of Psychology at Rhodes University, South Africa. He founded the Transcultural Psychosocial Organization (TPO), a relief organization in mental health and psychosocial care of (post)conflict and post-disaster populations in over 20 countries in Africa, Asia, and Europe. He worked part time as a psychotherapist and psychiatrist with immigrants and refugees in the Netherlands. His research interests focus on cultural psychiatry, public and global mental health, epidemiology, psychotraumatology, and medical anthropology.

Jeremy C. Kane, PhD, MPH is a psychiatric epidemiologist whose research is focused on measuring patterns of alcohol use, substance use, and related mental health problems among populations affected by HIV and violence in low- and middle-income countries and adapting, testing, and implementing evidence-based interventions for these problems.

Nancy H. Liu, PhD Assistant Clinical Professor, Department of Psychology, University of California, Berkeley.

Nancy is a clinical psychologist. Her expertise is in the clinical training and implementation of evidence-based psychological interventions for trauma, depression, and severe mental disorders. She teaches coursework in global mental health and clinical diagnosis, assessment, and interventions. She was a former Consultant with the WHO focusing on guidelines for reducing excess mortality in individuals with severe mental disorders.

Tej Mishra, MPH is an epidemiologist and researcher with the "Refugee Behavioral Health Program" at the Research Program on Children and Adversity at Boston College School of Social Work, Chestnut Hill, Massachusetts, USA.

Trudy Mooren, PhD is a clinical psychologist and senior researcher at ARQ Centrum'45 and Endowed Professor 'Family Functioning after Psychotrauma' at the Department of Clinical Psychology, Faculty of Social Sciences, Utrecht University. She studies the consequences of psychotrauma and forced migration for family functioning and is interested in assessment and interventions to support family resilience.

Kerim Munir, MD, MPH, DSc is Director of Psychiatry, University Center in Developmental Disabilities, Division of Developmental Medicine, Boston Children's Hospital, and Holmes Society Fellow in Global Health and Associate Professor of Psychiatry and Pediatrics, Harvard Medical School, Boston, USA.

Ramzi Nasir, MD, MPH is a Consultant Paediatrician in Developmental-Behavioral Paediatrics at the Royal Free London NHS Foundation Trust and the Portland Hospital, London, UK. He is involved in a variety of initiatives to promote the well-being of children with developmental disabilities in the humanitarian context.

Julia Oakley, LCSW is a mental health therapist and coordinator of the Program for Survivors of Torture and Severe Trauma at Northern Virginia Family Service's Multicultural Center in Falls Church, Virginia, USA. As part of a multilingual team offering mental health and immigration legal services, she works predominantly with asylum seekers, asylees, and refugees who are survivors of trauma. She earned a Master of Science in Social Work and a Master of International Affairs from Columbia University.

Yoke Rabaia, PhD conducts research related to mental and psychosocial health at the Community and Public Health Institute at Birzeit University, Palestine.

Ria Reis, PhD is a cultural anthropologist, specialized in religious and medical anthropology. Her research focus is on young people's health perceptions and strategies, the intergenerational transmission of vulnerabilities in contexts of inequality, and children's cultural idioms of distress. She is an expert in, and passionate about, the articulation of anthropological research within multidisciplinary (mental) health research and interventions.

Cécile Rousseau, MD is professor of the Division of Social and Cultural Psychiatry at McGill University. She has worked extensively with immigrant and refugee communities, developing specific school-based interventions and leading policy-oriented research. Presently her research focuses on intervention and prevention programs to address violent radicalization.

Leslie Snider, MD, MPH is a psychiatrist with over 20 years' experience in mental health and psychosocial support programs and research in diverse global settings. She serves as Director of the Global MHPSS Collaborative for Children and Families in Adversity, hosted by Save the Children Denmark. She began as a public mental health clinician while directing International Mental Health Studies for 10 years at Tulane Public Health School. Internationally, she collaborates with various UN agencies, governments, and NGOs in developing programs and quality care standards for children and families affected by disasters, conflict, HIV/AIDS, poverty and exploitation, and served as technical advisor to the US government, UNICEF, and others. She has over 40 publications, developed several widely used international resources for MHPSS in emergencies, and authored a children's book for children and caregivers affected by the Ebola crisis.

Suzan J. Song, MD, MPH, PhD is a double-board certified child/adolescent and adult psychiatrist and humanitarian mental health and psychosocial (MHPSS) consultant. Currently, she is Director of the Division of Child/Adolescent & Family Psychiatry and Associate Professor at George Washington University, spokesperson on Refugee Mental Health for the American Psychiatric Association, and subject matter expert to the US Department of Health and Human Services on refugee mental health and to the US State Department's Office to Monitor and Combat Trafficking in Persons. She has provided multiple testimonies to Congress on the mental health of unaccompanied minors and child trafficking. Her work as a humanitarian MHPSS consultant with UNHCR, UNICEF, the International Medical Corps, and the International Rescue Committee is informed by her clinical care of forcibly displaced children, adults, and families (survivors of torture, refugees, asylum seekers, unaccompanied minors, survivors of trafficking, and returned hostages) for over 10 years as medical director of two community clinics and in her current clinic. Dr. Song completed training from the University of Chicago, Harvard, Stanford, and the University of Amsterdam. Her two decades of global mental work span Sierra Leone, Liberia, Ethiopia, KwaZulu/Natal, Haiti, Burundi, Syria/Jordan, the D.R. Congo, and the USA as technical adviser to multiple refugee and survivor of torture programs.

Lindsay Stark, DrPH is an Associate Professor at Washington University in St. Louis' Brown School and an internationally recognized expert on the protection and well-being of women and children in situations of extreme adversity. Dr. Stark's particular area of expertise is measuring sensitive social phenomenon and evaluating related interventions that seek to reduce violence, abuse, and exploitation of women and children.

Peter Ventevogel, MD, PhD is a psychiatrist and a medical anthropologist. Since 2013, he has worked with UNHCR, the refugee agency of the United Nations, as their Senior Mental Health Officer based in Geneva. In this role he is responsible for providing guidance and technical support to the country operations of UNHCR worldwide. From 2008 to 2013 he was editor-in-chief of *Intervention, Journal for Mental Health and Psychosocial Support in Conflict Affected Areas*. He worked with the NGO HealthNet TPO in mental health projects in Afghanistan (2002–2005) and Burundi (2005–2008) and as their Technical Advisor Mental Health in the head office in Amsterdam (2008–2011). In 2011 and 2012 he also worked as psychiatrist with Arq Foundation, the national trauma expert center in the Netherlands. Peter regularly did consultancies for the World Health Organization and the UNHCR in Egypt, Jordan, Libya, Pakistan, Sudan, and Syria. He is involved in several academic short courses such the annual course Mental Health in Complex Emergencies (Fordham University, New York) and the Summer Institute Global Mental Health (Teachers College, Columbia University).

An Verelst, PhD is a clinical psychologist with a doctoral degree in Educational Sciences. Currently, An is project coordinator for Ghent University on a Horizon 2020 project called RefgueesWellSchool that evaluates the impact of six psychosocial interventions for young refugees and migrants in schools. Previously, she managed a psychosocial support center for children and communities affected by war in Eastern Congo where she also carried out her doctoral research on the psychosocial consequences of sexual violence during and after the armed conflict.

Sophie Vindevogel, PhD in educational sciences, has been working with populations affected by war and political violence for over ten years. Her research is situated at the intersection of strength-oriented, community-based, and transcultural approaches. It addresses stressors and resources in the context of stressful events and focuses primarily on how children, adolescents, families, and communities deal individually and collectively with various forms of adversity and what contributes to resilience and quality of life.

Michael Wessells, PhD is Professor at Columbia University in the Program on Forced Migration and Health. A long time psychosocial and child protection practitioner and researcher on the holistic impacts of war and political violence on children, he currently leads inter-agency, multi-country research on community-led child protection.

Part I

Theoretical Approaches to Comprehensive Understanding of Child, Adolescent, and Family Refugee Mental Health

Bridging the Humanitarian, Academic, and Clinical Fields Toward the Mental Health of Child and Adolescent Refugees

Peter Ventevogel and Suzan J. Song

Conceptual Debates in the Field of Child Refugee Mental Health

Many early publications on the effects of collective violence focused on posttraumatic stress disorder (PTSD), a diagnostic category that was only in 1980 enshrined in the third edition of the *Diagnostic and Statistical Manual* (DSM-III), the formal psychiatric classification system (DSM-III). While the concept was not completely new [26], the adoption by the DSM prompted major research efforts around PTSD. Increasingly, symptoms of PTSD were identified among children [90] including among resettled refugee children [3, 5, 36, 86]. However, from the beginning, there was a vocal group of critics who questioned the applicability of the concept among refugees. They argued that framing phenomena like recurrent memories, high vigilance, and loss of hope in refugees as symptoms of PTSD requiring medical treatment were an imposition of Western diagnostic categories. Doing so would ignore the social context that produces "symptoms" and as such only makes things worse by "pathologizing" reactions that could be better perceived as socially and culturally patterned adaptive reactions to adversity and loss [10, 21, 61].

Overall, the debate among mental health professionals around the presence of PTSD among refugees seems to have withered down over time, at least among mental health professionals working with refugees in high-income countries. In recent major publications around mental health of refugees and disaster-affected populations, the PSTD concept is not contested or seen as controversial anymore [28, 46, 82, 92].

P. Ventevogel
Public Health Section (Division of Resilience and Solutions), United Nations High Commissioner for Refugees, Geneva, Switzerland

S. J. Song (✉)
Department of Psychiatry, George Washington University, Washington, DC, USA
e-mail: suzan.song@post.harvard.edu

© Springer Nature Switzerland AG 2020
S. J. Song, P. Ventevogel (eds.), *Child, Adolescent and Family Refugee Mental Health*, https://doi.org/10.1007/978-3-030-45278-0_1

However, while the concept of PTSD has become widely accepted in refugee mental health care in "resettlement countries," concerns remain to be voiced around the overtly strong focus on treating *symptoms in the individual* rather than using systemic approaches that expand the focus from the individual to that of *the family and community* [30, 43, 51, 57].

Theoretical concepts that get increasing scholarly attention include resilience and the socio-ecological model of refugee mental health and well-being. These concepts are not novel, but attempts to bring these thoughts within mainstream refuge mental health care are relatively recent [58, 65]. Such concepts largely still lack operational translation into evidence-based intervention approaches, although important recent advances are made [6, 22, 23].

Conceptual Debates in Humanitarian Mental Health and Psychosocial Support

Similar debates around trauma-focused versus community-based approaches, and clinical versus socio-ecological approaches, have marred the field of "mental health and psychosocial support" (MHPSS) in humanitarian settings [76]. The field of MHPSS was, and to a large extent remains, theoretically influenced by community- and recovery-focused approaches formulated by social psychologists, social workers, and social scientists [8, 9, 11, 60, 83]. The needs in massive humanitarian crises are often so overwhelming and accompanied by major ruptures in supportive social systems and formal services that strong triage is required. Assistance cannot be solely dependent on specialized clinical mental health workers [55, 56].

Of pivotal importance was the publication of the *Inter-Agency Standing Committee (IASC) Guidelines for Mental Health and Psychosocial Support in Emergency Settings* [33] that led to a (rather fragile) consensus among policy makers and practitioners [1, 74, 84]. A key notion in these guidelines is that interventions need to be situated within a multilayered system that integrates approaches to foster recovery of emergency-affected communities through strengthening social support and rebuilding of community structures with more clinical approaches for those with severe or disabling mental health conditions [81]. The IASC MHPSS guidelines greatly contributed to the consolidation of MHPSS as a field for interventions [31]. The model has been adopted by almost all major humanitarian actors including the World Health Organization, UNICEF, the United Nations High Commissioner for Refugees, and the International Organization for Migration and provides a unifying framework, despite significant differences in programming of these organizations [34, 54, 67, 70, 73]. However, the impact of the IASC Guidelines outside humanitarian emergencies is limited. Many mental health professionals working in refugee mental health are unaware of the guidelines or feel unable to use them clinically, as the guidelines are written for massive humanitarian crises with limited human resources. Not very helpful in this regard is the conspicuous absence of reference to psychological trauma in the IASC guidelines, which has prompted critique from academic trauma researchers [12, 91]. Issues related to the utility of trauma-focused cognitive behavioral therapies in humanitarian contexts are unresolved and keep provoking heated discussions [47, 48, 75].

The Importance of Socio-ecological Approaches and Public Mental Health

Over the last decades, dozens of edited books about the mental health of refugees and other people affected by armed conflict have been published. Also, there are many books focusing on the mental health of children and young people affected by war. Some early precursors of this book address issues that are remarkably similar to the issues at stake in contemporary refugee mental health, such as the balance of psychosocial and mental health interventions, the importance of social support, the danger of addressing "symptoms" devoid of context [15], and the importance of social work and social policies [85]. A range of important publications in the early 2000s addressed the mental health consequences of collective violence in populations affected by armed conflict and incorporated the mounting critique on the way in which Western psychiatric categories were ascribed to refugee populations, while social, political, and economic factors that play a central role in refugees' experience were ignored [80]. In 2002, Joop de Jong [17] edited a book detailing work of the Transcultural Psychosocial Organization, a nongovernmental organization that he founded. The book details the pioneering approaches in the provision of mental health and psychosocial care for conflict-affected populations. His book does not specifically focus on refugees or children, but makes an important synthesis of the literature in the introduction chapter, placing interventions in a broad global public mental health perspective [16]. In the same period, Miller and Rasco [45] edited an important book that used a socio-ecological perspective in the conceptualization of mental health issues of refugees. It showcased, as in the book of de Jong, examples of how practitioners used such perspectives in their work. The books of de Jong and of Miller and Rasco made important theoretical contributions to the field and have deeply influenced our thinking. Several other books on the mental health of refugees or conflict-affected populations published in the same era either take more critical stances toward conventional paradigms in refugee mental health [8, 32] or use more conventional trauma-focused or clinical approaches [7, 38, 42, 87]. None of those books specifically focused on children, but publications on refugee and war-affected children see a similar oscillation around the same issues. There continues to be a lack of major breakthroughs despite re-emerging attention to the use of socio-ecological models of refugee mental health, incorporating resilience perspectives, considering the importance of daily stressors, and applying long-term perspectives [4, 25, 29, 35, 40, 59, 63, 64]. Overall, within the theory of child refugee mental health care, clinical and socio-ecological perspectives are gradually converging [79], but we have a long way to go to reach integration in programmatic praxis [44].

Why This Book?

We have learned much from the books and articles that we briefly referenced above. So, one could argue, why a new book? We feel the answer is in bringing together a variety of approaches within a single volume that is easily accessible to mental health practitioners. We distinguish five key features that, taken together, we hope gives this book an added value.

Using a Global Perspective

Academic texts often distinguish between child refugees in low- and middle-income countries and those in resettlement settings in high-income countries [24, 52]. There are good reasons to do this. For example, the situation of a South Sudanese child in a refugee camp in northern Uganda differs dramatically from the situation of a resettled South Sudanese refugee child in a country like Sweden: the problems are different. The available resources are different. The social context is different. But what about a South Sudanese refugee who lives for many years in the Egyptian metropolis of Cairo? Or a South Sudanese refugee child in a transit center in Southern Italy? In a globalizing and increasing interdependent world, the sharp distinctions between "here" and "there" are becoming blurred. The refugee in Uganda may well be in close touch with relatives in Egypt, Italy, or Sweden through social media and the Internet. Of more importance than being a refugee in a transit country or having arrived as an asylum seeker in a host country is the context in which children live. For example, keeping children in immigration detention leads to poorer mental health outcomes [18, 27, 39, 49, 53].

Borders are becoming blurred and porous, despite desperate attempts of governments to erect walls and fences. This book therefore chooses a global perspective: in all chapters the authors attempt to provide information that is useful *across settings* without sharply dividing the world simplistically into "low- and middle-income" or "pre-migration" on one side and "high-income countries" or "resettlement countries" on the other.

Blending Research Findings with Clinical Wisdom

Research into refugee mental health is booming. As described above, there are many systematic reviews on a range of relevant research topics such as mental health epidemiology and therapeutic interventions [24, 41, 50, 52]. These data are tremendously important and exciting, albeit sometimes written in rather dense and scholarly manners. There are also publications such as manuals, to assist clinicians in providing mental health care for child refugees [13, 19, 88, 89]. There are also practitioner reviews that provide a synthesis of key clinical issues to practitioners

[20, 37, 78] and policy- oriented programmatic guidance for work in humanitarian contexts [2, 33, 62]. In the current book, we aim to blend all these perspectives into a cocktail with many different ingredients that is easily digestible and, as we hope, gives the reader a taste for more.

Linking Treatment of the Individual with the Context of Family, Community, and Society

Mental health treatment is more than what happens between the walls of a consultation room and can also include activities within communities, schools, and people's homes. In humanitarian settings, MHPSS programs are often broadly conceptualized to include activities that can be done by nonspecialists in nonclinical settings [77]. The field of humanitarian MHPSS has developed strong intersectoral ways of working that we feel could be useful for high-income settings as well, particularly where refugee mental health in high-income settings is often dominated by trauma-focused approaches.

Considering a Range of Clinical Issues

A popular but erroneous assumption is that psychopathology of refugees is necessarily related to having experienced traumatic events and that the clinical issues are mainly related to psychological trauma. Another common erroneous assumption is that traumatic events predominantly occur in the country of origin. In our clinical experiences, refugee children struggle as much with issues that happened during the perilous journey to safety and after having arrived in presumably safe countries. Without a doubt, the horrific events that a sizeable group of refugee children went through have an important impact on their mental state. But other psychopathology is caused by, or mediated through, the current context in which refugee children live – often characterized by instability, socioeconomic hardships, marginalization, and loss of agency.

Therefore, refugee mental health should not be seen as a subsection of psychotraumatology. The whole spectrum of mental health conditions is relevant to refugees. The World Health Organization estimates that around 22% of adult populations exposed to collective violence develop clinically relevant mental health conditions [14]. Prevalence rates of PTSD but also of other anxiety disorders, depression, complicated grief disorder, and psychotic disorders increase significantly. These data are for adults, but we have no reason to believe the picture will be dramatically different for conflict-affected children. Therefore, we felt it was important to integrate information on a wide range of mental health issues such as grief, depression, anxiety disorders, severe mental disorders, substance use disorders, and developmental disabilities.

Making the Text Accessible for Nonspecialists

Regularly, we are approached by clinicians and aspiring researchers in the field who would like to get involved in working with refugee children. We feel that many of the extant literature is not very accessible to them because of the length of texts and the specialized focus of many. We felt an introductory text was needed that could provide readers who are relatively new to the subject a concise overview of the state of the art, without discussing topics so much in depth that readers would lose attention. The current book aims to synthesize current knowledge and good practices on the topic in a way that does not yet exist, as far as we know. What we had in mind is the kind of book that we wished we could have read when we started our work with child refugee mental health.

Defining the Core Concepts

What Is a Refugee?

An unprecedented 70.8 million people around the world are forcibly displaced from their homes due to armed conflict and situations of generalized violence [71]. Half of the 25.9 million refugees are under the age of 18 years old, making mental health of refugee children a major and growing public health problem.

Refugees are defined as persons who have been forced to leave their country to escape war, violence, conflict, or persecution and have crossed an international border to find safety in another country. The 1951 Refugee Convention is a major international legal document that defines a refugee as: "someone who is unable or unwilling to return to their country of origin owing to a well-founded fear of being persecuted for reasons of race, religion, nationality, membership of a particular social group, or political opinion" [68]. It is sometimes assumed that all refugees have fled war. However, people can also become refugees because they are political activists, have experienced sexual and gender-based violence, or were persecuted due to religion or sexual orientation. An asylum seeker is someone who requests international protection, but whose application still has to be processed. An internally displaced person is someone who is forcibly displaced within the borders of their country. This book focuses on refugees, asylum seekers, and internally displaced persons but not on migrants (i.e., persons who voluntarily cross borders in search for employment or education).

Many refugee children flee together with their parents, but others arrive as unaccompanied or separated children (UASC). "Separated children" are separated from both parents, or from their previous legal or customary primary caregiver, but not necessarily from other relatives. They may be accompanied by other adult family members. "Unaccompanied children" are separated from both parents and other relatives and, as consequence, are not cared for by an adult who, by law or by custom, is responsible for their care [72].

What Is a Child?

As explained in Chaps. 1 and 2 of this book, the definitions of who is considered a child and who is an adult vary considerably. In this book we use the United Nations definitions of childhood (see Box 1.1) for reasons of consistency within the text. The children and adults with whom we work may have different definitions, highlighting the notion that childhood is a cultural construct that has different meanings based on context and environment.

Box 1.1 Definition of Childhood Terms

Children	0–18 years old
Adolescents	10–19 years old
Youth	15–24 years old

Sources: [66, 69]

What Is the Migration Trajectory of a Refugee?

Just as the reasons for becoming a refugee are varied, so are their experiences of the journey to safety. Often the refugee trajectory is defined as a linear process of pre-migration (the baseline situation at home that is disturbed by violence or other causes), migration (flight from the home country to a new country, with transitory stays in a refugee camp), and resettlement. The trajectory of many refugees is, however, less straightforward, much more complex, and often nonlinear. First, only a minority of refugees ever get resettled in a third country. Many others stay for long periods in refugee camps, informal settlements, or in rented settlements in urban settings, therefore being a refugee or asylum seeker for years or decades. Resettlement is only one of the solutions, the others being local integration, or return to the country of origin when conditions have improved. The experience of many refugees includes multiple migrations and, sometimes, long-term detention by governments, such as happens with "offshore detention" of asylum seekers arriving by sea in Australia, or by smuggler, traffickers, and armed groups such as happens in the Sahara and Northern Africa. Another misconception is that the transitory phase of refugee is mostly through stays in refugee camps. In reality, most refugees live in urban settings or integrated in rural communities.

What Is Trauma?

There is a popular notion that all refugees are "traumatized" and victimized based on their experiences in their home country. Disorders such as PTSD, depression, and anxiety have shown to be high in this population, though with extremely variable prevalence rates and few longitudinal understandings of the mental health process over time. These disorders fail to encapsulate the acculturation stress, cultural bereavement, traumatic loss, despair, and hopelessness that people may experience, as well as the loss of social and cultural connectedness and a sense of belonging. The term "traumatized" or "victim" can be disempowering and stigmatizing for the child and family that have been exposed to potentially traumatic events. We therefore prefer the term "traumatic" as an adjective above "trauma" as a noun. Exposure to potentially traumatic events may lead to response that can be called "traumatic" in one child, but not in another. Moreover, the focus on potentially traumatic experiences that lead to refugee status may overlook and undervalue the importance of the attrition stressors that affect the mental health for the refugee child. Such stressors related to uncertainty about the future, legal status, loved ones, as well as discrimination, acculturative stress, and ambiguous loss of loved ones, play a large role in the development and maintenance of poor mental health for refugee children.

How This Book Is Organized

The book is set up in four main parts to provide a comprehensive approach to the understanding of child, adolescent, and family refugee mental health. The first part provides an overview of concepts that are fundamental to the care of child and adolescent refugees through a research and public health lens. Bennouna, Stark, and Wessells describe the population of refugee and war-affected youth from a socioecological framework. While multiple academic fields have agreed on the importance of the sociocultural context in the pathways to poor child and adolescent mental health, Reis, Crone, and Berckmoes critically examine how to unpack "context" and "culture" for refugee youth. Understanding how both context and culture can be used to support resilience in refugee youth and families can be useful in both practice and policy. Vindevogel and Verelst describe the use of a resilience framework for refugee youth in a humanitarian context. Since the strongest evidence for promoting the mental well-being of war-affected youth is on family-level variables, understanding the role of family as both sources of support and strain can be critical when working with refugee youth and families [63, 64].

The second section of the book shifts from academic and humanitarian public mental health approaches to integrating clinical, practical guidance on important principles to consider in the mental health assessment of refugee children, adolescents, and families. Song and Ventevogel and Song and Oakley use their clinical expertise to provide clinical guidance for practitioners. As many clinicians are working in humanitarian contexts, we also asked Snider and Hijazi to discuss the UNICEF operational guidelines on how to support community-based mental health and psychosocial support that can be scaled up based on current evidence for the implementation of programs in humanitarian settings.

The third part of the book discusses symptom clusters commonly seen in refugee children and adolescents. We are grateful to have seasoned clinicians that can discuss nuanced issues with this population. Jones uses her breadth of clinical care in humanitarian settings to help practitioners engage with grief and loss with refugee children and families; Rousseau and Gagnon discuss not only how to understand but also how to address the impact of stress and traumatic events on children; and Ventevogel and de Jong highlight the depression and despair that some youth and families may experience in their chapter on emotional disorders in refugee children. We also include chapters on topics that have a growing body of clinical research and are in dire need of clinical intervention. Greene and Kane provide a review of substance abuse in conflict-affected children. Cavallera, Nasir, and Munir give a practical guide to the assessment and management of children with developmental disabilities, particularly in humanitarian settings, and Liu and Chowdhary discuss severe mental illness and neuropsychiatric disorders among refugee children.

The fourth part of the book integrates the theory, research, and clinical approaches to provide practical examples of how to use a family- and strengths-based approach toward the assessment and care of mental health problems for refugee children. Dybdal describes an intervention by Save the Children in Denmark that enhances resilience in unaccompanied young men. Mooren, Bala, and Van der Meulen underscore the need for family-centered approaches with refugee youth and ways to engage family in humanitarian contexts; and Frounfelker, Mishra, Gautam, Berent, Abdi, and Betancourt are exemplary in their collaboration between researchers and community members in using family-centered approaches for child refugee populations.

What This Book Hopes to Accomplish

We hope this text will provide practical, clinical guidance on how to assess and manage mental health conditions in refugee children/adolescents and their families. Our wish is to introduce clinicians to new ways of thinking that combine the insights of a strengths-based and resiliency approaches and family-centered approaches with practical guidance for clinicians of various skill levels. We equally hope to remind researchers and policy makers of the clinical realities in working with refugee children. Finally, we hope that the book can contribute to a further advancement of the field of child refugee mental health care as it is our strong conviction that humanitarian workers, mental health clinicians, and researchers alike can benefit from using a framework that incorporates clinical approaches to mental health problems with notions of resilience, family-centered care, and awareness of context and culture.

References

1. Ager A. Consensus and professional practice in psychosocial intervention: political achievement, core knowledge-base and prompt for further enquiry. Intervention. 2008;6:261–4.
2. Alliance for Child Protection in Humanitarian Action. Standard 10: mental health and psychosocial distress. In Minimum standards for child protection in humanitarian action. Author; 2019. p. 131–138.
3. Almqvist K, Brandell-Forsberg M. Refugee children in Sweden: post-traumatic stress disorder in Iranian preschool children exposed to organized violence. Child Abuse Negl. 1997;21:351–66.

4. Apfel RJ, Bennet S. Minefields in their hearts: the mental health of children in war and communal violence. New Haven: Yale University Press; 1998.
5. Beiser M, Dion R, Gotowiec A, Hyman I, Vu N. Immigrant and refugee children in Canada. Can J Psychiatry. 1985;40:67–72.
6. Betancourt TS, Berent JM, Freeman J, Frounfelker RL, Brennan RT, Abdi S, et al. Family-based mental health promotion for Somali bantu and Bhutanese refugees: feasibility and acceptability trial. J Adoles Health. 2019; https://doi.org/10.1016/j.jadohealth.2019.1008.1023.
7. Bhugra D, Craig T, Bhui K, editors. Mental health of refugees and asylum seekers. Oxford: Oxford University Press; 2010.
8. Boothby N, Strang A, Wessells M, editors. A world turned upside down: social ecological approaches to children in war zones. Bloomfield: Kumarian Press; 2008.
9. Boyden J, De Berry J, editors. Children and youth on the front line: ethnography, armed conflict and displacement. New York: Berghahn Books; 2004.
10. Bracken PJ, Petty C, editors. Rethinking the trauma of war. London: Free Association Books; 1998.
11. Bragin M. The psychological effects of war on children: a psychosocial approach. In: Carll EK, editor. Trauma psychology: violence and disaster. Westport: Praeger; 2007. p. 195–230.
12. Cardozo BL. Guidelines need a more evidence based approach: a commentary on the IASC guidelines on mental health and psychosocial support in emergency settings. Intervention. 2008;6(3-4):252–4.
13. Cavallera V, Jones L, Weisbecker I, Ventevogel P. Mental health in complex emergencies. In: Kravitz A, editor. Oxford handbook of humanitarian medicine. Oxford: Oxford University Press; 2019. p. 117–53.
14. Charlson F, van Ommeren M, Flaxman A, Cornett J, Whiteford H, Saxena S. New WHO prevalence estimates of mental disorders in conflict settings: a systematic review and meta-analysis. Lancet. 2019;394:240–8.
15. Cole E, Espin OM, Rothblum ED, editors. Refugee women and their mental health: shattered societies, shattered lives. London: Routledge; 1992.
16. de Jong JT. Public mental health, traumatic stress and human rights violations in low-income countries. In: de Jong J, editor. Trauma, war, and violence: public mental health in socio-cultural context. New York: Kluwer Academic/Plenum Publishers; 2002. p. 1–91.
17. de Jong JT, editor. Trauma, war, and violence: public mental health in socio-cultural context. New York: Kluwer Academic/Plenum; 2002.
18. Dudley M, Steel Z, Mares S, Newman L. Children and young people in immigration detention. Curr Opin Psychiatry. 2012;25(4):285–92.
19. Eapen V, Graham P, Srinath S. Where there is no child psychiatrist: a mental healthcare manual. London: Royal College of Psychiatrists; 2012.
20. Ehntholt KA, Yule W. Practitioner review: assessment and treatment of refugee children and adolescents who have experienced war-related trauma. J Child Psychol Psychiatry. 2006;47(12):1197–210.
21. Eisenbruch M. From post-traumatic stress disorder to cultural bereavement: diagnosis of southeast Asian refugees. Soc Sci Med. 1991;33(6):673–80.
22. Ellis HB, Abdi S, Winer P. Mental health practice with immigrant and refugee youth; a socio-ecological framework. Washington, D.C.: American Psychological Association; 2019.
23. Fazel M, Betancourt TS. Preventive mental health interventions for refugee children and adolescents in high-income settings. Lancet Child Adoles Health. 2018;2:121–32.
24. Fazel M, Reed RV, Panter-Brick C, Stein A. Mental health of displaced and refugee children resettled in high-income countries: risk and protective factors. Lancet. 2012;379(9812):266–82. https://doi.org/10.1016/S0140-6736(11)60051-2.
25. Fernando C, Ferrari M, editors. Handbook of resilience in children of war. New York: Springer; 2013.
26. Gersons BP, Carlier IV. Post-traumatic stress disorder: the history of a recent concept. Br J Psychiatry. 1992;16:742–8.
27. Hodes M. The mental health of detained asylum seeking children. Eur Child Adolesc Psychiatry. 2010;19:621–3.

28. Hoven CW, Amsel LV, Tyano S, editors. An international perspective on disasters and children's mental health. Cham: Springer; 2019.
29. Hyman I, Vu N, Beiser M. Post-migration stresses among southeast Asian refugee youth in Canada: a research note. J Comp Fam Stud. 2000;31(2):281–93.
30. Hynie M. The social determinants of refugee mental health in the post-migration context: a critical review. Can J Psychiatry. 2018;63:297–303.
31. IASC Reference Group for Mental Health and Psychosocial Support. Review of the implementation of the IASC guidelines on mental health and psychosocial support in emergency settings. Geneva: IASC; 2015.
32. Ingleby D, editor. Forced migration and mental health: Rethinking the care of refugees and displaced persons. New York: Springer; 2004.
33. Inter-Agency Standing Committee. IASC guidelines on mental health and psychosocial support in emergency settings. IASC: Geneva; 2007.
34. International Federation Reference Centre for Psychosocial Support. Psychosocial interventions: a handbook. Copenhagen: International Federation of Red Cross and red Cresecen Societies; 2009.
35. Jordans MJ, Pigott H, Tol WA. Interventions for children affected by armed conflict: a systematic review of mental health and psychosocial support in low-and middle-income countries. Curr Psychiatry Rep. 2016;18(1):1–15.
36. Kinzie JD, Sack WH. Severely traumatized Cambodian children: research findings and clinical implications. In: Ahearn FL, Athey JL, editors. Refugee children: theory, research, and services. Baltimore: Johns Hopkins University Press; 1991. p. 92–105.
37. Kirmayer LJ, Narasiah L, Munoz M, Rashid M, Ryder AG, Guzder J, The Canadian Collaboration for Immigrant and Refugee Health (CCIRH). Common mental health problems in immigrants and refugees: general approach in primary care. Can Med Assoc J. 2011;183(12):E959.
38. Krippner S, McIntyre TM, editors. The psychological impact of war trauma on civilians: an international perspective. Westport: Praeger; 2003.
39. Kronick R, Rousseau C, Cleveland J. Mandatory detention of refugee children: a public health issue? Paediatr Child Health. 2011;16(8):e65–7.
40. Lau W, Silove D, Edwards B, Forbes D, Bryant R, McFarlane A, et al. Adjustment of refugee children and adolescents in Australia: outcomes from wave three of the Building a New Life in Australia study. BMC Med. 2018;16:157.
41. Lustig SL, Kia-Keating M, Knight WG, Geltman P, Ellis H, Kinzie JD, et al. Review of child and adolescent refugee mental health. J Am Acad Child Adolesc Psychiatry. 2004;43:24–36.
42. Martz E, editor. Trauma and rehabilitation after war and conflict: community and individual perspectives. New York: Springer; 2010.
43. Measham T, Guzder J, Rousseau C, Pacione L, Blais-McPherson M, Nadeau L. Refugee children and their families: supporting psychological well-being and positive adaptation following migration. Curr Probl Pediatr Adolesc Health Care. 2014;44:208–15.
44. Miller KE, Jordans MJD. Determinants of children's mental health in war-torn settings: translating research into action. Curr Psychiatry Rep. 2016;18(6):58.
45. Miller KE, Rasco LM, editors. The mental health of refugees. Ecological approaches to healing and adaptation. Mahwah/London: Erlbaum; 2004.
46. Morina N, Nickerson A. Mental health of refugee and conflict-affected populations: theory, research and clinical practice. Cham: Springer; 2018.
47. Mundt AP, Wünsche P, Heinz A, Pross C. Evaluating interventions for posttraumatic stress disorder in low and middle income countries: narrative exposure therapy. Intervention. 2014;12(2):250–66.
48. Neuner F, Schauer M, Elbert T. On the efficacy of narrative exposure therapy: a reply to Mundt et al. Intervention. 2014;12(2):267–78.
49. Newman LK, Steel Z. The child asylum seeker: psychological and developmental impact of immigration detention. Child Adolesc Psychiatr Clin N Am. 2008;17(3):665–83.
50. Newnham EA, Kashyap S, Tearne J, Fazel M. Child mental health in the context of war: an overview of risk factors and interventions for refugee and war-affected youth. In: Morina

N, Nickerson A, editors. Mental health of refugee and conflict-affected populations. Cham: Springer; 2018. p. 37–63.

51. Pain C, Kanagaratnam P, Payne D. The debate about trauma and psychosocial treatment for refugees. In: Simich L, Andermann L, editors. Refuge and resilience: promoting resilience and mental health among resettled refugees and forced migrants. Dordrecht: Springer; 2014. p. 51–60.

52. Reed RV, Fazel M, Jones L, Panter-Brick C, Stein A. Mental health of displaced and refugee children resettled in low-income and middle-income countries: risk and protective factors. Lancet. 2012;379(9812):250–65. https://doi.org/10.1016/S0140-6736(11)60050-0.

53. Reijneveld SA, de Boer JB, Bean T, Korfker DG. Unaccompanied adolescents seeking asylum: poorer mental health under a restrictive reception. J Nerv Ment Dis. 2005;193(11):759–61.

54. Schininà G, editor. Manual on community-based mental health and psychosocial support in emergency and displacement. Brussels: International Organization for Migration; 2019.

55. Silove D. The challenges facing mental health programs for post-conflict and refugee communities. Prehospital Disaster Med. 2004;19(1):90–6. Retrieved from http://www.ncbi.nlm.nih.gov/pubmed/15453165.

56. Silove D. Do conflict-affected societies need psychiatrists? Br J Psychiatry. 2012;201(4):255–7. https://doi.org/10.1192/bjp.bp.112.108480.

57. Silove D, Ventevogel P, Rees S. The contemporary refugee crisis: an overview of mental health challenges. World Psychiatry. 2017;16(2):130–9. https://doi.org/10.1002/wps.20438.

58. Simich L, Andermann L, editors. Refuge and resilience: promoting resilience and mental health among resettled refugees and forced migrants. Dordrecht: Springer; 2014.

59. Song SJ. Globalization and mental health: the impact of war and armed conflict on families. Amsterdam: University of Amsterdam; 2015.

60. Strang AB, Ager A. Psychosocial interventions: some key issues facing practitioners. Intervention. 2003;1(3):2–12.

61. Summerfield D. Childhood, war, refugeedom and 'trauma': three core questions for mental health professionals. Transcult Psychiatry. 2000;37:417.

62. The Sphere Project. Mental Healrth and psychosocial support. In: The sphere handbook: humanitarian charter and minimum standards in humanitarian response. Geneva: Sphere; 2018. p. 339–42.

63. Tol WA, Jordans MJ, Kohrt BA, Betancourt TS, Komproe IH. Promoting mental health and psychosocial well-being in children affected by political violence: part I – current evidence for an ecological resilience approach. In: Fernando C, Ferrari M, editors. Handbook of resilience in children of war. New York: Springer; 2013. p. 11–27.

64. Tol WA, Song S, Jordans MJ. Annual research review: resilience and mental health in children and adolescents living in areas of armed conflict–a systematic review of findings in low- and middle-income countries. J Child Psychol Psychiatry Allied Discip. 2013;54(4):445–60. https://doi.org/10.1111/jcpp.12053.

65. Ungar M. Practitioner review: diagnosing childhood resilience–a systemic approach to the diagnosis of adaptation in adverse social and physical ecologies. J Child Psychol Psychiatry Allied Discip. 2015;56(1):4–17. https://doi.org/10.1111/jcpp.12306.

66. United Nations. N.d. Youth: https://www.un.org/en/sections/issues-depth/youth-0/.

67. United Nations Children's Fund. Operational guidelines on community based mental health and psychosocial support in humanitarian settings: three-tiered support for children and families. New York: UNICEF; 2018.

68. United Nations General Assembly. Convention relating to the status of refugees. New York: United Nations; 1951. Available at: https://www.refworld.org/docid/3be01b964.html. Accessed 25 Nov 2019.

69. United Nations General Assembly. Convention on the rights of the child, vol. 1577 (3). New York: United Nations; 1989.

70. United Nations High Commissioner for Refugees. Operational guidance for mental health and psychosocial support programming in refugee operations. Geneva: United Nations High Commissioner for Refugees; 2013.

71. United Nations High Commissioner for Refugees. 2019. Figures at a glance: https://www.unhcr.org/figures-at-a-glance.html.
72. United Nations High Commissioner for Refugees. Child protection (vs 1.5). In Emergency handbook. Geneva: UNHCR; 2018. https://emergency.unhcr.org/entry/43381/child-protection.
73. van Ommeren M, Hanna F, Weissbecker I, Ventevogel P. Mental health and psychosocial support in humanitarian emergencies. East Mediterr Health J. 2015;21(7):498–502.
74. Ventevogel P. The IASC guidelines on mental health and psychosocial support in emergency settings, from discussion to implementation. Intervention. 2008;6(3-4):193–8.
75. Ventevogel P. The role of brief trauma focused psychotherapies (such as narrative exposure therapy) in areas affected by conflict. Intervention. 2014;12(2):244–9.
76. Ventevogel P. Interventions for mental health and psychosocial support in complex humanitarian emergencies: moving towards consensus in policy and action? In: Morina N, Nickerson A, editors. Mental health in refugee and post-conflict populations. Cham: Springer; 2018. p. 155–80.
77. Ventevogel P, Duchesne B, Hughes P, Whitney C. Mental health and psychosocial support (MHPSS). In: Abubakar I, Zumla A, editors. Clinical Handbook of Refugee Health. London: Taylor & Francis; 2020.
78. Ventevogel P, Pereira X, Verghis S, Silove D. Mental health of refugees. In: Allotey PA, Reidpath D, editors. The health of refugees: public health perspectives from crisis to settlement. 2nd ed. Oxford: Oxford University Press; 2019. p. 106–27.
79. Vostanis P. New approaches to interventions for refugee children. World Psychiatry. 2016;15:75–7.
80. Watters C. Emerging paradigms in the mental health care of refugees. Soc Sci Med. 2001;52(11):1709–18.
81. Weissbecker I, Hanna F, El Shazly M, Gao J, Ventevogel P. Integrative mental health and psychosocial support interventions for refugees in humanitarian crisis settings. In: Wenzel T, Drozdek B, editors. Uncertain safety: understanding and assisting the 21st century refugees. Cham: Springer; 2019. p. 117–53.
82. Wenzel T, Drozdek B, editors. An uncertain safety: understanding and assisting the 21st century refugees. Cham: Springer; 2019.
83. Wessells M. Do no harm: toward contextually appropriate psychosocial support in international emergencies. Am Psychol. 2009;64(8):842–54.
84. Wessells M, van Ommeren M. Developing inter-agency guidelines on mental health and psychosocial support in emergency settings. Intervention. 2008;6(3-4):199–218.
85. Westermeyer J. Mental health for refugees and other migrants: social and preventive approaches. Springfield: C.C. Thomas; 1989.
86. Westermeyer J. Psychiatric services for refugee children: an overview. In: Ahearn FL, Athey JL, editors. Refugee children: theory, research and services. Baltimore: Johns Hopkins University Press; 1991.
87. Wilson JP, Drozdek B, editors. Broken spirits: the treatment of traumatized asylum seekers, refugees and war and torture victims. New York: Routledge; 2004.
88. World Health Organisation. mhGAP Intervention Guide (mhGAP-IG) version 2.0 for mental, neurological and substance use disorders for non-specialist health settings. Geneva: WHO; 2016.
89. World Health Organization, & United Nations High Commissioner for Refugees. mhGAP Humanitarian Intervention Guide (mhGAP-HIG): clinical management of mental, neurological and substance use conditions in humanitarian emergencies. Geneva: WHO; 2015.
90. Yule W. Post-traumatic stress disorder. Arch Dis Childhood. 1999;80:107–9.
91. Yule W. IASC Guidelines–generally welcome, but…. Intervention. 2008;6(3–4):248–51.
92. Zipfel S, Pfaltz MC, Schnyder U, editors. Refugee mental health. Lausanne: Frontiers Media; 2019.

Children and Adolescents in Conflict and Displacement

2

Cyril Bennouna, Lindsay Stark, and Michael G. Wessells

Introduction

Armed conflict is increasingly encroaching upon the lives of children and adolescents around the globe. The stark images of girls and boys standing disoriented against the backdrop of concrete rubble in cities such as Damascus, Sana'a, Mosul, and Mogadishu have become too familiar over recent years. Such photographs attest to several alarming trends in armed conflict that are increasingly endangering the lives of civilians and young people in particular. The urbanization of today's armed conflicts means that attacks have a higher likelihood of directly harming civilians, compared to conflicts fought in less populated areas [28, 54]. Meanwhile, collateral damage to infrastructure and residential property—the rubble in the background—can have a range of secondary effects to public services and local economies. The continued use of landmines and increasing reliance on aerial bombing campaigns in many high-intensity conflicts greatly increase the likelihood of civilian harm [39, 52]. What is worse, armed forces and non-state armed groups alike have demonstrated profound disrespect for international humanitarian law, intentionally targeting civilians as a strategy of war. Horrifying examples include the Assad regime's repeated chemical weapons attacks on Syrian civilians, the Saudi Arabian

C. Bennouna
Political Science, Brown University, Providence, RI, USA

L. Stark (✉)
Brown School, Washington University in St. Louis, St. Louis, MO, USA
e-mail: lindsaystark@wustl.edu

M. G. Wessells
Program on Forced Migration and Health, Columbia University, New York, NY, USA

© Springer Nature Switzerland AG 2020
S. J. Song, P. Ventevogel (eds.), *Child, Adolescent and Family Refugee Mental Health*, https://doi.org/10.1007/978-3-030-45278-0_2

coalition's indiscriminate airstrikes and sieges of rebel-held Yemeni cities, and Boko Haram's abduction of hundreds of children [65, 80, 86, 111, 114].

These trends have dire implications when considering that some 357 million children and adolescents live in areas affected by armed conflict, up from some 200 million two decades ago [7]. Nearly one in six people under the age of 18 years old lives within 31 miles (50 km) of violence related to armed conflict. The dangers associated with conflict-affected areas have led to an unprecedented level of forced migration globally. Currently 68.5 million people are displaced due to armed conflict and persecution, and the numbers of forcibly displaced people has risen each year since 2012 [112]. Children and adolescents account for some 52 percent of refugees [112].

This chapter examines how the interplay of risk, protective, and promotive factors at different levels of the social environment, and at different points in time, influences the mental health and psychosocial well-being of children and adolescents.

Children, Adolescents, and Armed Conflict

Children and adolescents around the world encounter and respond to armed conflict in a variety of ways. Potentially traumatic events, such as experiencing an attack or torture, can cause significant psychological distress and can ultimately contribute to the development of post-traumatic stress disorder (PTSD), depression, and other adverse emotional and behavioral outcomes [23]. In addition, a host of daily stressors, from social isolation and discrimination to impoverishment, can have strong detrimental effects on young people's mental health and psychosocial well-being [61]. These daily stressors have a constant presence among those living in conflict-affected setting—and usually persist well after they have fled—compromising young people's coping systems and leaving them even more vulnerable to the effects of traumatic stress.

Researchers and practitioners alike have increasingly drawn on the social ecological framework to conceptualize the complexities of children and adolescents' experiences with armed conflict and its fallout [19, 27, 82, 102, 122]. Originally introduced by Urie Bronfenbrenner, and adapted to a wide range of applications thereafter, this framework subdivides children's social environments into several nested levels [22]. The exact terms used for each of these levels change, depending on how the framework is being applied.

The social ecological framework emphasizes that the social environment and the relationships within them challenge or support children's mental health and psychosocial well-being. In this chapter, we begin at the broadest level, by describing the societal influences of armed conflict on girls and boys. We then narrow in on factors at the community level, followed by the interpersonal and family level, before finally focusing on the ways that individual factors contribute to children and adolescents' experiences of armed conflict. In addition to distinguishing between these levels, the social ecological framework also emphasizes the importance of the interactions between them over time, which we highlight throughout the chapter. This approach avoids the historic tendency to view adverse mental health and psychosocial well-being outcomes almost exclusively in individual terms. Instead, the framework enables us to begin comprehending the dynamic ways in which social environments influence children/adolescents' adverse and adaptive responses to the extreme adversities of war.

Society

Children and adolescents are deeply embedded in the societal systems that are thrown into disarray in the lead up to armed conflict and thereafter. For this reason, it is critical that humanitarian practitioners consider how factors in children's social, economic, and political lives affect them in times of crisis. Today's wars were usually preceded by years, if not decades, of political turmoil. The Syrian civil war, for example, began in 2011 with demonstrators protesting the Assad regime's repressive use of force against civilians—including minors—institutional corruption and failed economic and environmental policies, which had lasted years [5]. Many of today's armed conflicts, in fact, follow numerous cycles of previous political violence, including, for instance, in Afghanistan, Yemen, the Central African Republic, and Myanmar. In such settings, the systems preserving social order—including those supporting child/adolescent mental health and psychosocial well-being, such as healthcare and education—became fragile well before the first gunshot, leaving populations all the more vulnerable to the effects of armed conflict. To assess children's exposure to adversity as a sole function of the present conflict in such circumstances would ignore crucial historical context.

Against this backdrop, the onset of armed conflict can have a range of influences on the social fabric of affected areas. Some of this influence depends on the narratives produced by the various parties to conflict and their sympathizers to justify their actions. Those who see themselves as oppressed by the state, for example, may find hope in the struggle for liberty, despite the dangers of fighting. Meanwhile, others may exploit ideological narratives, such as exclusionary nationalism or religious fundamentalism, to recruit supporters and vilify opponents. Members of historically persecuted minority groups may fear being scapegoated and targeted by the majority, which in turn can lead them to fight or flee. Researchers have found that how young people and their communities make sense of armed conflict plays a significant role in their mental health outcomes, as well as in the reintegration of former combatants and returnees following the cessation of hostilities [17, 18, 95, 121]. In turn, how a conflict is remembered or forgotten by a society has great bearing on whether the conflict recurs [115].

While civilian mortality often soars in the context of armed conflict, both from direct violence and from the collapse of these life-sustaining systems, those who remain struggle to preserve the routine and traditions of normal life and to make ends meet, usually beyond the reach of humanitarian assistance. Over time, as different armed forces and groups vie for control over territories and seek to impose their own brands of order on local populations, they can reshape local norms and practices. For example, Islamist militant groups, such as Ansar Dine, al-Shabaab, and the Islamic State of Iraq and Syria (ISIS), have at various times imposed their extreme interpretations of Sharia law in the territories they control, severely restricting the freedom of women and girls and banning certain forms of dress, cultural practices, and daily goods.

Confronted by this multitude of dangers, many are trapped, without the means or the freedom to leave. Millions of others leave their homes behind and take refuge in camps or settlements for internally displaced person (IDP), or seek asylum in other countries as refugees. For many, this means trading one form of marginalization for another. It is indicative that policymakers in host countries usually refer to hosting forced migrants as a "burden." In many cases, IDPs, asylum-seekers, and refugees are treated with fear, suspicion, or even outright hostility by local governments and/or host communities. The fact that developing countries host some 85 percent of the world's refugees certainly explains part of this tendency. Local populations in these host countries may feel underserved by their governments and therefore consider refugees a competition for limited resources and economic opportunity [112]. Most refugees and asylum-seekers in fact have no pathway to citizenship in these countries and have extremely limited rights to employment and local public services.

Recent years have seen a tremendous proliferation of negative attitudes toward refugees in high-income and traditionally tolerant countries, from Germany, Sweden, and the United Kingdom, to the United States, even as others in those countries work tirelessly to welcome newcomers. Across many parts of the world, politicians have denigrated refugees as invaders, job stealers, disease vectors, rapists, and terrorists. The growing hostility toward forced migrants means that, even when they have reached relative safety from acute warfare, children and adolescents must endure suspicion, prejudice, and lack of safety while simultaneously navigating the complexities of a new educational, linguistic, and religious environment and trying to obtain citizenship status [14, 15, 48, 71]. These post-displacement factors can have a number of detrimental effects on children and adolescents' acculturation and mental health and psychosocial well-being outcomes [34, 56, 100].

Community

Children and adolescents are active members of their communities. They contribute to public life not only as students but also as athletes, artists, activists, and aspiring adults, modelling but also challenging the behavior of the authority figures around them. To varying degrees, they are generally aware of the large issues facing society and especially as these issues manifest within the community. As such, children and adolescents can be highly attuned to the effects that armed conflict has on community life, even if they do not always understand them the same way as adults do. Furthermore, children—and adolescents in particular—sometimes play a sizeable role in conflict, whether through an association with armed groups or through engagement in peace processes. It is necessary to appreciate the variety of ways that children and adolescents not only encounter but also respond to armed conflict at the community level in order to devise appropriate approaches for improving their well-being.

Around the world, in rural and urban communities alike, education and health form the bedrock of children's public lives. Unfortunately, however, the importance of raising the next generation often does not safeguard schools and health facilities from the fallout of armed conflict in today's unconventional battlefields. An abundance of evidence suggests that armed forces and groups alike target civilian structures intentionally, including schools and health facilities, across many of the world's conflicts [11, 13, 38, 54, 83]. Combatants sometimes bomb schools and health facilities directly, as well as other civilian or "soft" targets, but their attacks can take more insidious forms as well, from occupying and using buildings for military purposes to threatening service providers and supply chains, to abducting students and patients and forcing them into hard labor, sex acts, marriage, and/or active participation in hostilities [10, 38]. Such insecurity frequently means that caregivers in conflict zones keep their girls and boys at home, contributing to school dropout and an underutilization of healthcare, even for acute needs [109]. In such circumstances, many schools and health facilities close, whether temporarily or permanently. In Yemen alone, some 27 percent of schools have closed, two million minors are out of school, and—as of late 2016—some 55 percent of health facilities were not functioning [83, 110].

In the midst of this insecurity and destruction, what is left of civil society erodes too, as community elders, neighborhood associations, grassroots activism groups, charities, and local media organizations disband or are forced to operate underground. Public safety and justice systems tend to also be compromised, enabling greater impunity for violations against young people [109, 124]. In addition to the shuttering of these and other public services, girls and boys also suffer from the erosion of local economies; the poverty, malnutrition, and disease that result from the confluence of these factors can have devastating effects on young people's mental health and psychosocial well-being. With limited resources, humanitarian actors do their best to reinforce local providers and replenish needed supplies, all the while combatants increasingly deny humanitarian actors access to the populations most affected by armed conflict, or attack aid workers outright [54].

Non-state armed groups also use community resources, such as schools and places of worship, to indoctrinate and ultimately recruit young people. An analysis of the UN Secretary General's annual *Children and Armed Conflict* reports, which tally grave violations that have been verified in select high-risk countries over the previous year, has found 49,640 cases of girls and boys being used by armed groups and forces between 2005 and 2016, whether through voluntary or forced recruitment [54]. The risks of becoming associated with combatants are by no means limited to young people from places directly experiencing armed conflict, however. The global reach of recruitment efforts has become painfully evident in recent years, with ISIS having recruited some 27,000–31,000 fighters from at least 86 different countries, as of a 2015 estimate [104]. Yet, non-state armed groups have been recruiting transnationally for years, both via social media and in person—for instance through abductions along migrant routes and refugee camps [78, 120, p. 31–56].

Armed groups and forces use children and adolescents of all ages as combatants but also as scouts, cooks, porters, laborers, recruiters, and a number of additional roles [69]. These roles are often fluid, with one person potentially serving multiple functions. In some contexts, girls and boys play the same or similar roles in combat and in supporting combatants, while, in others, each is recruited (or abducted) based on traditionally gendered roles. In many places, for instance, girls are forced to "marry" male soldiers and are disproportionately subjected to sexual violence [69]. Regardless of their role, young people associated with combatants face several risks to their physical and mental health, experience significant stigma, and tend to have trouble reintegrating into their communities well after the cessation of hostilities [17, 91, 107, 120, p. 107–53]. In addition to the risks of sexual violence and fatal injury, children and adolescents associated with armed conflict may be exposed to a barrage of daily stressors and traumatic life events, from hard labor and coerced substance use, to maiming, torture, and the forced murder of civilians.

Asylum-seekers and refugees encounter a tremendous amount of risks throughout the course of their displacement. The geography of today's conflicts means that, even if they are able to make it out of their countries alive, a large proportion of forced migrants must take refuge in countries that are themselves fragile. Parents frequently decide to migrate further, searching for a stable place of refuge, where their children can have a chance to recover and resume their education. Given the overwhelming number of obstacles involved in crossing international borders as a forced migrant, young people and their families must often place their faith—and their last remaining finances—in smugglers, who are not always capable, or willing, to broker their safe passage. Along the way, migrants are often targeted by opportunists trying to exploit their vulnerabilities. Intricate criminal networks have flourished along common migration routes around the world, often in connection with armed groups, local government officials, and smugglers [47, 105]. As a result, many young asylum-seekers are abducted into labor and sex trafficking operations or kidnapped for ransom. Others are captured by state forces and either placed in detention under cruel conditions or forcibly returned to their home country [59]. The complexity of risks that forced migrants face during their displacement not only demonstrates the interactions between factors at the community, family, and society levels, but also problematizes these terms altogether as they relate to such contexts. As young asylum-seekers move across international borders and the familiar web of community actors from home is replaced with border control officers, humanitarian actors, and agents of transnational smuggling or trafficking networks, it becomes clear that many have lost their communities altogether, at least temporarily.

Given the overwhelming dangers of growing up in a conflict-affected country, and the considerable risks that young people and their families take in fleeing, it is tempting to believe that conditions are much better once forced migrants have reached their destination. Considering the great diversity of contexts that forced migrants move through after they have left their home countries, it can be misleading to generalize about refugees as such. Nevertheless, if the ultimate goal for forced migrants is not only to survive but also to find a "durable solution," either through authorized local integration, resettlement in a third country, or voluntary repatriation, the steep majority do not actually reach their destination for a long time, if ever. UNHCR's records, for example, indicate that 667,400 refugees of all ages returned to their home countries in 2017, 102,800 were admitted for resettlement, and 73,400 were naturalized [112]. Meanwhile, some 3.1 million people were seeking asylum, and 25.4 million were already registered as refugees [112]. Although these figures are admittedly crude, they make the point that many more people (well over three times as many) in 2017 were trying to enter the refugee system than being successfully moved out of it. In a perpetual state of limbo, many young asylum-seekers and refugees move from camp, to informal settlement, to detention center, and back.

While young people are often better able to access basic services as refugees than in their country of origin, access to quality services varies widely across displacement contexts [68, 94]. Only 61 percent of registered child refugees attend primary school, and only 23 percent of adolescent refugees attend secondary school [113]. The rest struggle to find and keep work, if they are capable; some are unable to do much, owing to illness, malnutrition, injury, and/or adverse mental health conditions [55]. Access to services can be especially difficult for the 58 percent of refugees that are estimated to live in urban areas, not to mention for the asylum-seekers and undocumented forced migrants living in urban settlements [112]. Those who are fortunate enough to enroll in school and see a trained health provider on a reliable basis frequently experience discrimination by providers, and from their communities more broadly, whether based on their refugee status or their ethnicity, race, religion, gender, or language skills [100]. Children and adolescents resettled to high-income countries face similar challenges, especially in today's political climate of austerity and anti-immigration sentiment, leaving many with a feeling of isolation and alienation [33, 34, 58, 62].

Refugees and asylum-seekers often discover that the community-level insecurities they tried to escape back home have followed them across the border, albeit in different forms and degrees. In conflicts where ethnic or sectarian divisions play a significant role in the hostilities, refugees tend to find similar identity politics at work in camp settings. In Kenya's multinational Kakuma and Dadaab camps, for instance, several observers have documented fighting between rival ethnic groups that mirror conflicts in the sending country (e.g., between Sudanese Dinkas and Nuers), as well as emerging rivalries between different national groups (e.g., Somalis and Sudanese), and conflicts with host communities [26, 74 p. 88–101]. Non-state armed groups sometimes have a presence in refugee camps and informal settlements as well, taking advantage of the concentration of vulnerable people and resources to regroup, recruit, and refuel, or to mount attacks against perceived enemies [37]. The combination of these and other factors—such as underlying employment conditions in the host community and pressure from outside governments—often leads governments to securitize camps and official settlements, severely restricting refugees' freedom of movement and livelihood opportunities, while fanning the misperception of refugees as threats (e.g., "refugee warriors") [41, 79, 108]. In such situations, those who leave or avoid camps in order to find work opportunities in cities are vulnerable to arrest and deportation, exploitation by corrupt police, and further violence with local communities [37, 74, p. 181].

Refugee girls and boys may work for artificially low wages in a variety of industries, both in the formal and informal economies, from agriculture, construction, and trade crafts, to sex work [3, 31]. Even in the formal economy, such work is often illegal, depending on the child's age, the duration or danger of their work, or simply because they are not citizens; each of these infractions can be a cause for arrest. While much of this labor can indeed have a series of negative effects on child/adolescent safety and health, it also attests to their vital importance to their family and community's ability to cope following displacement [21]. Children as young as 5 overcome grievous risks on a daily basis in factories and in the streets to earn a living for their households and for their families back in their home countries [53].

Beyond the economy, girls and boys of all ages contribute to the resilience of their communities in several important ways [118]. Children and adolescents draw on their boundless energy and creativity to practice the traditional arts and crafts of their home countries while learning and building upon those of their new communities. They hold sports competitions, plays, and concerts; write poetry and journalism; and paint murals. They also band together to dream of better lives, and in so doing, they tend the hope of peace. As 16-year-old Hamza Almustafa wrote in a piece for *Ritsona Kingdom Journal*, a youth-run online magazine published in Greece' Ritsona refugee camp:

> *And I promise the people, one day we will be safe. We will light candles. We will not cry anymore. We are going to build. We are going to do. And all the people will be brothers and sisters. There will be no difference between colours and religions. There will be no more weapons. There will be love, hugs and kisses.* [2]

This tenacious hope for rebuilding is crucial for a community's ability to continue enduring hardship and to eventually overcome it. What is more, when young people are allowed the opportunity, they act on their aspirations by forming organizations and starting movements that have a hand in reconstituting not only their communities but also their societies more broadly. Recent years have seen growing attention to the roles that adolescents play in peacebuilding during conflict and displacement, whether by advancing peace education with peers, promoting reconciliatory dialogue between rivaling factions, campaigning against the drivers of violence and insecurity, contributing to truth and reconciliation processes, or creating groups that serve as alternatives to non-state armed groups [40, 89, 126]. For these reasons and more, children and adolescents have been referred to as "the missing peace" [89].

Interpersonal Relationships and Family

Healthy relationships with relatives and friends are foundational to children's development and well-being. In times of crisis, children and adolescents draw on these relationships as a shield against adversity. Caregivers can mediate many of the effects of armed conflict through supportive parenting and the maintenance of a safe home environment [106]. Family members also monitor young people's health and connect them with services and support when they need it. Family cohesion has been associated with greater service utilization and psychological outcomes [36]. In turn, girls and boys play significant roles in taking care of one another. They draw on siblings and peers for information, advice, and consolation but also for humor and fun in spite of the hardships that surround them. Youngsters also support their families and friends emotionally and help them to integrate culturally, economically, and technologically in contexts of displacement and resettlement.

Unfortunately, armed conflict disrupts many facets of childhood relationships, both before displacement and thereafter [11]. Girls and boys often feel the breakdown of societal and community systems reverberate throughout their home lives, as their caregivers lose their livelihoods and sense of security and are forced to move into more crowded households. Over time, such stressors tend to wear on relationships within the family, potentially exacerbating underlying tensions. As armed conflict intensifies, many parents and older relatives leave home to fight, or bring the conflict home by holding military or political meetings, stockpiling arms and ammunition, or hosting combatants or displaced persons. Relatives may take different sides in the conflict or disagree about how to protect their families in such uncertain times. The inability to provide basic resources and protection for their families can harm caregivers' sense of self-worth and authority, which may in turn contribute to harsher parenting styles [16, 32, 88]. In contexts where masculinity is constructed around notions of being "the provider," the sense of emasculation sometimes drives men to use violence against their partners and children, perhaps in part explaining high rates of intimate partner violence and family violence in emergency settings [76, 82, 96, 99, 101]. Exposure to traumatic events, moreover, can compromise caregivers' mental health, sometimes contributing to substance use and further perpetration of violence, all of which increase the risk of harmful outcomes for girls and boys [60, 63, 91].

In order to keep their daughters and sons safe, caregivers sometimes tighten controls over their children's relationships and community lives. For many youngsters, this means not only staying home from school, as mentioned above, but also being cut off from social and recreational opportunities. Teenagers may rebel against these proscriptions, increasing family tensions. Caregivers in several contexts tend to focus their efforts at control on girls more often than boys. In the eastern DRC and refugee camps in Ethiopia and Rwanda, for example, caregivers worried particularly about older girls, who they saw as vulnerable to sexual pressure, participation in transactional sex, rape, and early pregnancy [16, 90]. With the hope of protecting their daughters, caregivers used narratives of fear and shame to limit their mobility and interaction with males.

Concerns over the ability to provide for, and protect, their daughters lead some parents to arrange marriages for them earlier than they would have otherwise [9]. In Jordan, for instance, Save the Children reports that registered marriages among Syrian refugee girls under 18 doubled from 12 percent in 2011 to 25 percent by 2013 [84]. Unfortunately, early marriage may actually increase girls' risk of victimization, as intimate partners have been disproportionately responsible for perpetrating violence against women and girls in many contexts of conflict and displacement [96, 97]. Early marriage can also have deleterious effects on child/adolescent sexual and reproductive health and educational outcomes and has been associated with suicidality [103, 119]. Of course, young people sometimes decide to leave their family home of their own volition, whether because of family stressors, romantic relationships, or otherwise [16]. However, owing to the loss of property and income and the collapse of traditional institutions, children and adolescents frequently cannot afford to marry. Where marriage is seen as a rite of passage into adulthood, the inability to marry can suspend child/adolescent social growth, delegitimize (and criminalize) their relationships and children, and potentially result in further unrest [44, 85].

A familiar refrain among conflict-affected populations is that "everyone has lost someone." The sustained rates of high mortality from violence and morbidity in places like South Sudan and Syria create the conditions in which the loss of a parent, sibling, or other close relation is all too common an experience for children and adolescents [49]. In such settings, however, death is not the only kind of loss. For example, in Syria, tens of thousands have been disappeared by the regime and abducted by non-state armed groups, leaving spouses and children to wonder about their fate indefinitely [4]. Bereavement is among the most agonizing experiences a person can endure. Much more than a single traumatic event, the loss of a caregiver or sibling during childhood often feels recurrent. As girls and boys mourn the memory of a central figure in their lives, they must also learn to cope without that person's critical caregiving relationship and protection. Having already lost their homeland, community, and sense of stability, the death or disappearance of such a vital relationship can be catastrophic for young forced migrants. The intensity of this suffering can precipitate depression, prolonged grief reactions, and any number of additional idioms of distress [42, 64, 67]. How individuals grieve is both deeply personal and culturally bounded. For many forced migrants, fleeing home also means losing the ability to fulfil the cultural and spiritual rites of mourning that are so fundamental to the grieving and healing process [125].

Some families make it out of the conflict-affected countries intact, only to be separated in flight by any number of factors, from armed attack and police raids to natural disasters. As a result, some children and adolescents are displaced without their parents. Sometimes, these girls and boys remain in the care of adult relatives, but too often they are entirely unaccompanied by a caregiving adult. In fact, some families intentionally send their children to seek asylum alone, whether because they have limited resources to pay smugglers, or because they expect the child will have more favorable chances of receiving asylum as an "unaccompanied minor." In an ill-conceived and inhumane effort at deterrence, many countries, from Australia to Greece to the United States, have at times adopted policies of holding unaccompanied, asylum-seeking minors in detention and then often deporting them [20]. In the United States, the Trump Administration even resorted to forcibly separating child and adolescent asylum-seekers from their families as a matter of policy, leading to much public outcry [81, 98]. Without the protective and promotive benefits of family relationships, children and adolescents that have become separated, unaccompanied, and/or detained face an especially high risk of poor mental health and psychosocial well-being outcomes [36, 117].

Individual

Through its multifarious effects on societies, communities, families, and interpersonal relationships, armed conflict severely limits the degree of agency that individuals can exert on their own lives. Yet, individual factors still play an important part in the child/adolescent experience of, and recovery from, armed conflict and displacement. First, as seen above, the social construction of individual identity, such as race, gender, and religious affiliation, informs the ways in which children encounter and interpret armed conflict and its effects at each ecological level. In turn, these individual characteristics have some bearing on child/adolescent's physical and mental health. For example, several studies have found that girls affected by armed conflict have a higher risk than boys of presenting with internalizing disorders, such as depression [75]. Male forced migrants, by contrast, are reportedly more prone to externalizing behaviors, such as alcohol and substance use. Child/adolescent age at exposure to violence and displacement, and the length of their exposure, may also affect their mental health and psychosocial well-being outcomes, with younger individuals and those with shorter durations of exposure often having better outcomes [36, 75]. Likewise, younger refugees may benefit from learning the language of their new communities more readily than their older counterparts, as well as spending more time in school before joining the labor market [43].

It can be difficult to assess the degree to which the relationships between individual identity factors and mental health symptomology are influenced by a priori neurobiological differences as opposed to differences in exposure to stressors, in caregiver support and utilization of services, and in rates of symptom disclosure, each of which may relate to different ecological factors [57]. Symptom disclosure and care-seeking, however, also vary according to individual-level factors, such as confidence in the availability of care and support, language skills, mental health literacy, and personal beliefs [29, 35]. Gender may affect symptom recognition and care-seeking as well, though more research is needed to characterize this relationship [35]. It goes without saying that those who are able to recognize their psychological distress symptoms and to seek care are more likely to receive the support they need, whether from mental health professionals or individuals in their community.

A range of additional psychological and cognitive factors at the individual level has been found to be protective or promotive in contexts of armed conflict and displacement. Coping styles, for example, may influence the degree to which stressors associated with armed conflict and displacement affect child/adolescent mental health and psychosocial well-being. Girls and boys deploy a variety of coping strategies [6]. When faced with a problem, a teenager may approach and actively resolve it, or may withdraw and try to avoid the problem altogether. Another may try to distract themselves from the problem, or to seek support from relatives or peers. Each of these approaches has cognitive, behavioral, emotional, and social dimensions, and none is thought to be more effective than the others across the board. To the contrary, coping strategies that combine these different approaches in accordance with the type of risk or problem at hand appear to be more effective [72]. For instance, a refugee may benefit from using an active coping style to respond to a mutable problem, such as a language barrier. In this case, studying the new language is likely to be more adaptive than withdrawing exclusively to the individual's home language. On the other hand, actively trying to solve a problem over which the refugee has little or no influence, such as the aerial bombing campaign of a foreign government, may exacerbate the individual's psychological distress. Indeed, the effectiveness of coping strategies is highly context- and symptom-specific [106]. Political ideology and religious faith can also have protective effects on young people's mental health and psychosocial well-being, perhaps by enabling them to make meaning out of their experiences and by promoting membership in broader communities and shared practices [8, 87]. The degree to which factors like political affiliation and activity may contribute to resilience, however, is also context-dependent [106].

Other cognitive factors that may influence child/adolescent recovery from their experiences of armed conflict and displacement include intelligence, self-regulation, cognitive flexibility, agency, personality, and self-efficacy [57]. These qualities contribute to children's ability to develop healthy relationships, make use of resources and services, and seize opportunities. When girls and boys take refuge in other countries, moreover, they must draw on each of these attributes to learn the rules and skills necessary to adapt to the new society they have entered. Likewise, the amount of education that children have had prior to displacement can also influence how they make meaning of armed conflict and how they respond to adversity. For their part, pre-existing physical and mental health conditions—such as severe psychiatric disorders, disability, and HIV/AIDS—can undermine child/adolescent adaptive processes, though more research is needed to further document and understand this relationship (Cavallera, Chap. 12, this volume; [36, 50, 70, 75]). By the same token, adverse physical and mental health outcomes resulting from conflict and displacement may cascade into further stressors, contributing to additional adverse outcomes [57]. Over time, the accumulation of adverse events erodes child/adolescent adaptive capacities and can have altogether disastrous effects on their neural development, physical well-being, and mental health [45].

Conclusion

The complex interplay of factors affecting children and adolescents in contexts of armed conflict and forced migration precludes simple solutions. Because armed conflicts compromise the ability (and sometimes the willingness) of states to meet the needs of their populations, humanitarian assistance from local and international organizations is often necessary. Over the past decade, humanitarian actors have made strides in developing more effective programs for children and adolescents [51, 73, 123]. However, efforts to improve the protection and well-being of these girls and boys continue to be limited by a weak evidence base. A recent study conducted by the Alliance for Child Protection in Humanitarian Action, for example, found that child protection experts largely felt the need for more evaluations of existing interventions [16]. In order to strengthen programs for young people affected by armed conflict and their families sufficiently, it will be critical to invest more deeply in improving the evidence regarding which approaches work best and how factors at different ecological levels, such as age, gender, ethnicity, citizenship, conflict dynamics, and cultural concepts of health, contribute to program effectiveness [77]. Enriching the evidence base will necessitate speaking with children and adolescents more often and listening to their experiences and opinions during needs assessments as well as program evaluations [1, 12, 92, 93, 116]. The more that humanitarian actors listen to the voices of young girls and boys—and engage them meaningfully in program planning and delivery—the more programs will be able to not only meet their needs but also reinforce their strengths.

Overall, this chapter suggests a need for greater context-specificity in interventions for children and adolescents affected by armed conflict and displacement. The sheer diversity of child/adolescent experiences, capacities, and preferences described above cautions against the kind of one-size-fits-all approach that has too often characterized humanitarian programming. Designing and delivering context-specific interventions is far from easy. In order to address the full scale of factors influencing risks and resilience, humanitarian actors will need to take a more holistic approach, bringing together the disciplines that are traditionally fragmented into sectors and mobilizing them into programs that are at once more agile and comprehensive [11, 123]. Following the Intervention Pyramid of the Inter-Agency Standing Committee (IASC) Guidelines for

MHPSS, such an approach should not only be multisectoral but also multitiered, starting with prevention at the base and then delivering increasingly specialized programming according to risk and need [30, 46, 127]. These principles are nothing new, but realizing them is increasingly urgent. As conflicts persist indefinitely in places such as Syria and Nigeria, Yemen, and South Sudan and the historic level of forced migration continues to rise year after year, the millions of girls and boys caught in the fray deserve humanitarian care that reaches for the highest standards and advances best practice.

References

1. Ager A, Blake C, Stark L, Daniel T. Child protection assessment in humanitarian emergencies: case studies from Georgia, Gaza, Haiti and Yemen. Child Abuse Negl. 2011;35(12):1045–52.
2. Almustafa H. Refugee. J Ritsona Kingdom. 2017;3:19. https://pub.lucidpress.com/280d6c46-6399-47a6-9ce0-a34d732f8b10/#!_RpvqjIacp1.
3. Amisi B. An exploration of the livelihood strategies of Durban Congolese refugees. Geneva: United Nations High Commissioner for Refugees Evaluation and Policy Analysis Unit; 2006. Available from https://www.refworld.org/pdfid/4ff15e542.pdf. Cited 2019 Jan 17.
4. Amnesty International. Between prison and the grave: Enforced disappearances in Syria. London: Amnesty International; 2015. Available from https://www.amnesty.org/download/Documents/MDE2425792015ENGLISH.PDF. Cited 2018 May 11.
5. Asher-Schapiro A. The young men who started Syria's revolution speak about Daraa, where it all began. Vice News. 2016. Available from https://news.vice.com/article/the-young-men-who-started-syrias-revolution-speak-about-daraa-where-it-all-began. Cited 2018 Apr 25.
6. Ayers TS, Sandier IN, West SG, Roosa MW. A dispositional and situational assessment of children's coping: testing alternative models of coping. J Pers. 1996;64(4):923–58.
7. Bahgat K, Dupuy K, Ostby G, Rustad SA, Strand H, Wig, T. Children and armed conflict: What existing data can tell us. Oslo: Peace Research Institute Oslo (PRIO); 2017. Available from https://www.prio.org/utility/DownloadFile.ashx?id=1550&type=publicationfile. Cited 2018 Apr 18.
8. Barber BK. Political violence, social integration, and youth functioning: Palestinian youth from the Intifada. J Community Psychol. 2001;29(3):259–80.
9. Bartels SA, Michael S, Roupetz S, Garbern S, Kilzar L, Bergquist H, et al. Making sense of child, early and forced marriage among Syrian refugee girls: a mixed methods study in Lebanon. BMJ Glob Health. 2018;3(1):e000509.
10. Bennouna C, Ali I, Nshombo M, Karume G, Roberts L. Improving surveillance of attacks on children and education in South Kivu: a knowledge collection and sensitivity analysis in the DR Congo. Vulnerable Children Youth Stud. 2016;11(1):69–77.
11. Bennouna C, Fischer HT, Wessells M, Boothby N. Rethinking child protection in emergencies. Int J Child Health Nutr. 2018;7(2):39–46.
12. Bennouna C, Mansourian H, Stark L. Ethical considerations for children's participation in data collection activities during humanitarian emergencies: a Delphi review. Confl Health. 2017;11(1):5.
13. Bennouna C, van Boetzelaer E, Rojas L, Richard K, Karume G, Nshombo M, et al. Monitoring and reporting attacks on education in the Democratic Republic of the Congo and Somalia. Disasters. 2018;42(2):314–35.
14. Bennouna C, Khauli N, Basir M, Allaf C, Wessells M, Stark L. School-based programs for Supporting the mental health and psychosocial wellbeing of adolescent forced migrants in high-income countries: A scoping review. Social Science and Medicine. 2019;112558.

15. Bennouna C, Ocampo MG, Cohen F, Basir M, Allaf C, Wessells M, Stark L. Ecologies of care: mental health and psychosocial support for war-affected youth in the US. Confl Health. 2019;13(1):47.
16. Bermudez LG, Parks L, Meyer SR, Muhorakeye L, Stark L. Safety, trust, and disclosure: a qualitative examination of violence against refugee adolescents in Kiziba Camp, Rwanda. Soc Sci Med. 2018;200:83–91.
17. Betancourt TS, Agnew-Blais J, Gilman SE, Williams DR, Ellis BH. Past horrors, present struggles: the role of stigma in the association between war experiences and psychosocial adjustment among former child soldiers in Sierra Leone. Soc Sci Med. 2010;70(1): 17–26.
18. Betancourt TS, Khan KT. The mental health of children affected by armed conflict: protective processes and pathways to resilience. Int Rev Psychiatry. 2008;20(3):317–28.
19. Betancourt TS, Meyers-Ohki MSE, Charrow MAP, Tol WA. Interventions for children affected by war: an ecological perspective on psychosocial support and mental health care. Harv Rev Psychiatry. 2013;21(2):70.
20. Bochenek MG. Children behind bars: the global overuse of detention of children. Human Rights Watch. 2016. Available from https://www.hrw.org/sites/default/files/supporting_resources/children_behind_bars.pdf. Cited 2018 May 11.
21. Boyden J. Children's experience of conflict related emergencies: some implications for relief policy and practice. Disasters. 1994;18(3):254–67.
22. Bronfenbrenner U. Toward an experimental ecology of human development. Am Psychol. 1977;32(7):513.
23. Bronstein I, Montgomery P. Psychological distress in refugee children: a systematic review. Clin Child Fam Psychol Rev. 2011;14(1):44–56.
24. Brown FL, Graaff AM, Annan J, Betancourt TS. Annual research review: breaking cycles of violence–a systematic review and common practice elements analysis of psychosocial interventions for children and youth affected by armed conflict. J Child Psychol Psychiatry. 2017;58(4):507–24.
25. Child Protection Working Group. Guidelines on the integration of child protection issues into multi-sectorial & other humanitarian assessments. CPWG. 2015. Available from http://cpwg.net/?get=010488%7C2016/02/Guidelines-on-Integration-of-CP-into-Multi-sectorial-Assessments_03-2015.docx. Cited 2018 May 18.
26. Crisp J. A state of insecurity: the political economy of violence in Kenya's refugee camps. Afr Aff. 2000;99(397):601–32.
27. Cummings EM, Merrilees CE, Taylor LK, Mondi CF. Developmental and social–ecological perspectives on children, political violence, and armed conflict. Dev Psychopathol. 2017;29(1):1.
28. Dathan J. Explosive truths: monitoring explosive violence in 2016. Action on Armed Violence. 2017. Available from https://aoav.org.uk/wp-content/uploads/2017/05/AOAV-Explosive-Monitor-2017v9single-pages.pdf. Cited 2018 Apr 18.
29. De Anstiss H, Ziaian T, Procter N, Warland J, Baghurst P. Help-seeking for mental health problems in young refugees: a review of the literature with implications for policy, practice, and research. Transcult Psychiatry. 2009;46(4):584–607.
30. de Jong JT, Berckmoes LH, Kohrt BA, Song SJ, Tol WA, Reis R. A public health approach to address the mental health burden of youth in situations of political violence and humanitarian emergencies. Curr Psychiatry Rep. 2015;17(7):60.
31. De Vriese M. Refugee livelihoods: a review of the evidence. Geneva: United Nations High Commissioner for Refugees Evaluation and Policy Analysis Unit; 2006. Available from https://www.unhcr.org/en-my/4423fe5d2.pdf. Cited 2019 Jan 17.
32. El-Khani A, Ulph F, Peters S, Calam R. Syria: the challenges of parenting in refugee situations of immediate displacement. Intervention. 2016;14(2):99–113.
33. Ellis BH, Abdi SM, Lazarevic V, White MT, Lincoln AK, Stern JE, Horgan JG. Relation of psychosocial factors to diverse behaviors and attitudes among Somali refugees. Am J Orthopsychiatry. 2016;86(4):393.

34. Ellis BH, MacDonald HZ, Lincoln AK, Cabral HJ. Mental health of Somali adolescent refugees: the role of trauma, stress, and perceived discrimination. J Consult Clin Psychol. 2008;76(2):184.

35. Ellis BH, Miller AB, Baldwin H, Abdi S. New directions in refugee youth mental health services: overcoming barriers to engagement. J Child Adolesc Trauma. 2011;4(1):69–85.

36. Fazel M, Reed RV, Panter-Brick C, Stein A. Mental health of displaced and refugee children resettled in high-income countries: risk and protective factors. Lancet. 2012;379(9812):266–82.

37. Fisk K. One-sided violence in refugee-hosting areas. J Conflict Resol. 2016; https://doi.org/10.1177/0022002716656447.

38. Global Coalition to Protect Education from Attack (GCPEA). Education under attack 2018. New York: GCPEA; 2018. Available from http://www.protectingeducation.org/sites/default/files/documents/eua_2018_full.pdf. Cited 2018 May 10.

39. Guha-Sapir D, Schlüter B, Rodriguez-Llanes JM, Lillywhite L, Hicks MHR. Patterns of civilian and child deaths due to war-related violence in Syria: a comparative analysis from the violation documentation center dataset, 2011–16. Lancet Glob Health. 2018;6(1):e103–10.

40. Hamber B, Gallagher E, Ventevogel P. Narrowing the gap between psychosocial practice, peacebuilding and wider social change: an introduction to the special section in this issue. Intervention. 2014;12(1):7–15.

41. Hanafi S, Long T. Governance, governmentalities, and the state of exception in the Palestinian refugee camps of Lebanon. J Refug Stud. 2010;23(2):134–59.

42. Heeke C, Stammel N, Knaevelsrud C. When hope and grief intersect: rates and risks of prolonged grief disorder among bereaved individuals and relatives of disappeared persons in Colombia. J Affect Disord. 2015;173:59–64.

43. Hou F, Beiser M. Learning the language of a new country: a ten-year study of English acquisition by South-East Asian refugees in Canada. Int Migr. 2006;44(1):135–65.

44. Hudson VM, Matfess H. In plain sight: the neglected linkage between brideprice and violent conflict. Int Secur. 2017;42(1):7–40.

45. Hughes K, Bellis MA, Hardcastle KA, Sethi D, Butchart A, Mikton C, et al. The effect of multiple adverse childhood experiences on health: a systematic review and meta-analysis. Lancet Public Health. 2017;2(8):e356–66.

46. Inter-Agency Standing Committee. The IASC guidelines on mental health and psychosocial support in emergency settings. Geneva: IASC; 2007. Available from https://interagencystandingcommittee.org/system/files/guidelines_iasc_mental_health_psychosocial_with_index.pdf. Cited 2018 May 18.

47. International Organization for Migration (IOM). Addressing human trafficking and exploitation in times of crisis: evidence and recommendations for further action to protect vulnerable and mobile populations. Geneva: IOM; 2015. Available from https://publications.iom.int/system/files/addressing_human_trafficking_dec2015.pdf. Cited 2018 May 2.

48. Joly D. Haven or hell?: asylum policies and refugees in Europe. London: Springer; 2016.

49. Jones L. Grief and loss in displaced and refugee families. In: Child, Adolescent and Family Refugee Mental Health. A Global Perspective. 2020;123–50.

50. Jones L, Asare JB, El Masri M, Mohanraj A, Sherief H, Van Ommeren M. Severe mental disorders in complex emergencies. Lancet. 2009;374(9690):654–61.

51. Jordans MJ, Pigott H, Tol WA. Interventions for children affected by armed conflict: a systematic review of mental health and psychosocial support in low-and middle-income countries. Curr Psychiatry Rep. 2016;18(1):9.

52. Khan A, Gopal A. The uncounted. New York Times Magazine. 2017. Available from https://www.nytimes.com/interactive/2017/11/16/magazine/uncounted-civilian-casualties-iraq-airstrikes.html. Cited 2018 Apr 18.

53. Khoury L. Special report: 180,000 young Syrian refugees are being forced into child labor in Lebanon. Vox. 2017. Available from https://www.vox.com/world/2017/7/24/15991466/syria-refugees-child-labor-lebanon. Cited 2018 May 7.

54. Kirollos M, Anning C, Fylkesnes GK, Denselow J. The war on children. Save the Children International. 2018. Available from https://www.savethechildren.org/content/dam/usa/reports/advocacy/war-on-children-report-us.PDF. Cited 2018 May 2.
55. Küppers B, Ruhmann B. "Because we struggle to survive": child labour amoung refugees of the Syrian conflict. Osnabrueck: Terre des Hommes International Federation; 2016. Available from https://reliefweb.int/sites/reliefweb.int/files/resources/TDH-Child_Labour_Report-2016-ENGLISH_FINAL_0.pdf. Cited 2018 May 7.
56. Liamputtong P, Kurban H. Health, social integration and social support: the lived experiences of young Middle-Eastern refugees living in Melbourne, Australia. Child Youth Serv Rev. 2018;85:99–106.
57. Masten AS, Narayan AJ. Child development in the context of disaster, war, and terrorism: pathways of risk and resilience. Annu Rev Psychol. 2012;63:227.
58. McCleary JS, Chaudhry S. Ethical considerations for social workers working with Muslim refugees. Soc Work Public Health. 2017;32(8):521–8.
59. Menjívar C, Perreira KM. Undocumented and unaccompanied: children of migration in the European Union and the United States. J Ethn Migr Stud. 2017;45:197.
60. Meyer SR, Steinhaus M, Bangirana C, Onyango-Mangen P, Stark L. The influence of caregiver depression on adolescent mental health outcomes: findings from refugee settlements in Uganda. BMC Psychiatry. 2017;17(1):405.
61. Miller KE, Rasmussen A. War exposure, daily stressors, and mental health in conflict and post-conflict settings: bridging the divide between trauma-focused and psychosocial frameworks. Soc Sci Med. 2010;70(1):7–16.
62. Montgomery E, Foldspang A. Discrimination, mental problems and social adaptation in young refugees. Eur J Pub Health. 2007;18(2):156–61.
63. Mootz JJ, Stark L, Meyer E, Asghar K, Roa AH, Potts A, Bennouna C. Examining intersections between violence against women and violence against children: perspectives of adolescents and adults in displaced Colombian communities. Conflict and Health. 2019;13(1):25.
64. Morina N, Von Lersner U, Prigerson HG. War and bereavement: consequences for mental and physical distress. PLoS One. 2011;6(7):e22140.
65. Motaparthy P. Bombing businesses: Saudi coalition airstrikes on Yemen's civilian economic structures. Human Rights Watch. 2016. Available from https://www.hrw.org/sites/default/files/report_pdf/yemen0716web.pdf. Cited 2018 Apr 18.
66. Murray J, Landry J. Placing protection at the centre of humanitarian action: study on protection funding in complex humanitarian emergencies. Global Protection Cluster. 2013. Available from https://reliefweb.int/sites/reliefweb.int/files/resources/protection-funding-study-final-report-1.pdf. Cited 2018 May 18.
67. Nickerson A, Liddell BJ, Maccallum F, Steel Z, Silove D, Bryant RA. Posttraumatic stress disorder and prolonged grief in refugees exposed to trauma and loss. BMC Psychiatry. 2014;14(1):106.
68. Norredam M, Mygind A, Krasnik A. Access to health care for asylum seekers in the European Union—a comparative study of country policies. Eur J Public Health. 2005;16(3):285–9.
69. O'Neil S. Trajectories of children into and out of non-state armed groups. In: O'Neil S, Van Broeckhoven K, editors. Cradled by conflict: child involvement with armed groups in contemporary conflict. United Nations University. 2018. pp. 38–79. Available from https://collections.unu.edu/eserv/UNU:6409/Cradled_by_Conflict.pdf. Cited 2018 May 2.
70. Pearce E, Paik K, Robles OJ. Adolescent girls with disabilities in humanitarian settings: "I am not worthless", I am a girl with a lot to share and offer. Girlhood Studies. 2016;9(1):118.
71. Pittaway E, Bartolomei L. Refugees, race, and gender: the multiple discrimination against refugee women. Refuge Can J Refugees. 2001;19(6):21.
72. Punamäki RL, Muhammed AH, Abdulrahman HA. Impact of traumatic events on coping strategies and their effectiveness among Kurdish children. Int J Behav Dev. 2004;28(1):59–70.

73. Purgato M, Gross AL, Betancourt T, Bolton P, Bonetto C, Gastaldon C, et al. Focused psychosocial interventions for children in low-resource humanitarian settings: a systematic review and individual participant data meta-analysis. Lancet Glob Health. 2018;6(4):e390–400.
74. Rawlence B. City of thorns: nine lives in the world's largest refugee camp. New York: Picador; 2016.
75. Reed RV, Fazel M, Jones L, Panter-Brick C, Stein A. Mental health of displaced and refugee children resettled in low-income and middle-income countries: risk and protective factors. Lancet. 2012;379(9812):250–65.
76. Rees S, Thorpe R, Tol W, Fonseca M, Silove D. Testing a cycle of family violence model in conflict-affected, low-income countries: a qualitative study from Timor-Leste. Soc Sci Med. 2015;130:284–91.
77. Reis R, Crone MR, Berckmoes LH. Unpacking culture and context in mental health pathways of child and adolescent refugees. In: Child, Adolescent and Family Refugee Mental Health. A Global Perspective. 2020;37–52.
78. Revkin M. "I am nothing without a weapon": understanding child recruitment and use by armed groups in Syria and Iraq. In: O'Neil S, Van Broeckhoven K, editors. Cradled by conflict: child involvement with armed groups in contemporary conflict. United Nations University. 2018. pp. 104–41. Available from https://collections.unu.edu/eserv/UNU:6409/Cradled_by_Conflict.pdf. Cited 2018 May 2.
79. Riley A, Varner A, Ventevogel P, Taimur Hasan MM, Welton-Mitchell C. Daily stressors, trauma exposure, and mental health among stateless Rohingya refugees in Bangladesh. Transcult Psychiatry. 2017;54(3):304–31.
80. Rodriguez-Llanes JM, Guha-Sapir D, Schlüter B, Hicks MH. Epidemiological findings of major chemical attacks in the Syrian war are consistent with civilian targeting: a short report. Confl Heal. 2018;12:16.
81. Rogers K, Stolberg SG. Trump resisting a growing wrath for separating migrant families. The New York Times. 2018. Available from https://www.nytimes.com/2018/06/18/us/politics/trump-immigration-germany-merkel.html. Cited 2018 July 18.
82. Rubenstein BL, Stark L. The impact of humanitarian emergencies on the prevalence of violence against children: an evidence-based ecological framework. Psychol Health Med. 2017;22(Suppl 1):58–66.
83. Rubenstein L, Bales C, Spitzer W, editors. Impunity must end: Attacks on education in 23 countries in conflict in 2016. Safeguarding Health in Conflict Coalition. 2017. Available from https://www.safeguardinghealth.org/sites/shcc/files/SHCC2017final.pdf. Cited 2018 May 2.
84. Save the Children. Too young to wed: the growing problem of child marriage among Syrian girls in Jordan. London: Save the Children UK; 2014. Available from https://www.savethechildren.org.uk/content/dam/global/reports/education-and-child-protection/too-young-to-wed.pdf. Cited 2018 May 11.
85. Schlecht J, Rowley E, Babirye J. Early relationships and marriage in conflict and post-conflict settings: vulnerability of youth in Uganda. Reprod Health Matters. 2013;21(41):234–42.
86. Segun M, Muscati S. "Those terrible weeks in their camp": Boko Haram violence against women and girls in northeast Nigeria. Human Rights Watch. 2014. Available from https://www.hrw.org/sites/default/files/reports/nigeria1014web.pdf. Cited 2018 Apr 18.
87. Silberman I. Religion as a meaning system: implications for the new millennium. J Soc Issues. 2005;61(4):641–63.
88. Sim A, Fazel M, Bowes L, Gardner F. Pathways linking war and displacement to parenting and child adjustment: a qualitative study with Syrian refugees in Lebanon. Soc Sci Med. 2018;200:19–26.
89. Simpson G. The missing peace: independent progress study on youth and peace and security. United Nations General Assembly and United Nations Security Council, A/72/761-S/2018/86. 2018. Available from https://reliefweb.int/sites/reliefweb.int/files/resources/Progress%20Study%20on%20Youth%2C%20Peace%20%26%20Security_A-72-761_S-2018-86_ENGLISH_0.pdf. Cited 2018 May 10.

90. Sommer M, Munoz-Laboy M, Wilkinson Salamea E, Arp J, Falb KL, Rudahindwa N, Stark L. How narratives of fear shape girls' participation in community life in two conflict-affected populations. Violence Against Women. 2018;24(5):565–85.

91. Song SJ, Tol W, Jong J. Indero: intergenerational trauma and resilience between Burundian former child soldiers and their children. Fam Process. 2014;53(2):239–51.

92. Song S, Ventevogel P. Principles of the Mental Health Assessment of Refugee Children and Adolescents: In: Child, Adolescent and Family Refugee Mental Health. A Global Perspective. 2020;69–80.

93. Song S, Oakley J. Conducting the Mental Health Assessment for Child and Adolescent Refugees. In: Child, Adolescent and Family Refugee Mental Health. A Global Perspective. 2020;81–100.

94. Spiegel PB. The humanitarian system is not just broke, but broken: recommendations for future humanitarian action. Lancet. 2017; https://doi.org/10.1016/S0140-6736(17)31278-3.

95. Stark L. Cleansing the wounds of war: an examination of traditional healing, psychosocial health and reintegration in Sierra Leone. Intervention. 2006;4(3):206–18.

96. Stark L, Ager A. A systematic review of prevalence studies of gender-based violence in complex emergencies. Trauma Violence Abuse. 2011;12(3):127–34.

97. Stark L, Asghar K, Yu G, Bora C, Baysa AA, Falb KL. Prevalence and associated risk factors of violence against conflict–affected female adolescents: a multi–country, cross–sectional study. J Glob Health. 2017;7(1):010416.

98. Stark L, Bennouna C. If not family separation or family detention, then what. The Hill. 2018. Available from http://thehill.com/opinion/immigration/394022-if-not-family-separation-or-family-detention-then-what. Cited 2018 July 19.

99. Stark L, Landis D. Violence against children in humanitarian settings: a literature review of population-based approaches. Soc Sci Med. 2016;152:125–37.

100. Stark L, Plosky WD, Horn R, Canavera M. 'He always thinks he is nothing': the psychosocial impact of discrimination on adolescent refugees in urban Uganda. Soc Sci Med. 2015;146:173–81.

101. Stark L, Roberts L, Wheaton W, Acham A, Boothby N, Ager A. Measuring violence against women amidst war and displacement in Northern Uganda using the 'neighborhood method'. J Epidemiol Community Health. 2009;64(12):1056.

102. Strang A, Wesseells MG, editors. A world turned upside down: social ecological approaches to children in war zones. Sterling: Kumarian Press; 2006.

103. Svanemyr J, Chandra-Mouli V, Raj A, Travers E, Sundaram L. Research priorities on ending child marriage and supporting married girls. Reprod Health. 2015;12(1):80.

104. The Soufan Group. Foreign fighters: an updated assessment of the flow of foreign fighters into Syria and Iraq. New York City: The Soufan Group; 2015. Available from http://soufangroup.com/wp-content/uploads/2015/12/TSG_ForeignFightersUpdate3.pdf. Cited 2018 May 2.

105. Taub B. The desperate journey of a trafficked girl. The New Yorker. 2017. Available from https://www.newyorker.com/magazine/2017/04/10/the-desperate-journey-of-a-trafficked-girl. Cited 2018 May 2.

106. Tol WA, Song S, Jordans MJ. Annual research review: resilience and mental health in children and adolescents living in areas of armed conflict–a systematic review of findings in low-and middle-income countries. J Child Psychol Psychiatry. 2013;54(4):445–60.

107. Tonheim M. Repair, stigmatisation or tolerance? Former girl soldiers' experience of their 'homecoming'. Conflict Security Develop. 2017;17(5):429–49.

108. Turner L. Explaining the (non-) encampment of Syrian refugees: security, class and the labour market in Lebanon and Jordan. Mediterranean Politics. 2015;20(3):386–404.

109. UNICEF, United Nations, Office of the Special Representative of the Secretary-General for Children, & Armed Conflict. Machel study 10-year strategic review: children and conflict in a changing world. UNICEF. 2009. Available from https://childrenandarmedconflict.un.org/publications/MachelStudy-10YearStrategicReview_en.pdf.   Cited 2018 May 15.

110. UNICEF. If not in school: The paths children cross in Yemen. UNICEF. 2018. Available from https://reliefweb.int/sites/reliefweb.int/files/resources/IF%20NOT%20IN%20 SCHOOL_March2018_English.pdf. Cited 2018 May 2.
111. United Nations General Assembly and Security Council. Report of the United Nations mission to investigate allegations of the use of chemical weapons in the Syrian Arab Republic on the alleged use of chemical weapons in the Ghouta area of Damascus on 21 August 2013. United Nations, A/67/997-S/2013/553. 2013. Available from https:// undocs.org/A/67/997. Cited 2018 Apr 18.
112. United Nations High Commissioner for Refugees (UNHCR). Global trends: forced displacement in 2017. Geneva: UNHCR; 2018. Available from http://www.unhcr. org/5b27be547.pdf. Cited 2018 July 30.
113. United Nations High Commissioner for Refugees (UNHCR). Left behind: refugee education in crisis. Geneva: UNHCR; 2018. Available from http://www.unhcr.org/59b696f44. pdf. Cited 2018 May 2.
114. United Nations Security Council. Letter dated 26 January 2018 from the Panel of Experts on Yemen mandated by Security Council resolution 2342 (2017) addressed to the President of the Security Council. United Nations, S/2018/68. 2018. Available from http://www.un.org/en/ga/search/view_doc.asp?symbol=S/2018/68. Cited 2018 Apr 18.
115. United Nations and World Bank. Pathways for peace: inclusive approaches to preventing violent conflict. Conference edition. Washington, D.C.: World Bank; 2018. Available from https://openknowledge.worldbank.org/handle/10986/28337. Cited 2018 May 14.
116. Ventevogel P, Jordans M, Reis R, de Jong J. Madness or sadness? Local concepts of mental illness in four conflict-affected African communities. Confl Heal. 2013;7(1):3.
117. Vervliet M, Lammertyn J, Broekaert E, Derluyn I. Longitudinal follow-up of the mental health of unaccompanied refugee minors. Eur Child Adolesc Psychiatry. 2014;23(5):337–46.
118. Vindevogel S, Verelst A. Supporting Mental Health in Young refugees: A Resilience Perspective. In: Child, Adolescent and Family Refugee Mental Health - A Global Perspective. 2020;53–66.
119. Walker JA. Early marriage in Africa–trends, harmful effects and interventions. Afr J Reprod Health. 2012;16(2):231–40.
120. Wessells MG. Child soldiers: from violence to protection. Cambridge: Harvard University Press; 2006.
121. Wessells M. Community reconciliation and post-conflict reconstruction for peace. In: Handbook on building cultures of peace. New York: Springer; 2009. p. 349–61.
122. Wessells MG. Children and armed conflict: introduction and overview. Peace Conflict. 2016;22(3):198.
123. Wessells MG. Children and armed conflict: interventions for supporting war-affected children. Peace Conflict. 2017;23(1):4.
124. Wessells MG, Lamin DF, King D, Kostelny K, Stark L, Lilley S. The limits of top-down approaches to managing diversity: lessons from the case of child protection and child rights in Sierra Leone. Peace Conflict. 2015;21(4):574.
125. Wessells M, Monteiro C. Psychosocial interventions and post-war reconstruction in Angola: interweaving Western and traditional approaches. Peace, conflict, and violence: peace psychology for the 21st century. Upper Saddle River, NJ: Prentice Hall/Pearson Education; 2001. pp: 262–75.
126. Wessells M, Monteiro C. Psychosocial assistance for youth: toward reconstruction for peace in Angola. J Soc Issues. 2006;62(1):121–39.
127. Wessells M, van Ommeren M. Developing inter-agency guidelines on mental health and psychosocial support in emergency settings. Intervention. 2008;6(3):199–218.
128. World Bank. The toll of war: the economic and social consequences of the conflict in Syria. Washington, D.C.: World Bank Group; 2016. Available from http://www.world-bank.org/en/country/syria/publication/the-toll-of-war-the-economic-and-social-consequences-of-the-conflict-in-syria. Cited 2018 Apr 27.

Unpacking Context and Culture in Mental Health Pathways of Child and Adolescent Refugees

Ria Reis, Mathilde R. Crone, and Lidewyde H. Berckmoes

Introduction

There is increasing awareness among scientists, clinicians, and policy makers that understanding the role of context in pathways to mental health and illness is key to the development of effective support and interventions for individuals, families, and communities [17, 76]. In disadvantaged populations, mental ill health intertwines with a multitude of physical and complex social problems [47]. This is especially relevant for children and adolescents who develop in interaction with the contexts that surround them. Children growing up in deprived circumstances disproportionally suffer from mental health problems (e.g., [5, 16, 49]). Exposure to violence and traumatic events in childhood or adolescence has a particularly detrimental effect on children's mental well-being [4, 19, 39]. Accumulating exposure to risk factors disproportionally increases the probability of mental health problems [3, 24, 35]. In adolescents, poor mental health is strongly intertwined with lower educational achievements, substance abuse, violence, and poor reproductive and sexual health

R. Reis (✉)
Department of Public Health & Primary Care, Leiden University Medical Center (LUMC),
Leiden, The Netherlands

Department of Anthropology, University of Amsterdam, Amsterdam, The Netherlands

Amsterdam Institute for Global Health and Development (AIGHD),
Amsterdam, The Netherlands

The Children's Institute, School of Child and Adolescent Health, University of Cape Town,
Cape Town, South Africa
e-mail: r.reis@lumc.nl

M. R. Crone
Department of Public Health & Primary Care, Leiden University Medical Center (LUMC),
Leiden, The Netherlands

L. H. Berckmoes
African Studies Centre, Leiden University, Leiden, The Netherlands

© Springer Nature Switzerland AG 2020
S. J. Song, P. Ventevogel (eds.), *Child, Adolescent and Family Refugee Mental Health*, https://doi.org/10.1007/978-3-030-45278-0_3

[48, 73]. For young refugees, displacement adds extra complexity to this accumulation process. Already at risk by the conditions causing flight, the process of flight, and the long periods in refugee settlements or under asylum-seeking procedures, the few children and adolescents who are resettled into third countries face stressors related to marginalization, discrimination, and other post-migration stressors, which all increase children's vulnerabilities [26, 27, 43]. Furthermore, ongoing tension in the home country may continue to negatively affect refugee children and their families [50, 63].

The cultural environment has particular salience in the interaction of biological, psychological, social, and environmental factors that determine vulnerability for and resilience to mental health problems [12, 46, 72, 76]. Cultural values underpinning family and community cohesion, positive parenting practices, peer and school support, and neighborhood connectedness may protect children from the negative effects of adverse events [8, 39, 66, 67, 68, 71]. In environments marked by conflict and flight, such protective resources are often severely damaged, e.g., due to broken family and community structures [7, 15, 40].

Agreement on the importance of the socio-cultural contexts in pathways to child mental (ill) health has led to an abundance of studies from intersecting fields of (cultural) psychology and psychiatry, public and global mental health, and health social science, including medical anthropology. Yet there is no agreement on how to unpack "context" or "cultural context." Context may be operationalized by quantifiable determinants. For instance, to understand how the context of war impacts on children's mental health, the number of experienced traumatic events may quantify "exposure," and an epidemiological study may show how higher levels of exposure are associated with increased vulnerability for mental health problems (e.g., [70, 75]). A qualitative researcher may argue that the mental health impact of living in a war context can only be understood by investigating all contextual dimensions – ecological, historical, political, social, economic, and cultural – that shape children's experiences and mental well-being, including their own perspectives and those of other stakeholders. Epistemological and methodological differences hinder the development of a unified language to discuss the role of context and culture and of interdisciplinary theories and methodologies to study cultural contexts in ways that could inform interventions.

This chapter describes how to conceptualize context and culture in relation to causal pathways in mental health of young refugees. After brief definitions, two common paradigms that operationalize cultural context will be discussed. The first considers human society as a system in which the different parts function together to sustain the whole. In this paradigm, cultural context refers to how people's worldview supports their institutions and practices, and value theories may be useful to explore the role of culture in pathways to (ill) mental health. The second, ecological paradigm conceptualizes context as component of a dynamic process involving interactions between an individual child's capabilities on one hand and the environment in which the child is embedded. Here, the cultural context is not a system with specific functions next to other systems, but overarches all other system levels. Cultural values embedded in institutions at the macro level operate at different ecological levels in shaping or withholding opportunities to individual children. An ecological paradigm is useful to understand how certain values may impact children's resourcefulness and mental health. We will describe which approaches may help identify cultural contexts and investigate cultural processes influencing mental health problems.

Defining "Context"

Despite general agreement that context matters, there is no single accepted definition. In Latin, *contextere* means "a weaving/joining together." In common discourse, context conveys the interrelated conditions – the setting – in which something exists or occurs.[1] Theoretically, "context" in children's pathways to mental (ill) health refers to the dynamic social, cultural, and environmental surroundings against which children's biological and psychological development can be profiled. A small excursion into cognitive linguistics may clarify why it is futile trying to map such context as a whole. Porto Requejo provides the example of the concept "FINGER," which.

> ... *can only be appropriately interpreted if profiled against another concept, HAND, which acts as a base. Thus, both base and profile together conform the meaning of the lexical item FINGER. This means that no linguistic unit can be understood isolatedly because all lexical concepts presuppose others. Congruently all our knowledge of the world can be seen as a huge network of interconnected concepts; a word is actually (...) just the starting point of the process of meaning construction. The range of possible associations that can be made during the process is potentially infinite.* [51]

How then do we pragmatically operationalize cultural context to understand young refugee's pathways to (ill) mental health? What approach helps contextual exploration of the most relevant associations with young refugees' mental (ill) health so that locally salient and optimally effective interventions may be developed?

Culture as a Social System

Context is often specified by adjectives: we speak of historical, political, economic, cultural, and medical contexts, among others. Dividing context in such components seems logical for institutional bodies governing our societies. For instance, the political context incorporates how authority is developed, which is supported by rules of government and institutions. Similarly, medical context refers to the health system: the way in which people, institutions, and resources are organized to promote, restore, or maintain a population's health. Policy documents often reflect such

---

[1] https://www.merriam-webster.com/dictionary/context; https://www.etymonline.com/word/context, retrieved 14–10-18

a systematic view on context. For instance, in relation to humanitarian emergencies, the WHO/UNHCR toolkit recommends a structure for desk studies, whereby general context is composed of demographic, historical, political, religious, economic, gender, and family aspects, cultural aspects, and general health aspects [77: 61].

From a practical perspective, defining context in terms of components based on institutional realities can help inform policy and practice. It is important for humanitarian workers to understand the contextual opportunities and obstacles faced by the children whose needs they address. For instance, some refugee children may be found missing from care because they lack birth certificates or are lost to follow-up not because of willful non-adherence but because they are forced to move to another setting. Mapping how the legal system facilitates and/or hampers a refugee child's access to care may help psychosocial workers in identifying points for action and intervention at system level (cf. [65]). Developing alternative modes of legal registration for refugee children born during flight can answer the host nation's duty to fulfill article 7 of the Convention on the Right of the Child that pronounces a child's right to a name. Similarly, the medical system may be put under scrutiny how it can adapt its procedures to refugee children's mobile lives (cf. [57]). Within an environment dominated by institutions, defining context in terms of its social functions and in-depth knowledge of the institutions that represent them may be pragmatically sound.

Philosophical Approach

Definitions of context in terms of the social functions of its components (e.g., governing, health, justice) are supported by a notion of human society as an organism in which the different parts function together to sustain the whole. In terms of its social functions, "cultural context" refers to people's worldview, their shared systems of knowledge, values, norms, roles, and attitudes, as they are embedded in and reinforce cultural institutions and practices. From a philosophical perspective, culture can be understood to provide answers to universal ontological questions, questions on what it means to be human. Five domains of human existence can be discerned: (a) the intra-human (mind–body); (b) the inter-human (social interactions); (c) the super-human (e.g., ancestors, god, embodied entities and forces); (d) extra-human (ecology, nature, cosmos, animals); and (e) time (the relationship between the past, present, and future).[2] Societies differ in the answers they provide and use these answers to structure their institutions, hence the wide differences in cultural contexts. For instance, the mind–body dualism characteristic for Western European thought has led to boundaries between neurology and psychiatry reflected in the organization of hospitals, training of specialists, and journals that publish advances in science.

---

[2] The first four dimensions form a philosophical framework the first author acquired while growing up, the original roots of which are proved hard to establish but have been applied pragmatically, for instance, in Dutch educational policy (e.g., [36]).

Culture thus structures how people live their lives and deal with others and the world around them. A framework in terms of culture as a social system may help reflect on cultural differences in how human suffering is given meaning and acted upon in various medical traditions. For instance, in biomedicine – including psychiatry – the intra-human usually receives most attention, even though a biopsychosocial approach may be propagated that pays attention to a person's social relations. In African healing, what transpires in the individual body/mind is often immediately interrelated with social and spiritual dimensions, for instance, when a healer attributes a woman's infertility to ancestor wrath over societal conflict. De Jong and Reis [20] show how a philosophical model may help compare how different local healing resources (including psychiatry or psychology) address mental health problems.

Value Theories

In epidemiologically oriented (cultural) psychology and psychiatry, cultural context is only considered a useful construct if it can be measured. Therefore, operational definitions are needed in terms of variables, so that factors can be identified that effect an outcome, for instance, mental health. Value theories are popular frameworks to operationalize cultural context in quantitative designs. Hofstede's theory distinguishes five value dimensions on which all nations vary and can be scored: (1) collectivism–individualism, (2) power distance, (3) uncertainty avoidance, (4) masculinity–femininity, and (5) long-term versus short-term orientation [30]. The model was meant to be applicable to nationally prevalent styles of organization. Critics, mostly the field of international management and organizational anthropology, demonstrated flawed methodologies, lack of empirical evidence to substantiate the model, lack of attention to cultural change, and an ethnocentric and deterministic mind frame underlying its assumptions (e.g., [21, 42]). Notwithstanding these critiques, the theory is still used and referred to, for instance, in the field of cross-cultural nursing (e.g., [44]).

In Schwartz' less controversial value theory, and more in line with the philosophical perspective outlined above, three core dilemmas are postulated that societies universally need to solve, pertaining to: (1) the relation between the individual and society (embeddedness versus autonomy), (2) the social order (hierarchy versus egalitarianism), and (3) people's relationship to the natural and social world (harmony versus mastery). Schwartz [61] emphasizes that all values are circularly interrelated and they have explanatory power only in combination. Heim et al. [29] apply this theory in a recent study on the relation between cultural values and mental disorders and claim to have found a clear and consistent relation of affective disorders with cultural values [29: 103].

Fraser and colleagues warn us, however, that it is not possible to evaluate cultural values outside of their relevant context. There is cross-cultural variation of what behavior is adaptive and normative. Certain values may cause unique risks to certain populations, and cultural risk and protective factors may operate differently for children in different cultural groups. Also, among migrant populations both low and high levels of acculturation to the culture of the host country are associated with mental health problems [28: 26–27]. Paraphrasing Boyden and De Berry [12], cultural factors can render the individual stronger or weaker depending on the specific context.

Clinical Approach

The problem is that the notion of value systems as coherent wholes belies that cultures are open and dynamic. Approaching the cultural context as a social system with specific functions risks neglecting individual agency – how adults and children perceive and intentionally act upon themselves, others, and the world – and cannot explain conflict and social change. Although cultural variables may carry relevance as determinants for mental health at the level of a population – e.g., refugee children – they may lead to unhelpful stereotypes at the level of an individual living in specific contexts, e.g., an Iraqi child living in a refugee setting in the Netherlands [9, 10, 31].

> June 2019. The youth health service of a municipality in the Netherlands received a case about a "cultural conflict" between a refugee family from Iraq and a local school. The family's youngest son had kicked his female teacher in an angry outburst in class and the school asked for advice on how to deal with religious values that might be implicated in the disrespect shown to his teacher. Careful analysis revealed that the conflict had started with the parents' fierce resistance to the school's advice to enroll their eldest son in special education, leading to the boy not going to school for months. The refugee parents, highly educated with prosperous positions before their flight, were deeply concerned about the educational opportunities for their children. Unfamiliar with the educational system in the Netherlands, they interpreted special education as an obstacle to what they saw their son's only way out from an otherwise bleak refugee situation, rather than how it was meant, to allow the child more time and support to catch up with schooling. Mounting tensions between the family and the school culminated in the youngest child expressing the family's distress in an angry outburst with a teacher he had a good relationship with.

Although value theories may sensitize practitioners to potential cultural differences, in clinical practice they need to understand the specific cultural context of illness experience of their clients for effective diagnostic assessment and clinical management [2]. The Cultural Formulation Interview (CFI), part of a chapter on Culture in the DSM-V, was developed in answer to this need [2]. Although the focus is on discerning cultural factors, the CFI does not aim to measure cultural traits; it provides practitioners with a semi-structured format for exploring the social-cultural context around a client and his or her mental health problem. Culture is defined as sets of values and orientations that individuals derive from membership in diverse social groups, aspects of an individual's background, developmental experiences, and current social contexts that may affect his or her perspective and the client's social network. These broad definitions are further operationalized in 16 open questions over 4 domains:

1. Cultural definition of the problem
2. Cultural perceptions of cause, context, and support
3. Cultural factors affecting self-coping and past help seeking
4. Cultural factors affecting current help seeking

The CFI has been evidenced to support clinicians to base their therapeutic interventions with migrant or displaced clients on accurate and culturally valid diagnoses [38]. In a case study, La Roche and Betz Bloom [37] show that the CFI is also applicable to (refugee) young children. They also observe, however, that the CFI relies much on language, among other shortcomings, and is not able to tap into young children's own cultural views. They plead for the development of a supplementary module for young children that would encourage children to communicate through creative means their views about themselves and their significant contexts. Interestingly they describe children's contexts or worlds in terms of self, home/family, school, and neighborhood [37]. This brings us to ecological notions of context and culture.

Cultural Context in an Ecological Mode

Frameworks tailored to assessing risk and protective factors for mental health often fail to capture how pathways to mental (ill) health unfold in constant interaction between individual children and the context in which they grow up. Epidemiological frameworks in particular usually pay little attention to the way in which people make sense of their experiences and how intentional actions based on such appraisals play a role in these pathways. Ecological theory offers an important alternative way to theorize context, including cultural context. Instead of focusing on risk and protective factors, an ecological approach conceptualizes children's resilience as a dynamic process operating across the lifespan [59] involving interactions between children's capabilities on one hand and the environment in which they are embedded. Capabilities include children's social skills and potential to work toward goals relevant to them [56, 71].

Individual children vary in their abilities to convert resources into valuable outcomes and their freedom to choose the kind of lives they have reason to value [62, 71]. Children's capabilities in themselves are shaped and influenced by the contexts in which they grow up. Self-regulation skills allow children to appropriately respond to their environment [13], but vary between individuals. Incorporating one or more self-regulation components in interventions has been shown to be successful in enhancing positive mental health outcomes [13]. In an ecological framework, cultural context is framed as an "opportunity structure," bolstering or restricting the capabilities of children to negotiate the resources they need [71: 28].

Like any other person, children are active participants in shaping their environments. For instance, cultural values centering around respect may prevent children from expressing their negative emotions openly ([55]; cf. [1]). At the same time, around the world, children in deprived communities collectively use and reshape the locally salient idioms of distress available to them, in ways that force adults to pay heed to children's suffering.

Cultural idioms of distress are shared, culturally distributed sets of symbols, behaviors, language, or meanings that are used by people to express, explain, and/or transform their distress and suffering [32]. For instance, in Northwest Uganda, the belief in *cen*, haunting spirits of the dead, allows internally displaced children in Northwest Uganda to express their bereavement and feelings of guilt and anxiety [54]. Similarly, in the first decade of this century, asylum-seeking children in Europe started to exhibit life-threatening withdrawal behavior that embodied and expressed the state of helplessness and hopelessness of their social situation and could only be effectively treated when psychiatric care was matched with legal interventions ensuring their families refugee status [53]. Children's power to disturb may engage adults in unexpected ways. Our example of a young Iraqi child acting out his family's distress over a conflict with the school in kicking his favorite teacher is a case in point. It is important to remember that context comes first: how children navigate and negotiate resources depends first on the opportunity structures available to them and second on their capabilities as they are informed by these structures [71: 27]. For example, poor access to mental health services leads to less negotiation power to protect themselves from abuse and neglect (cf. [41]).

The Cultural in Socio-Ecology

How we unpack "cultural context" depends on our definition of culture. Above, culture refers to people's worldview, their shared systems of knowledge, values, norms, roles, and attitudes, embedded in and reinforcing cultural institutions and practices. In ecological models, for instance, in Bronfenbrenner's framework, children are thought to develop in interaction with immediate and more remote environments, ranging from micro- to macro-system levels, nested layers that differ in proximity and strength of influence on the individual child [64]. In these models culture usually pertains to the macro-system level: to cultural blueprints overarching and influencing all other system levels [46, 68]. Cultural values embedded in institutions at the macro level operate at different ecological levels in shaping or withholding opportunities to individual children. Bronfenbrenner's "chrono-system ecological theory" captures the important dimension of time. Capabilities of children to negotiate resources and how they are enabled or restricted by their environment are influenced by the social continuities and changes occurring over time through the life course *and* the historical period during which the person lives. History affects all other levels [14]. This dynamic process leads to different and sometimes conflicting values active at the macro level, complicating a systematic representation in terms of a value system [46].

Case Example

Like some 300 other asylum-seeking children in the Netherlands, 2 Armenian asylum-seeking children (aged 12 and 13 years old) lived in the Netherlands for a decade unsuccessfully applying for refugee status, despite widespread public support for their appeals. When they lost their final legal bid and deportation was planned for the next day, they ran away from their foster home overnight. The police appeal to the public to help them locate the missing children was met with a public outcry: offers of hiding places circulated the media with explicit references to the resistance to German occupation during the second world war. The next day the Dutch government granted them the right to stay after all, allegedly because of concerns for their safety. This event has fostered hope for children in similar circumstances. As we speak, Christian ministers are guiding a continuous service relay race in a church that shelters an Armenian asylum-seeking family to prevent them from being deported. In the dilemma between obedience to the authorities and the fundamental value of compassion, they navigate the law that forbids the police to enter during church service.[3] The children's decision to go into hiding resonated with deeply embedded values regarding civil resistance.

The overarching cultural context is not a static and harmonious system, but a continuously changing chaotic and contested field fraught with ambivalences and contradictions. These characteristics complicate systematic descriptions of the cultural resources that may be converted by children into outcomes they have reason to value.

Struggles with different and competing values may also occur because of contrasts between pre-flight, flight, and settlement contexts [50]. Children may then be confronted with competing values at home versus at school, for instance. Frequently occurring changes in family structures due to conflict and displacement may also disturb values underpinning the roles of children and their caretakers. For example, the government or the United Nations High Commissioner for Refugees (UNHCR) may take over parental tasks of providers [60] or children may be asked to assume adult roles, e.g., as translator for their parents [40]. At the individual level, "culture" does not refer to remote macro-structures but to socially inflected, shared, learned, and internalized dispositions to oneself, others, and the world that structure and give meaning to how one lives one's life. How children feel and think about themselves and the world takes shape as specific desires that are culturally constituted [32, 45: 63–64]. In ecological theory, "meaning" is recognized as an important and indispensable element in the process of resilience. On one hand, meaning determines the resources their family, school, community, and nation

---

[3] https://nationalpost.com/news/child-asylum-seekers-go-into-hiding-before-dutch-deportation; https://www.volkskrant.nl/nieuws-achtergrond/estafette-kerkdienst-in-den-haag-om-uitzetting-armeense-familie-te-voorkomen-ik-heb-nog-twee-meter-preken-op-de-plank-liggen-~b85071a6/

provide. On the other hand, meaning also determines the decisions that people make regarding the resources they value [71: 22]. In other words, the cultural context not only shapes what resources are available for children and their actual abilities to convert resources into valuable outcomes but also the kind of lives children have reason to value. Anthropological research has shown that refugee children may suffer both personal and cultural bereavement or, in terms of psychopathology, individual trauma and historical trauma [22]. Their strategies may be tailored more to the suffering of others than their own suffering. For instance, Akello et al. [1] describe how internally displaced children in Gulu may hide their distress in an attempt to prevent triggering distress in others. Likewise, Tize, in her study about Palestinian refugee families in Berlin, shows how the eldest girls in the family disrupt their education to support their parents in taking care of the youngest children, as the parents are too busy trying to procure income. Moreover, as the children are witnesses to their parents' stress and resulting ill health, the girls silence their own suffering in the household [66].

Researching Cultural Context in an Ecological Approach

To understand the role of culture in the processes and mechanisms that lead to children's mental problems or resilience, it is senseless to try and map all cultural resources theoretically available to children. In reality, many theoretical possibilities do not exist for specific children in specific circumstances. Contextual exploration of the most relevant associations of culture with young refugees' mental (ill) health must start with young refugees themselves. This agrees with anthropological findings on how employing child-actor perspectives and participatory approaches in humanitarian contexts may provide insight in how children and adolescents navigate their volatile environments [6, 11, 12, 33].

Cultural context can be explored as an opportunity structure. Values related to parenting practices, peer group dynamics, educational programming, neighborhood connectedness, and family and community cohesion may be assessed by indicators associated with individual outcomes. Rapid participatory assessments using key informant interviews, focus groups, observation, and in-depth case studies have been shown to help make surveys more culturally relevant, for instance, by informing research instruments with contextually specific questions (e.g., [25, 74]).

However, to understand the processes that lead to mental (ill) health and to identify the causal mechanisms at stake, methodologies are needed that can capture how pathways unfold in time. Paying attention to life course dynamics may help identify culturally patterned exposures and experiences during development and understand how vulnerabilities for mental ill health vary and may accumulate over the lifespan and how time, context, human agency, or social circumstances and sensitive periods and critical events may lead to turning points in a child's mental well-being [18, 23, 34, 52]. Life course research may incorporate longitudinal quantitative designs as well as qualitative approaches that study in depth children's own worldview and cultural dispositions, their capabilities, and their experiences in navigating the cultural resources that are available to them.

Panter-Brick and Eggerman's [46] longitudinal research in Afghanistan offers an excellent example of how mental health surveys can be combined with qualitative enquiries in different mixed-methods designs to allow for cultural contextualization of quantitative findings and inform interpretation. By combining standard checklists enquiring into traumatic events with open-ended questions asking for respondents' appraisals of the relevance of these events in their lives, they were able to identify the importance of everyday violence. Further surveys and in-depth qualitative work with children provided understanding of the relevance of family relationship quality for children's outcomes and how the value of keeping children in school is an expression of hope and resilience in a high-risk environment. Their findings also revealed how cultural values governing life course norms (e.g., secure a good marriage or job) may lead to "cultural entrapment" and negative mental health outcomes in an environment lacking the opportunity structures needed for the expression of such values in their lives.

Interventions Incorporating an Ecological Approach

A life course perspective may help develop interventions that take into account the dynamics that govern children's developing capabilities, their constantly changing environments, and the complex negotiation process between children's capabilities and their immediate and more remote contexts. It can do so by informing our understanding of how to identify and implement prevention programs appropriate for the different (cultural) contexts and life stages [58]. Development of effective prevention strategies requires the translation of modifiable risk factors over the lifespan into programs and policies, particularly parenting and school-based interventions [18]. An approach that recognizes the importance of historical events and the timing of events over the life course is of pertinent value for addressing the mental health need of young refugees.

Conclusion

In our chapter we distinguished two broad approaches to operationalize cultural context. The first considers culture as a social system with specific functions to provide people with answers to ontological questions, help structure their social relations and interactions, and shape their institutions. We discussed how in this approach value theories may help explore how cultural orientations play out in pathways to (ill) mental health. Such theories are critiqued for the lack of substantiation at the population level and irrelevance at the individual level. However, their cultural dimensions and variables might be used as sensitizing concepts to help practitioners explore cultural differences and the role of the cultural context around a child's mental health problem. The Cultural Formulation Interview is a tool to help professionals to base their therapeutic interventions with migrant or displaced clients on accurate and culturally valid diagnoses. In the second approach, the cultural context is considered to overarch and interact with all other ecological system levels. At the macro level, culture operates as a dynamic and contested field fraught with ambivalence and contradiction. More than others, refugee children and adolescents may be confronted with competing values, and these confrontations may offer them new opportunities but also accumulate their vulnerabilities to mental ill health. Theoretically, the cultural context is as unbounded as the range of possible associations that give meaning to a word. In the real lives of young refugees, cultural context emerges as resources and restrictions manifested and negotiated in their interaction with immediate and more remote environments as these evolve and change over their life course. By exploring children's pathways to mental (ill) health from an ecological life course perspective, taking culture seriously as it is expressed in resources as well as resourcefulness, effective strategies may be developed to prevent the negative accumulations that may spiral children and adolescents into mental ill health.

References

1. Akello G, Reis R, Richter A. Silencing distressed children in the context of war in northern Uganda: an analysis of its causes and its health consequences. Soc Sci Med. 2010;71(2):213–20.
2. American Psychiatric Association (APA). Diagnostic and statistical manual of mental disorders (DSM-5). Washington, D.C.: American Psychiatric Association Publishing; 2013.
3. Appleyard K, Egeland B, van Dulmen MH, Sroufe LA. When more is not better: the role of cumulative risk in child behavior outcomes. J Child Psychol Psychiatry. 2005;46(3):235–45.
4. Attanayake V, McKay R, Joffres M, Singh S, Burkle F Jr, Mills E. Prevalence of mental disorders among children exposed to war: a systematic review of 7,920 children. Med Confl Surviv. 2009;25(1):4–19.
5. Axinn WG, Scott KM, Chardoul SA. The demography of mental health. In: Friedman H, editor. Encyclopedia of mental health. 2nd ed. New York: Academic Press; 2015. p. 18–25.
6. Berckmoes LH. Elusive tactics: urban youth navigating the aftermath of war in Burundi. Doctoral thesis. Amsterdam: VU University; 2014.
7. Betancourt TS, McBain RK, Newnham EA, Brennan RT. Context matters: community characteristics and mental health among war-affected youth in Sierra Leone. J Child Psychol Psychiatry. 2014;55:217–26.
8. Betancourt T, Abdi S, Ito B, Lilienthal G, Agalab N. We left one war and came to another: resource loss, acculturative stress, and caregiver-child relationship in Somali refugee families. Cult Divers Ethn Minor Psychol. 2015;21(1):114–25.
9. Brewer P, Venaik S. On the misuse of national culture dimensions. Int Mark Rev. 2012;29(6):673–83.
10. Brewer P, Venaik S. The ecological fallacy in national culture research. Organ Stud. 2014;35(7):1063–86.
11. Boyden J. Children's experience of conflict related emergencies: some implications for relief policy and practice. Disasters. 1994;18(3):265–72.
12. Boyden J, de Berry J. Children and youth on the frontline: ethnography, armed conflict and displacement. New York: Berghahn; 2005.
13. Bronson MB. Self-regulation in early childhood. New York: Guildford Press; 2000.
14. Bronfenbrenner U, Morris P. The ecology of developmental processes. In: Lerner RM, editor. Theoretical models of human development. Handbook of Child Psychology, vol. 1. 5th ed. New York: Wiley; 1998. p. 993–1028.
15. Catani C. War at home: a review of the relationship between war trauma and family violence. Verhaltenstherapie. 2010;20:19–27.
16. Costello EJ, Compton SN, Keeler G, Angold A. Relationship between poverty and psychopathology. JAMA. 2003;290:2023–9.

17. Cummings EM, Merrilees CE, Taylor LK, Mondi CF. Developmental and social-ecological perspectives on children, political violence, and armed conflict. Dev Psychopathol. 2017;29:1–10. https://doi.org/10.1017/S0954579416001061.

18. D'Arcy C, Meng X. Prevention of common mental disorders: conceptual framework and effective interventions. Curr Opin Psychiatry. 2014;27(4):294–301.

19. De Jong JTVM, Berckmoes LH, Kohrt BA, Song SJ, Tol WA, Reis R. A public health approach to address the mental health burden of youth in situations of political violence and humanitarian emergencies. Curr Psychiatry Rep. 2015;17(7):60.

20. De Jong JT, Reis R. Collective trauma resolution: mass dissociation as a way of processing post-war traumatic stress in West Africa. Transcult Psychiatry. 2013;50(5):645–62.

21. d'Iribarne P. National cultures and organisations in search of a theory. J Cross-Cult Manag. 2009;9(3):309–21.

22. Eisenbruch M. The mental health of refugee children and their cultural development. Int Migr Rev. 1988;22(2):282–300.

23. Elder GH Jr. The life course as developmental theory. Child Dev. 1998;69(1):1–12.

24. Evans GW, English K. The environment of poverty: multiple stressor exposure, psychophysiological stress, and socioemotional adjustment. Child Dev. 2002;73(4):1238–48.

25. Eyber C, Ager A. Researching young people's experiences of war: participatory methods and the trauma discourse in Angola. In: Boyden J, de Berry J, editors. Children and youth on the frontline: ethnography, armed conflict and displacement. New York: Berghahn; 2005. p. 189–208.

26. Fazel M, Stein A. The mental health of refugee children. Arch Dis Child. 2002;87:366–70.

27. Fazel M, Reed RV, Panter-Brick C, Stein A. Mental health of displaced and refugee children resettled in high income countries: risk and protective factors. Lancet. 2012;379:266–82.

28. Fraser MW, Kirby LD, Smokowski PR. Risk and resilience in childhood. In: Fraser M, editor. Risk and resilience in childhood: an ecological perspective. 2nd ed. Washington, D.C.: NASW press; 2004. p. 13–66.

29. Heim E, Wegmann I, Maercker A. Cultural values and the prevalence of mental disorders in 25 countries: a secondary data analysis. Soc Sci Med. 2017;189:96–104.

30. Hofstede G. Culture's consequences: comparing values, behaviors, institutions, and organizations across nations. 2nd ed. Thousand Oaks: SAGE; 2001.

31. Højholt C. Situated inequality and the conflictuality of children's conduct of life. In: Scraube E, Højholt C, editors. Psychology and the conduct of everyday life. East Sussex: Routledge; 2016. p. 13–66.

32. Hollan D. Self systems, cultural idioms of distress, and the psycho-bodily consequences of childhood suffering. Transcult Psychiatry. 2004;41(1):62–79.

33. Honwana A, De Boeck F, editors. Makers & breakers: children & youth in postcolonial Africa. Oxford: James Currey; 2005.

34. Koenen KC, Rudenstine S, Susser E, Galeo S. A life course approach to mental disorders. Oxford: Oxford University Press; 2014.

35. Kolthof HJ, Kikkert MJ, Dekker J. Multiproblem or multirisk families? A broad review of the literature. J Child Adoles Behav. 2014;2:4. https://doi.org/10.4172/2375-4494.1000148.

36. Lagerweij NAJ. Naar een nieuw school concept voor de jaren negentig. Unpublished conference lecture. Woudschoten; 1990.

37. La Roche MJ, Betz Bloom J. Examining the effectiveness of the cultural formulation interview with young children: a clinical illustration. Transcult Psychiatry. 2018; https://doi.org/10.1177/1363461518780605.

38. Lewis-Fernández R, Krishan Aggarwal N, Lam PC, Galfalvy H, Weiss MG, Kirmayer LJ, et al. Feasibility, acceptability and clinical utility of the cultural formulation interview: mixed-methods results from the DSM-5 international field trial. Br J Psychiatry. 2017;210:290–7.

39. Masten AS, Narayan AJ. Child development in the context of disaster, war, and terrorism: pathways of risk and resilience. Annu Rev Psychol. 2012;63:227–57.

40. McFarlane CA, Kaplan I, Lawrence JA. Psychosocial indicators of wellbeing for resettled refugee children and youth: conceptual and developmental directions. Child Indic Res. 2011;4:647–77.

41. Meinck F, Cluver LD, Boyes ME, Mhlongo EL. Risk and protective factors for physical and sexual abuse of children and adolescents in Africa: a review and implications for practice. Trauma Violence Abuse. 2015;16(1):81–107.

42. McSweeney B. Hofstede's identification of national cultural differences: a triumph of faith a failure of analysis. Hum Relat. 2002;55(1):89–118.

43. Montgomery E. Long-term effects of organized violence on young middle eastern refugees' mental health. Soc Sci Med. 2008;67(10):1596–603.

44. Ong-Flaherty C. Critical cultural awareness and diversity in nursing: a minority perspective. Nurse Lead. 2015;13(5):58–62.

45. Ortner SB. Anthropology and social theory. Culture, power and the acting subject. Durham: Duke University Press; 2006.

46. Panter-Brick C, Eggerman M. Understanding culture, resilience, and mental health: the production of hope. In: Ungar M, editor. The social ecology of resilience. A handbook of theory and practice. New York: Springer; 2012. p. 369–86.

47. Patel V, Saxena S, Lund C, Thornicroft G, Baingana F, Bolton P, et al. The lancet commission on global mental health and sustainable development. Lancet. 2018;392:1553–98.

48. Patton GC, Azzopardi P, Kennedy E, Coffey C, Mokdad A. Global measures of health risks and disease burden in adolescents. Chapter 5. In: Bundy DAP, de Silva N, Horton S, Jamison DT, Patton GC, editors. Child and adolescent health and development. Washington, D.C.: The World Bank; 2017.

49. Pinto-Meza A, Moneta MV, Alonso J, Angermeyer MC, Bruffaerts R, Caldas de Almeida JM, et al. Social inequalities in mental health: results from the EU contribution to the world mental health surveys initiative. Soc Psychiatry Psychiatr Epidemiol. 2013;48(2):173–81.

50. Porter M, Haslam N. Predisplacement and postdisplacement factors associated with mental health of refugees and internally displaced persons. A meta-analysis. JAMA. 2005;294(5):602–12.

51. Porto Requejo MD. The role of context in word meaning construction: a case study. Int J English Stud. 2007;7(1):169–79.

52. Power C, Kuh D. Life course and developmental origins of adult health and disease, British Medical Association. 2016. Retrieved from bma.org.uk.

53. Reis R. Depressive devitalization and pervasive refusal syndrome: new child idioms of distress? In: Tankink M, Vysma M, editors. Roads and boundaries. Travels in search of (re)connection. Diemen: AMB Publishers; 2011. p. 176–86.

54. Reis R. Child idioms of distress as a response to trauma: therapeutically beneficial, and for whom? Transcult Psychiatry. 2013;50(5):623–44.

55. Reis R. Children's idioms of distress. In: Manderson L, Cartwright E, Hardon A, editors. The Routledge handbook of medical anthropology. London: Routledge; 2016. p. 36–42.

56. Robeyns I. The capability approach in practice. J Polit Philos. 2006;14(3):351–76.

57. Rossell N, Salaverria C, Hernandez A, Alabi S, Vasquez R, Bonilla M, et al. Community resources supporting adherence to treatment appointments reduce abandonment of treatment in childhood cancer in El Salvador. J Psychosoc Oncol. 2018;16:1–14.

58. Rudenstine S, Galea S. Preventing brain disorders: a framework for action. Soc Psychiatry Psychiatric Epidemiol. 2015;50(5):833–41.

59. Rutter M. Resilience: Causal pathways and social ecology. In: Ungar M (ed.). The social ecology of resilience. A handbook of theory and practice. New York: Springer; 2012. pp. 33–42.

60. Ruzibiza Y, Berckmoes LH, Neema S, Reis R. Lost in freedom: the double face of freedom in the context of sexuality among young Burundians living in Nakivale refugee settlement, Uganda. Forthcoming.

61. Schwartz, S.H. (2012). An overview of the Schwartz theory of basic values. Online Read Psychol Cult 2(1):2307.

62. Sen A, Nussbaum M. The quality of life. Oxford: Oxford University Press; 1993.

63. Bennouna C, Stark L, Wessells M. Children and Adolescents in Conflict and Displacement. In: Song SJ, Ventevogel P, editors. Child, adolescent & family refugee mental health. New York: Springer Nature; 2020;17–36.

64. Song SJ, Ventevogel P. Child, adolescent & family refugee mental health. New York: Springer Nature; in press.
65. Spronk-van der Meer SI. The right to health of the child: an analytical exploration of the international normative framework. Antwerp: Intersentia Publishing; 2014.
66. Tize C. Living in permanent temporariness: the multi-generational ordeal of living under Germany's toleration status. J Refugee Studies; 2020. https://doi.org/10.1093/jrs/fez119.
67. Tol WA, Jordans MJD, Reis R, De Jong JTVM. Ecological resilience: working with child-related psychosocial resources in war-affected communities. In: Brom D, Pat-Horenczyk R, Ford J, editors. Treating traumatized children: risk, resilience, and recovery. New York: Routledge/Taylor & Francis Group; 2009. p. 164–82.
68. Tol WA, Song SJ, Jordans MJD. Resilience in children and adolescents living in areas of armed conflict: a systematic review of findings in low- and middle-income countries. J Child Psychol Psychiatry. 2013;54:445–60.
69. Tol WA, Jordans MJD, Kohrt BA, Betancourt TS, Komproe IH, Fernando C, Ferrari M. Promoting mental health and psychosocial wellbeing in children affected by political violence: part II-expanding the evidence base. In: Ferrari M, Fernando C, editors. Handbook of resilience in children of war. New York: Springer; 2013.
70. Tol WA, Komproe IH, Jordans MJD, Ndayisaba A, Ntamutumba P, Sipsma H, De Jong JTVM. School-based mental health intervention for children in war-affected Burundi: a cluster randomized trial. BMC Med. 2014;12:56. https://doi.org/10.1186/1741-7015-12-56.
71. Ungar M, editor. The social ecology of resilience. A handbook of theory and practice. New York: Springer; 2012.
72. Ventevogel P, Jordans MJD, Eggerman M, van Mierlo B, Panter-Brick C. Child mental health, psychosocial well-being and resilience in Afghanistan: a review and future directions. In: Fernando C, Ferrari M, editors. Handbook of resilience in children of war. New York: Springer; 2013. p. 51–79.
73. Weaver LJ, Mendenhall E. Applying syndemics and chronicity: interpretations from studies of poverty, depression, and diabetes. Med Anthropol. 2014;33:92–108.
74. Weiss W, Bolton P, Shakar A. Rapid assessment procedures (RAP): addressing the perceived needs of refugees & internally displaced persons through participatory learning and action. 2nd ed. Baltimore: Johns Hopkins University, School of Public Health; 2000.
75. Wilker S, Pfeiffer A, Kolassa S, Koslowski D, Elbert T, Kolassa I-T. How to quantify exposure to traumatic stress? Reliability and predictive validity of measures for cumulative trauma exposure in a post-conflict population. Eur J Psychotraumatol. 2015;6:28306. https://doi.org/10.3402/ejpt.v6.28306.
76. WHO. A practical toolkit for professionals going to work in humanitarian emergencies. Geneva: Author; 2012.
77. WHO & UNHCR. Assessing mental health and psychosocial needs and resources: toolkit for humanitarian settings. Geneva: Author; 2012.

Supporting Mental Health in Young Refugees: A Resilience Perspective

4

Sophie Vindevogel and An Verelst

Forced Migration Stressors

Migration usually occurs amidst complexly entangled push and pull factors that are experienced, perceived or anticipated. It is sometimes a well-deliberated but often an impulsive decision – wavering between choice and coercion. There is a huge variation in the degrees of freedom people experience to make a genuine decision. Many of today's cases can be labelled as forced migration, whereby people have no choice but to move in order to live a dignified life or even stay alive. Over half of the refugees worldwide are under the age of 18 years [37]. Unaccompanied refugee minors are often seen as particularly vulnerable to depriving living conditions and violence before, during and after the flight [6].

With the marked increase in forced migration worldwide, there has been an expansion of research on the mental health consequences of war and displacement stressors. Typically, these studies are centred around measuring symptoms and syndromes like post-traumatic stress, depression and anxiety, as these appear to be most prevalent among refugee populations [12]. These research lines have led to the production of a vast knowledge base on the mental health impact of exposure to stressful living conditions and subsequent involuntary movement in dire circumstances. It has also contributed importantly to the understanding of migration stressors and their influence on the mental health, development and functioning of refugee youths.

However, such research has been grounded in victimology and psychopathology frameworks that shape the discourse around refugees' mental health and when overly used lead to the social construction of refugees as traumatized victims who

S. Vindevogel (✉)
Department of Social Educational Carework, University of Applied Sciences and Arts Ghent, Gent, Belgium
e-mail: sofie.vindevogel@hogent.be

A. Verelst
Department of Social Work and Social Pedalogy, Ghent University, Gent, Belgium

© Springer Nature Switzerland AG 2020
S. J. Song, P. Ventevogel (eds.), *Child, Adolescent and Family Refugee Mental Health*, https://doi.org/10.1007/978-3-030-45278-0_4

are weak, powerless, harmed and in dire need for extensive and specialized mental health support [27]. This has cultivated the public belief that mental health issues like 'trauma', for instance, are essential to the refugee experience. Furthermore, normal distress under abnormal circumstances has been framed as psychopathological, which has also led to a global imposition of Western views and interventions onto culturally diverse populations [41]. The representation of refugees as traumatized victims has been repeatedly criticized by scholars, practitioners and activists who argue that people engage in an active and social way with the adversities they encounter [33]. These arguments have been substantiated by epidemiological studies documenting that only a minority of people with a refugee history is found to develop lasting or disabling psychological distress [24, 30].

In this chapter, we depart from the transition framework to show that the potential impact of migration on the mental health of refugees reaches further than what is typically captured within a victimology and psychopathology perspective and opens up space for considering positive transformation. The chapter then continues by promoting a social ecological approach to resilience, drawing on topical theoretical frameworks in combination with supportive evidence and our own research in this field.

Transition: Being, Belonging and Becoming in the Face of Migration

'Transition' is generally defined as a change process occurring at specific periods or turning points during the life course, entailing a chain of consecutive events that culminate in a multilayered and often a multi-year process of change and adaptation [45]. The forced migration process can be considered as a complex transition whereby people move from their society of origin to one or more societies of (temporary) resettlement. This move involves (repeatedly) altered settings, frameworks of reference, role expectations and living conditions, which instil disequilibrium and necessitate adaptation. Young refugees thus need to redefine their lives in strongly altered contexts where previously assumed roles, social positions, functions and occupations are challenged. Their sense of self may become fragmented with previous identities eroding, subordinating to that of being a refugee. Such experiences may also significantly compromise their sense of belonging and future orientation.

Moreover, forced migration is typically characterised by unremitting unpredictability and uncertainty [28], as life becomes spatially and temporally undetermined. Young refugees often experience a state of liminality, as they are situated betwixt and between the life they left behind and their pending or aspired life [1, 10]. Even after years of pursuing stability and integration in the resettlement context, altering situations like family reunification may bring along challenging changes in the lives of young refugees. Many resettling youths face relational struggles caused by intergenerational gaps, different integration speeds and changing family roles, among other things [23, 8, 16]). Illustrative is the story of Deng, a South Sudanese unaccompanied refugee minor in northern Uganda (Box 4.1).

Transition in the context of forced migration thus refers to the prolonged, mutual and transformative processes wherein refugees are involved after they leave their homes.

Box 4.1: Deng's Experience in Northern Uganda

Deng entered northern Uganda as an unaccompanied refugee minor of 15 years soon after the onset of the war in South Sudan. He was placed in a section with other people from the Dinka ethnic community, but soon learned that he needed to be self-reliant. Even though it had never been his decision to stay there, he tried to move on and managed to make a living by seeking employment as a farmer outside the settlement. Although this wasn't the job that Deng had pursued in life, it was one of the few employment possibilities in this context and every extra shilling was welcome to survive in the settlement. Because he was fluent in English, he also became a well-respected spokesperson for his settlement section, in relation to aid agencies and management. While Deng was proud of these achievements, he often felt like an outsider in these interactions with Ugandan civilians and aid workers. Sometimes the loneliness and worries about his relatives almost made him return home, but he realized that he was in a safer place now. After 5 years, his mother fled too and came to live with him. Deng talks of this period with ambivalence. He experienced how this reunification, although being a source of joy for him, also brought a huge responsibility to facilitate his mother's settlement as a newcomer and prevented him from moving on with his activities. Her stories of how his sister was raped and killed and his father disappeared without any trace evoked so much anger that he sometimes couldn't control. As he was acting out his distress, his valued position and role in the settlement section became threatened. While he was hoping to return to South Sudan soon, that future perspective became doubtful when his only remaining relative now joined him in the refugee settlement.

What this transition framework adds to the predominant psychopathology and victimology frameworks is a broader lens to understand that the mental health impact of migration reaches well beyond the emotional processing of trauma but equally involves dealing with fragmentized senses of being, belonging and becoming. The transition framework enables us to look beyond the anticipated post-traumatic symptoms in young refugees and to see the broader challenges that continue to influence them during and long after resettlement. It then becomes clear that refugees have a sense of who they are, where they belong and what their future entails for them, often strongly impacted upon by an accumulation of experiences linked to the migration process. Because of the disconnection, dissonance and adaptation involved in the passage over different societies, transition may be distressing and lead to mental health disturbances [28].

Yet, when successfully dealt with, transitions can offer opportunities that may lead to positive transformation and growth [19, 45]. Aversive and severely distressing experiences may transform the individual in a positive way, in spite of temporary mental health challenges and support needs. Indeed, it has been argued that the manifestation of mental health symptoms in refugees "is one aspect of the metamorphosis to a new state of equilibrium" [27, p. 280]. Many refugee youths have transcended the impact of their life-changing flight experiences and the protracted uncertainty in their lives and continued pursuing significant life projects like having romantic relationships and graduating [32]. In studying and supporting such new equilibrium and positive transformation, the resilience paradigm has gained momentum.

Facilitating Adaptation and Positive Transformation: The Resilience Framework

The resilience paradigm is grafted on the observation that many people in stressful situations are doing surprisingly well and seeks to understand and support what enables people to deal with adversity. A contemporary, widely adopted definition of resilience is: "In the context of exposure to significant adversity, resilience is both the capacity of individuals to navigate their way to the psychological, social, cultural and physical resources that sustain their wellbeing, and their capacity individually and collectively to negotiate for these resources to be provided and experienced in culturally meaningful ways" [36, p.225].

This suggests that resilience should be understood in terms of person-environment interactions, involving multilevel dynamics in the larger social ecology. For instance, a recent study shows that a strong social network is conducive to active coping strategies in stressful situations, but that in turn active coping strategies are also conducive to the development of a strong social network that collectively tries to cope with the stressful situation[17]. This emphasizes the strong contextual determination of individual responses and the individual contribution to the collective process that takes shape in response to challenging situations. In spite of these insights on the person-environment dynamics, studies, policies and programmes for war-affected youths continue to draw predominantly upon an individualistic approach. Although a number of resilience-promoting interventions are implemented at the level of schools, for instance, they chiefly target individual capacities and more specifically cognitive-emotional functioning [9, 22].

Individual conceptions and applications of resilience have been criticized for risking the individualized responsibility of problems and for resulting in non-interventionism, because they tend to come down to the promotion of self-reliance [29], self-determination, self-responsibility and self-help [43]. That implies that the onus to display adaptive functioning and mental health is principally on the individual and not on the environment. Policy and practice initiatives foregrounding the resilience approach have not always sufficiently acknowledged or emphasized the importance of an enabling environment, granting access to resources that allow refugees to become resilient [29]. Moreover, these initiatives have often shunned the responsibility at the multiple environmental layers including migration, refugee and asylum policy, where such access to resources is granted or denied [29]. Stories of young South Sudanese refugees in northern Uganda, like Deng (Box 4.1), show how a resilience and self-reliance policy complemented with a strategic reduction of actual support results in structural limitations for these youngsters to actually resettle and build their future lives in the context of the settlement [29]. All too often, overcoming the impact of an inherently social phenomenon like armed conflict, human rights violation, persecution, flight or another man-made disaster has been portrayed as an individual matter, concealing its sociogenesis and inflicting a huge responsibility on the people affected by it. In what follows, we therefore promote a dynamic and social-ecological notion of resilience. By doing so, we deliberately reposition resilience and successful transition processes of refugee youth where they belong: in the social sphere.

Social-Ecological Approaches to Resilience

A central premise of this social-ecological framework is that the context co-defines the strategies employed by individuals to work their way through transition. To render the transition a positive transformation, one is challenged to rethink and renegotiate the identity, social role and future perspectives in relation to the new situation, through the use of renewed frameworks and resources [42]. White [48] conceptualized this process as a 'migration of identities'. By exploring and adopting alternative perspectives on oneself and one's situation, people's strengths and possibilities may become more strongly foregrounded, which is imperative to assume a coherent sense of self and orientation to the future [2, 14]. These perspectives are strongly influenced by context and culture, which shape the development of a positive self-image and what is considered as meaningful social roles and valuable pursuits in life. Since context and culture may drastically change with the migration process, new frameworks may give renewed meaning to one's identity, social role and future goals. Context and culture also determine whether the strategies to gain control over their situation, explore new territories of identity, establish new meaningful roles and develop life purpose are considered adaptive. Individual coping strategies, for instance, may differ cross-culturally, since culture influences the appraisal of stress and the preference for certain coping strategies [5]. Similarly, being trustful in relationships may be valued positively and regarded as a sign of adaptation, whereas distrust may be very functional for refugees in contexts of uncertainty, violence and abuse as well as be protective in the process of adaptation in the country of arrival [27]. In restrictive contexts such as detention centres, refugees' expressions of resistance or their active contesting of rules can be valued negatively, yet form a meaningful expression of their resilience to withstand stressful living conditions [26]. It may lead them to encounter their own agency and impact as well as to explore alternative identity dimensions and become milestones in their transition process. Resources, to be fostering resilience, should therefore be meaningful to the person using them. It is exactly the interaction between the person's capacities, agency and motivation to seek those resources that may promote his/her wellbeing and the contextual responsiveness to provide resources or negotiate access to them that leads to meaningful support [34].

Another basic tenet of social-ecological approaches is that professional interventions aim to build on and strengthen existing processes of support to boost the extant resource reservoir and build the capacity of people and communities to deal with adversity. It would be wrong to impose highly specialized and professionalized support without taking stock of how people naturally respond to stressful experiences and of what basic supports are present in their context [3, 39]. Of course, the existence of informal support processes and resources does not imply that professional interventions are not required, but that these need to build on what is already there in order to be efficient and sustainable [47].

This social-ecological approach to resilience reveals further how the full unfolding and maximal expression of human potentialities may be restrained when the environment is not responsive to people's needs and may be oppressing their resilience. Diverse agents and agencies in the social ecology may act as vehicles that facilitate or inhibit access to a communal resource reservoir [15]. In case of inhibition of access to resources, human rights violations and social injustice may (re-) occur. While resettlement societies are expected to fight against social injustice, refugees face increased risk of violence, hate crime, sexual violence or even police violence [11]. It is therefore important to conceptualise resilience as the process of not only coping with adversity and injustice but also opposing their existence before, during and after migration [25]. Support to refugee youths will not effectively be put in place without paying attention to social injustice processes preventing them to fully benefit from it [35].

The impact of conflict-driven displacement is mediated strongly by contexts of migration and resettlement [12, 31], implying that society can alleviate suffering or worsen it by magnifying the impact of previous war and displacement experiences. Refugee policies and support programmes can foster resilience by assuring that the systems with which refugee youths interact can (continue to) foster adaptive functioning and provide necessary resources to sustain wellbeing in challenging times. These systems are threatened or even disrupted by processes of collective violence and injustice, similar to the protracted armed conflicts that many refugee youths fled from [7]. Community systems, social networks, family ties and ethnic bonds can be severely affected, often implying the loss of significant sources of protection against mental health risks and of guidance in the context of injustice [44].

This social-ecological approach is also enshrined in the United Nations Refugee Agency's definition of resilience in refugee contexts, by conceptualizing it as "the ability of individuals, households, communities, national institutions and systems to prevent, absorb and recover from shocks, while continuing to function and adapt in a way that supports long-term prospects for sustainable development, peace and security, and the attainment of human rights" [38, p. 2]. This approach reinforces the view that supporting resilience is about so much more than avoiding or mitigating the mental health impact of the human-made disaster. It also entails the fostering of an orientation towards the future and is preoccupied with increasing the capacity to live and live together in the face of taxing circumstances while at the same time trying to improve those circumstances. This implies that the development of resilience also includes social and more structural interventions aimed at increasing the social capital and supportive capacity of the context in which these refugees reshape their sense of self and their lives.

Supporting Resilience in Refugee Youths: A Multilevel Approach

Following from the above analysis of forced migration as a transition process and the major challenges that lie within for refugee youths, as well as from the research on resilience as a transactional process involving mutually interactive and interdependent systems, some clear principles for resilience-supportive approaches can be foregrounded. These principles are supported by the striking consistency in findings on what fosters resilience [21, 35], which provide multilevel entryways to support refugee youths.

Strengthening Refugee Youths

In support provided to refugee youths, irrespective of the setting, it is crucial to work towards decreasing daily stressors, sources of vulnerability, barriers to support and the mental health impact of stressful experiences before, during and after the migration trajectory. It is also critical to work towards the affirmation of their strengths, personal agency, motivation and sense of mastery to identify and utilize what can help them towards a positive transition in the post-migration context. Supporting resilience thus goes past offering remedial interventions. Both pathways are necessary to help youths deal with challenging living conditions and the effects on their mental health and daily functioning and to regain control over their lives [6]. Overall, youths with a refugee background should be supported to (re-)establish a coherent sense of self, to truly resettle and connect with others and their surroundings and to cultivate a future orientation that provides direction in times and spaces of protracted uncertainty. While certain organizations will offer rather general services facilitative of resilience and other organizations will provide more specialized and clinical interventions focused on enhancing mental health, this kind of mental health support should always be part of any service supporting youths with a refugee background [40].

Because refugee youths are often categorized on the basis of their refugee status – only one dimension of their identity – it is of utmost importance to keep seeing them as unique persons and to maintain a holistic perspective on their situation. They often enter services with a particular question related to, e.g. legal-administrative, financial, medical, housing, employment, shelter or mental health difficulties they experience. For professionals, it is straightforward to focus on resolving that particular issue. However, broadening their scope by exploring what is underlying these particular difficulties and how they interconnect with other life domains, as well as how the person and his environment already deal with it, allows professionals to look at the person and their own role in a different way. Working holistically also implies considering the interwovenness of the past, present and future of young refugees. It implies working with the connections and tensions of living in or between two societies with their particular cultures, frameworks of reference, expectations, etc. Then, additional or alternative identities and roles can be explored in connection with the past and aspirations for the future. The latter can be supported by helping them to obtain realistic goal setting, identifying proactive coping strategies and negotiating for the resources that may support them in working towards what is a meaningful future. This goes beyond helping them to reach typical 'milestones' in the integration trajectory, like learning the new language, graduating from school, obtaining a job or living independently. These milestones may be supportive for transition, but it is important to take stock of what is valuable for each individual [34, 35].

A resilience lens invites professionals to become better aware of the representations they make of young refugees and of the frameworks influencing their understanding of support needs throughout the migration trajectory. Do we consider young persons with a refugee background generally as vulnerable and needy, or as strong and capable? What public discourses and professional frameworks influence our perception and approach of a particular young refugee in our support service? The dynamic and contextual frameworks on mental health in the context of forced migration, as discussed above, reveal that our understanding will always be partial, relational and situated in time and place.

Building Supportive Environments Around Refugee Youths

The social-ecological approach points to the importance of supportive capacities in the youths' environment. This includes a role for professionals in helping to make community resources available and accessible and deconstructing barriers to support. Barriers may be due to limited or fragmented social support networks, difficulty in accessing professional services or discrimination on the housing or job market, among other things. Especially in the (perceived) absence of a social network, it is crucial to create a supportive environment around refugees directly upon arrival in a host society [4].

Creating a supportive environment implies providing or negotiating (access to) the resources that can help young refugees in healing from earlier harm inflicted upon them, in developing resilience as they forge future avenues for themselves in society and in easing integration through facilitating connection with their broader social context on which their wellbeing so strongly depends. That supportive environment may encompass other youths and families; religious, ethnic or cultural communities; volunteers and experts by experience; (mental) health-promoting services; and local community networks and civil society organisations among others. For Manzor, a young Afghan refugee in Belgium (Box 4.2), the strong collaboration between the public centre for social welfare and the Afghan community-based organisation helped to strengthen existing resources and build new ones from a preventive perspective. Also child-friendly spaces, for example, usually mobilize the entire community for the wellbeing and protection of children amidst armed conflict [18]. Also the school can offer a setting to support resilience of refugee youths [13], where peer relationships and sense of belonging can be fostered and access to a range of services can be facilitated [46]. Further, resources from the home country or the flight experience should not be overlooked in resilience sup-porting programmes. Through the use of various (social) media, these distal resources can transcend borders and become very meaningful, for professionals too, in bolstering resilience of young refugees.

Apart from these informal support systems, it is likely that multiple professional services will enter the lives of young refugees at one point in their migration trajec-tory. Because the challenges refugees have to deal with are situated on multiple life domains, their support needs are inevitably multifaceted and complex which ren-ders referral to other services often indicated. In the referral process, barriers to those services can be experienced for multiple reasons, e.g. waiting list, language barrier and rigid consultation hours. Barriers are sometimes also established during the first contacts due to opposing viewpoints on the situation or mismatching expec-tations, hence failing to create a trusting relationship and engagement for a mean-ingful person-centred support trajectory. A crucial aspect of promoting resilience is to build structural bridges to other services and jointly tackle often invisible exclu-sion mechanisms and stressors in support systems. This also challenges profession-als from different sectors to think about how we can better support young refugees by setting up coordinated trajectories around them. Creating a supportive environ-ment hence goes beyond offering stand-alone, short-term resilience interventions. In order to be efficient and sustainable, it is imperative to embed any service in an integrated support system around young refugees [40]. This continuum of care should not only be comprised of professional support but equally involve the infor-mal support provided by caretakers or community systems [38].

Advocacy

The literature is starting to document that changes to youths' disadvantageous envi-ronments can have a greater impact on their mental health and functioning than focused and specialized interventions on these youths individually, especially for youths facing more severe challenges [25, 34]. Consequently, promoting resilience of refugee youths implies questioning and altering stressful or otherwise disadvan-tageous policies and practices in the resettlement society. Refugee-specific policies and programmes should be embedded within a socially inclusive society that offers accessible resources and real opportunities for refugee youths [4]. Supportive soci-eties create opportunities and support for young refugees to grow and continue developing themselves into competent, functional citizens. Promoting resilience is hence about providing a warm and supportive reception context in which refugee youths and their families can find true asylum. It is about designing or rethinking current policies and institutional support systems for refugees from a mental health and resilience lens. This is obviously at odds with current practices like isolation in detention centres, long asylum procedures or multiple forced relocations of refugees. These procedures all too often impede the rebuilding of lives, social networks and futures, which is so central to positive transition.

It is vital for professionals to offer resistance towards the often predominant objectifying, individualizing, problematizing and guilt-inducing discourses on refugees in their societies. When confronted with the cracks in the system through their interactions with refugee youths, professionals can choose to stand with them and give recognition to the injustices, power and privileges that may affect these youths deeply [20]. In addition, professionals can advocate for a resilience-promoting policy by monitoring the realisation of human rights and social justice for refugees, enforcing real opportunities for social integration and denouncing social and structural processes increasing young refugees' vulnerability.

Box 4.2: Manzor's Experience in Belgium

Following a long, risky journey from Afghanistan through the Middle East and Europe in very precarious circumstances, a protracted asylum procedure and relocation to different collective reception centres, Manzor (18 years) found a private apartment in a Flemish municipality, with help from the public centre for social welfare. While he recalls this step to independent living as marking a hopeful milestone, he also remembers the loneliness and fear of living in a strange environment where he knew nothing and no one. Because he arrived as an unaccompanied minor and did not know anyone in that municipality, the social assistant proposed to connect Manzor to an Afghan community-based organisation in the nearest city. Volunteers affiliated to that organization work in the region to connect newcomers with citizens and public facilities, introduce them to the nearest mosque and its associations, support them with translation and administration, provide homework support, etc. The public centre for social welfare collaborates closely with this organization to identify and report challenges, like discrimination of newcomers on the housing market, to the local council. Together they support the council in developing and implementing a supportive policy for newcomers, and asylum seekers with a precarious legal status in particular. Through this collaboration, Manzor got to know many people in his neighbourhood, got connected to peers whom he shares similar struggles and aspirations with, was able to identify the services he could utilize to get the support needed, was donated supplies to furnish his apartment and found courage to endeavour on a school career.

Conclusion

In this chapter, we documented how refugee youths' mental health responses are complex, dynamic and contextual in nature, implying that to understand resilience we need to understand the supportive dynamics between these youths and their surroundings. The social-ecological approach to resilience compels to look beyond representations of the traumatized victim who needs to overcome his trials of life, to recognize that forced migration is a collective challenge that requires the fostering of an adaptive and supportive environment. To realise this, it is key to work on multiple ecological levels: to strengthen youths with a refugee background in (further) developing a coherent sense of identity, belonging and purpose; to increase availability and accessibility of informal and professional resources for them; and to advocate for the realisation of human rights, social justice and real opportunities for social integration. Despite these clear anchoring principles for resilience-supporting interventions, evidence-based knowledge on the effectiveness of resilience interventions in general is nascent. Consequently, more research should be conducted to extend evidence on which approaches work best for refugee youths and their families. Especially interventions on the family, school, community or societal level require more investigation to supplement the current understanding of how mental health and resilience of refugee youths can be promoted in the daily living contexts.

Bibliography

1. Agier M. Managing the undesirables: refugee camps and humanitarian government. Cambridge: Polity Press; 2011.
2. Becker G. Disrupted lives: How people create meaning in a chaotic world. Berkeley/Los Angeles/London: University of California Press; 1999.
3. Boothby N, Strang A, Wessells M. A world turned upside down. Bloomfield: Kumarian Press; 2006.
4. Correa-Velez I, Gifford SM, Barnett AG. Longing to belong: social inclusion and wellbeing among youth with refugee background in the first three years in Melbourne, Australia. Soc Sci Med. 2010;71:1399–408.
5. De Jong JT. Public mental health and culture: disasters as a challenge to Western mental health care models, the self, and PTSD. In: Wilson JP, Drozdek B, editors. Broken spirits, the treatment of traumatized asylum seekers, refugees, war and torture victims. New York: Brunner-Routledge; 2004. p. 159–78.
6. Derluyn I, van Ee E, Vindevogel S. Psychosocial wellbeing of 'vulnerable' refugee groups in (post-)conflict contexts: an intriguing juxtaposition of vulnerability and resilience. In: Wenzel T, Drozdek B, editors. An uncertain safety. Cham, Switzerland: Springer International Publishing; 2019. p. 213–31.
7. Derluyn I, Vindevogel S, De Haene L. Towards a relational understanding of the reintegration and rehabilitation processes of former child soldiers. J Aggress Maltreat Trauma. 2013;22(8):869–86.
8. Deng SA, Marlowe JM. Refugee resettlement and parenting in a different context. J Immigr Refug Stud. 2013;11:416–30.
9. Diab M, Peltonen K, Qouta SR, Palosaari E, Punamäki RL. Effectiveness of psychosocial intervention enhancing resilience among war-affected children and the moderating role of family factors. Child Abuse Negl. 2015;40:24–35.

10. El-Sharaawi N. "Everything here is temporary": psychological distress and suffering among Iraqi refugees in Egypt. In: Hinton D, Hinton A, editors. Genocide and mass violence: memory, symptom, and recovery. Cambridge: Cambridge University Press; 2014. p. 195–211.
11. European Union Agency for Fundamental Rights. Fundamental rights report 2018. Geneva: European Union Agency for Fundamental Rights; 2018.
12. Fazel M, Reed R, Panter-Brick C, Stein A. Mental health of displaced and refugee children resettled in high-income countries: risk and protective factors. Lancet. 2012;379:266–82.
13. Fazel M, Betancourt TS. Preventive mental health interventions for refugee children and adolescents in high-income settings. Lancet Child Adolesc Health. 2018;2(2):121–32.
14. Grimes RL. Deeply into the bone: Re-inventing rites of passage. Berkeley/Los Angeles/London: University of California Press; 2002.
15. Hollifield M, Gory A, Siedjak J, Nguyen L, Holmgreen L, Hobfoll S. The benefit of conserving and gaining resources after trauma: a systematic review. J Clin Med. 2016;5(11):1–15.
16. Hynie M, Guruge S, Shakya YB. Family relationships of Afghan, Karen and Sudanese refugee youth. Can Ethn Stud. 2013;44(3):11–28.
17. Iacoviello BM, Charney DS. Psychosocial facets of resilience: implications for preventing posttrauma psychopathology, treating trauma survivors, and enhancing community resilience. Eur J Psychotraumatol. 2014;5(1):23970.
18. Kostelny K, Wessells M. Child friendly spaces: Promoting children's resiliency amidst war. In: Handbook of resilience in children of war. New York, NY: Springer; 2013. p. 119–29.
19. Layne CM, Beck CJ, Rimmash H, Southwick JS, Moreno MA, Hobfoll SE. Promoting 'resilient' posttraumatic adjustment in childhood and beyond. 'Unpacking' life events, resources, and interventions. In: Brom D, Pat-Horenczyk R, Ford JD, editors. Treating traumatized children. Risk, resilience and recovery. New York: Routledge/Taylor & Francis Group; 2009. p. 13–47. Lee PL. Making now precious: working with survivors of torture and asylum seekers. Int J Narrat Ther Commun Work. 2012;5:1–9.
20. Lee PL. Making now precious. Working with survivors of torture and asylum seekers. Int J Narrat Ther Commun Work. 2013;1:1–10.
21. Masten A. Global perspectives on resilience in children and youth. Child Dev. 2014;85:6–20.
22. McMullen J, O'Callaghan P, Shannon C, Black A, Eakin J. Group trauma-focused cognitive-behavioural therapy with former child soldiers and other war-affected boys in the DR Congo: a randomized controlled trial. J Child Psychol Psychiatry. 2013;54:1231–41.
23. McCleary JS. The impact of resettlement on Karen refugee family relationships: A qualitative exploration. Child Fam Soc Work. 2017;22(4):1464–71.
24. Miller KE, Rasmussen A. The mental health of civilians displaced by armed conflict: an ecological model of refugee distress. Epidemiol Psychiatr Sci. 2017;26(2):129–38.
25. Prilleltensky I. Wellness as fairness. Am J Community Psychol. 2012;49(1–2):1–21.
26. Ramadan A. Spatialising the refugee camp. Trans Inst Br Geogr. 2013;38(1):65–77.
27. Rousseau C, Measham TJ. Posttraumatic suffering as a source of transformation: a clinical perspective. In: Kirmayer LJ, Lemelson R, Barad M, editors. Understanding trauma: integrating biological, clinical and cultural perspectives. Cambridge: Cambridge University Press; 2007. p. 275–94.
28. Schiltz J. Encountering uncertainty. Everyday camp life and futures of South Sudanese refugee youth in Northern Uganda. Ghent: Ghent University; 2018.
29. Schiltz J, Derluyn I, Vanderplasschen W, Vindevogel S. Resilient and self-reliant life: South Sudanese refugees imagining futures in the Adjumani refugee setting, Uganda. Child Soc. 2018;33(1):1–14.
30. Silove D, Ventevogel P, Rees S. The contemporary refugee crisis: an overview of mental health challenges. World Psychiatry. 2017;16(2):130–9.
31. Siriwardhana C, Ali SS, Roberts B, Stewart R. A systematic review of resilience and mental health outcomes of conflict-driven adult forced migrants. Confl Heal. 2014;8:1–14.
32. Sampson RC, Gifford SM, Taylor S. The myth of transit: the making of a life b asylum seekers and refugees in Indonesia. J Ethn Migr Stud. 2006;42(7):1135–52.
33. Summerfield D. War and mental health: a brief overview. BJM. 2000;321(7255):232–5.

34. Ungar M. Working with children and youth with complex needs. 20 skills to build resilience. New York: Routledge; 2015.
35. Ungar M. What works. A manual for designing programs that build resilience . Nova Scotia: Resilience Research Centre; 2018.
36. Ungar M. Resilience across cultures. Br J Soc Work. 2008;38:218–35.
37. UNHCR. Global Trends. Forced discplacement in 2018. UNHCR, Geneva; 2019. https://www.unhcr.org/5d08d7ee7.pdf.
38. United Nations High Commissioner For Refugees. Resilience and self-reliance from a protection and solutions perspective. 2017. https://www.unhcr.org/excom/standcom/58ca4f827/resilience-self-reliance-protection-solutions-perspective.html.
39. Van Ommeren M, Wessells M. Inter-agency agreement on mental health and psychosocial support in emergency settings. Bull World Health Organ. 2007;85(11):822.
40. Ventevogel P. Interventions for mental health and psychosocial support in complex humanitarian emergencies: moving towards consensus in policy and action? Theory, research and clinical practice. In: Morina N, Nickerson A, editors. Mental health of refugee and conflict-affected populations. Cham: Springer; 2018. p. 155–80.
41. Ventevogel P, Jordans M, Reis R, de Jong J. Madness or sadness? Local concepts of mental illness in four conflict-affected African communities. Confl Health. 2013;7(1):3.
42. Vindevogel S. From military to civilian life: challenges and resources in the transition of former child soldiers from military to civilian life. Gent: Academia Press; 2013.
43. Vindevogel S. Resilience in the context of war: a critical analysis of contemporary conceptions and interventions to promote resilience among war-affected children and their surroundings. Peace Conflict J Peace Psychol. 2017;23(1):76–84.
44. Vindevogel S, De Schryver M, Broekaert E, Derluyn I. Challenges faced by former child soldiers in the aftermath of war in Uganda. J Adolesc Health. 2013;52:757–64.
45. Vogler P, Crivello G, Woodhead M. Early childhood transitions research: A review of concepts, theory and practice. Working Paper 48: Studies in Early Childhood Transitions. The Hague: Bernard van Leer Foundation; 2008.
46. Ward C, Geeraert N. Advancing acculturation theory and research: The acculturation process in its ecological context. Curr Opin sychol. 2016;8:98–104.
47. Wessells M. Psychosocial wellbeing and the integration of war-affected children: toward a community resilience approach. In: Derluyn I, Mels C, Parmentier S, Vandenhole W, editors. Re-member. Rehabilitation, reintegration and reconciliation of war-affected children. Cambridge, England: Intersentia; 2012. p. 57–75.
48. White M. Re-authoring lives: Interviews and essays. Adelaide, South Australia: Dulwich Centre Publications; 1995.

Part II

Mental Health Assessment of Refugee Children

Principles of the Mental Health Assessment of Refugee Children and Adolescents

Suzan J. Song and Peter Ventevogel

Introduction

Mental health workers and other clinicians evaluate children and adolescents for psychological disturbance that can manifest in emotional, physical, cognitive, or behavioral issues that create social or academic difficulties. When performing a mental health assessment of refugee children, awareness of the complexities of needs that they face is important, as these children have often been exposed to multiple risks, and complex needs may not be addressed through a single perspective, agency, or intervention [9, 14]. A mental health assessment for refugee children should therefore incorporate the various contexts and settings through a developmental, cultural, and socio-ecological lens. Such an assessment is strongly multidisciplinary. When sufficient human resources are available, input from staff with a background in social science (social work, anthropology) can be very useful. This chapter is thus not only for clinical psychiatrists, psychologists, and therapists but also for caseworkers, protection workers, counselors, and legal aid providers who are asked to be involved in mental health assessment for refugee children. Consider the following examples:

- A physician or nurse in a health center is asked to evaluate an adolescent's mental health state in order to initiate clinical care.
- A case manager is asked to interview a refugee family with multiple problems to identify how to help the children in the family.

S. J. Song (✉)
Department of Psychiatry, George Washington University, Washington, DC, USA

P. Ventevogel
Public Health Section (Division of Resilience and Solutions), United Nations High Commissioner for Refugees, Geneva, Switzerland

© Springer Nature Switzerland AG 2020
S. J. Song, P. Ventevogel (eds.), *Child, Adolescent and Family Refugee Mental Health*, https://doi.org/10.1007/978-3-030-45278-0_5

- A protection worker is asked to interview an unaccompanied minor in a refugee camp in order to assess the protection risks and specific threats to emotional well-being.
- A school counselor is concerned about a child's emotional state as a recently resettled refugee in a new school.
- A lawyer is conducting a forensic evaluation for an adolescent seeking asylum and is not sure if his/her mental health state warrants further care.

The purpose of a mental health assessment for refugee children is to

1. Determine, in ways that are sensitive to culture and context, if a child has a serious social, emotional, or behavioral problem that is impairing his or her functioning to impact one's normal developmental trajectory.
2. Determine whether an intervention is necessary.
3. Identify and evaluate personal, cultural, and social strengths and sources of support.
4. Develop intervention recommendations and a plan to help the child and family engage in treatment, inclusive of building on youth and family strengths and available resources.

Engaging the Sociocultural Context

The Role of the Socio-Ecological Context in an Assessment

Psychological well-being and functioning of children are highly interwoven into the family, peer, and school setting in which they live [4]. A child must be assessed in relation to the multiple spheres of influence surrounding them, including the agencies, communities, and cultures in which they are embedded. A full mental health assessment will therefore require obtaining information not only from the child but also from the supports around them such as caretakers or family, teachers, or health workers such as pediatricians, family doctors, or general practitioners. If a refugee child is being assisted by social services (e.g., a resettlement office, a community-based organization, or a protection agency), information from records and caseworkers can be invaluable, especially in cases of unaccompanied or separated asylum-seeking and refugee children. However, obtaining previous records and history can be a particular challenge for this group as the mental health assessment may be their first contact with an agency in the country.

Unpacking Emotional and Behavioral Distress

Culture and context are at the core of identity formation of refugee children and strongly influence the manifestation and expression of emotions. Understanding relevant cultural concepts of mental illness, as well as idioms of distress that are often "embodied" – expressed through the body and not expressed through language – can help clinicians and providers better understand the child's emotional experience and prevent the imposition of labels that do not have relevance or meaning for the child and his or her social surroundings. Engaging with such local expressions of distress can help clinicians to better understand the views of the refugee child and their social network around the putative causes of distress and the expected course and, moreover, can help in setting shared therapeutic targets and increase therapeutic empathy and treatment adherence [17]. The exploration of local idioms of distress is not something that many mental health professionals are familiar with. Cultural brokers may have a role in documenting the perspectives of the refugee child and family and explore the cultural and contextual factors that may play a role in the development of symptoms and the help-seeking behavior.

Standard classification systems such as the *Diagnostic and Statistical Manual* (DSM-V) and the *International Statistical Classification of Diseases and Related Health Problems* (ICD-11) have been critiqued for their reductionist perspective that minimizes personal complexities and overlooks the sociocultural context in which symptoms are produced [3, 28]. A multilevel, ecosocial approach and ethnographic understanding of mental distress for refugee children may serve as a complement to provide a well-informed assessment that positions mental health conditions within a wider sociocultural context [18]. Despite considerable epistemological challenges with standard categorizations of mental health problems, using such classifications is more or less inevitable and has many purposes – for refugee registration, communication among practitioners, coordinating collaborative care, and health financing. While certainly not ideal, it is the best model we have at the current moment and can function as a guide for clinicians in selecting treatment options.

Dimensional Approach to Mental Health Problems

Global mental health practitioners have shown the utility and success of combining biomedical and local explanatory models of illness experiences into contextually appropriate interventions [1, 15]. Related to the divide with global mental health between conventional clinical approaches and ecosocial approaches, the Lancet Commission on Global Mental Health (2018) has recommended that the global mental health agenda incorporates a staged approach to understanding of and responding to mental health problems. Such an approach would replace a binary classification (with someone "having the disease" or not) with a staged, dimensional approach and would converge social and biological determinants of mental health problems throughout one's life course [20].

Role of Culture and Context in Shaping "Normal"

Understanding the child's cultural and social context is essential for a useful, accurate, and relevant assessment. Different sociocultural contexts influence the roles of children in their families and communities, including how they are expected to interact interpersonally. Clinicians should be mindful of the role of cultural and social factors in shaping what is normal in child development. Industrialized societies in North America and Europe may prioritize individualism and empowerment, using concepts that flow out of such values such as "lacking boundaries," "enmeshment," or "dependent personality." These may not be accurate and may instead be misleading for children from societies that highly value interpersonal reliance and dependency [7]. For example, American clinicians may prioritize the individuation of an adolescent from his/her parents [21], but this may not be appropriate for the family who prioritizes family interdependence.

Case Study

Abdi, an 11-year-old refugee boy, arrives from a remote part of an Eastern African country* to the USA with his mother, seeking asylum due to religious persecution and related domestic violence. Mother reports that her husband was physically and emotionally abusive, threatening her life multiple times. She was 10 years old at time of marriage, and her husband was 25 years old. One year ago, the sister of Abdi was killed in a family conflict. Due to financial difficulties, the boy was living with his aunt, while mother visited on weekends. They are now reunited after 6 months. They have been in the USA for less than a year, and the boy does not listen to anyone. He is involved in all aspects of mother's life, including setting her up on romantic dates to find a new husband. He interprets for her in the session. She says, "He is my everything." He is failing in school, has multiple arguments with students and teachers, and shows general disrespect toward his mother, stating he does not need to listen to anyone. Mother explains that in her culture, boys are adults at an early age, sometimes as early as 8 years old, and often have more power than the mother. She feels she cannot, and should not control him, and does not know how to best manage him. The clinician is therefore left with the mother's reported cultural norm of the role of a child as an adult and the child's negative behavior and ability to function in this new setting.

(source: clinical notes from first author. Details of the case have been changed to prevent recognition)

This case illustrates that the cultural norms around childhood and masculinity in the country may be at odds with norms in the host country. The absence of a large supportive social network and the dire economic circumstance makes that in this case the responsibilities surpass the capacities of the boy causing major behavioral problems and affecting his social and educational functioning.

A helpful tool to obtain a "quick scan" of cultural factors in the life of the person is the 'Cultural Formulation Interview" (CFI) which provides a framework to systematically explore areas such as the cultural definition of the problem, perceptions of causes and course, cultural identity of the person, ways the person is coping in the present and past, and help-seeking strategies used [19]. The CFI is particularly useful for work with refugees [22]). Additional information on cultural and contextual factors related to mental health of refugees can be found in desk reviews that have been prepared for Somalian refugees [6], Syrian refugees [11], and Rohingya refugees from Myanmar [24].

Developmental Understanding

The Role of Development in Understanding Mental Health Problems

Prior to conducting a mental health assessment, clinicians must have a good understanding of normal child development. This includes a developmental framework that is sensitive to what is normal in the culture and context of the child (refer to Chap. 3). For refugee children, it is important to situate symptoms in the actual context of the refugee and to evaluate how the interplay between various external factors affects symptom expression. A mental health assessment should explore to what extent the symptom or behavior is a normal reaction to one's socio-ecological situation, as well as to identify whether changing the environment could significantly alter symptoms. Developmental factors can affect how emotional and behavioral symptoms manifest in children. For example, behavioral problems in children such as bedwetting or tantrums could be developmentally normal for toddlers, but not for primary school-aged children (6–15 years old). A clinician needs to understand the child's symptoms or difficulties as compared to the acceptable range of behaviors at various developmental ages and the manifestations of problems in each developmental phase.

Role of Development and Communication Style

Practitioners should also be mindful of the impact of development on a child's ability to communicate their feelings and experiences. Younger children may not trust unfamiliar people and may not have the cognitive maturity to understand, let alone discuss, their internal emotional states. Adolescents may perceive adults as judging them. Developmental factors also play a role in the manifestation and expression of mental health symptoms, such as the response to exposure to traumatic events. Toddlers who have witnessed or experienced war in their home country may show fears of the dark or tantrums. However, toddlers who have not experienced war or trauma may also frequently experience fears of the dark or exhibit tantrums with yelling and crying, which are not necessarily a sign of psychopathology. The label of being a "refugee" should not divert our attention from other elements of their social roles, development, and personal identity. Therefore, understanding normal child/adolescent development in a cultural context is imperative, as well as using observation and evaluation of a child's current level of social, emotional, and behavioral functioning in relation to his/her peers (age and stage of development).

Case Example
In a refugee camp in Jordan, a humanitarian child protection worker noticed a 14-year-old Syrian boy screaming and crying alone outside of his tent. The worker approached and found that the boy was angry that his parents would not let him wander by himself to the main entrance gate. He was bored, felt trapped, and missed his friends, family, and life back in Syria. On further discussion, he revealed his unease whenever a plane flew above, felt alone, thinking his parents did not understand him, and was both angry and scared after witnessing two families physically and verbally assaultive at the water and sanitation station. The worker understood how hard social isolation and change from one's main supports were on the developmental need of someone in early adolescence. Even though the child's emotional reactions were possibly a normal response to his refugee-related experience, he still needed further assessment and support. The worker introduced him to a mental health counselor, who met with the child and parents, provided psychoeducation about the potential adverse mental health consequences that can follow from the experience of displacement from one's home and culture, and provided potential coping strategies to manage anger and anxiety, as well as connected him with adolescent-friendly spaces and programs to feel more a sense of belonging since developmentally, adolescents may seek peer support.
  (source: clinical notes from first author. Details of the case have been changed to prevent recognition)

Working with Interpreters

Considerations in Working with Interpreters

Language barriers may necessitate the use of interpreters. While it may be difficult to find professional interpreters, especially in the case of rare languages, the use of family members as interpreters should be avoided, due to the significant pressures it can place on the client and interpreting family member. The translation of phrases implies making choices on how and what to translate, making interpretation rarely neutral, particularly when terms from one language cannot be easily translated into another. The influence of an interpreter during an assessment; therefore, goes beyond the translation of words. The presence of a third person in the room changes the dynamics of the experience. Some refugees may see the role of an interpreter as a co-therapist, particularly when the same interpreter is present over multiple sessions [2]. The position of an adult interpreter in a child interview has potential to create an imbalance of power, which can unwittingly lead to silencing, distorting, or influencing the voice of the child with what the child tells [16]. When the interpreter is from the same country as the child, issues of trust and confidentiality can arise. An interpreter from the same community or background can increase the feeling of being at home and understood but can also lead to isolation and mistrust if the child is concerned that the interpreter may share information with others in the community.

Persistent Language Barriers

Sometimes the use of an interpreter still does not solve language barriers. Refugee children may have a rare local language as their "mother tongue," while the interpreter may speak the national language or standard dialect of the country. For example, the Democratic Republic of Congo and South Sudan have dozens of local languages. Official interpreters often speak the larger "national" language that functions as a lingua franca in a country or region, such as Lingala, kiSwahili, or Juba Arabic. A refugee child may be able to sufficiently master such a language sufficiently to communicate for daily survival, but not enough to discuss in-depth emotional issues. Moreover, some English terms do not have a clear equivalent term in the child's primary language, as may be the case for terms indicating emotions, such as the nuances between "anxiety," "fear," "irritation," and "anger" [27].

Interpreters as Cultural Mediators

After the session, debriefing with the interpreter can be useful to ascertain how the interpreter judges the child's use of language and any cultural nuances that can help inform the contextual and developmental understanding of the child. In this way, interpreters can act as "cultural mediators," particularly if the interpreter and child share a similar (sub)cultural background that is markedly different from the clinician's background. The clinician can ask the interpreter to provide background information about cultural issues that may have arisen in the session [26].

Box 1 Tips for Working with Interpreters During Mental Health Assessment of Refugee Children and Adolescents (Based on Flores [10] and Tribe and Morrisey [26])
- Instruct interpreters to translate with minimal editing and tell-inform you if they do not understand something the child has said.
- Clearly explain the purpose of the session to the child; why the interpreter is present; and what his/her role is.
- Emphasize confidentiality among everyone in the room, including the interpreter,
- Use simple sentence construction and appropriate pauses.

- Work slowly so the interpreter, child, and clinician can easily understand each other.
- Avoid using proverbs and metaphors that are often culture-specific and ambiguous.
- Verify whether interpreter and child/adolescent have understood.
- Pay careful attention to nonverbal cues.

Building an Alliance

Understanding Confidentiality

Child refugees may not have had a mental health interview before, and therefore may not be accustomed to the seemingly intrusive questioning about one's emotional or behavioral state. The role of a mental health professional and the goal of the assessment may not be clearly understood and should be explained in simple terms [13]. In case of an unaccompanied child, it can be helpful to involve their caseworker or foster care parent in the initial assessment [8]. Being clear about the limitations of confidentiality are important, as youth and caretakers are likely not aware of the extent to which information may be transferred to legal or state authorities. For example, it is possible that community-based agencies will ask to view mental health assessments. In most countries, legal and the medical regulations state that medical reports cannot be shared with others (including other medical institutions) unless the involved person (or the legal custodian) has given explicit permission. There may be a need to make exceptions, such as when there is an imminent danger to self or to others, in which case a psychiatrist is obliged to share information in order to save lives. Therefore, confidentiality should be explained without reassurance or promises that cannot be guaranteed, so as not to damage trust with children.

Showing Respect to Refugee Children

Building an alliance with children incorporates showing respect and displaying genuine interest. When children feel heard, supported, and validated, they may be more likely to provide honest responses about their experiences and feelings. Clinicians should tell children that they will be taking notes during the interview because they want to ensure they are understanding the child's perspective and to highlight that notes are for the clinician's use and will not be shared with authorities. In some cultures, people may not feel comfortable being interviewed or having so much attention focused on them and feel suspicious about the attention. Care can be taken to both acknowledge the difficulty in talking about oneself and to kindly invite children to be participants in the conversation.

It is important to be reflective on how we are being perceived by refugee children, since many may feel confused or scared with a clinician's questions and concern. A warm, supportive, yet professional environment can help a child or adolescent feel more comfortable. When a child appears embarrassed or ashamed, we can try to relay a nonjudgmental approach to their situation and instead convey that we have heard them and want to understand their experience. Sometimes first talking about topics that are not as sensitive can be helpful, such as questioning about favorite ways to spend free time, favorite games, or practical information. A combination of questions and statements can help youth not feel interrogated. Clinicians should always be mindful of the goal of the assessment, to only ask questions about potentially traumatic events or sad experiences if required to reach a sufficiently robust conclusion about one's life history and pathology. Clinicians should also be mindful of their own reasons behind inquiries. Refugee children often have experienced persecution and violence, much of which may be interesting to the clinician. However, intricate details about potentially traumatic experiences are not always necessary, and if the child does not feel comfortable sharing, they should not be pressured to do so. Oftentimes, children may need multiple sessions before feeling comfortable sharing various triggering or scary past experiences.

Incorporating the Effects of Potentially Traumatic Experiences on Child/Adolescent Refugees

The Role of Potentially Traumatic Events in a Refugee Child's Life

The refugee experience is diverse: some youth have experienced war, while others have experienced sexual- and gender-based violence or persecution due to political and religious beliefs and related behaviors or sexual orientation. Part of the assessment can incorporate an evaluation of whether an adverse event was traumatic or not. Individuals can place different meanings and give different emotional valence to the same adversity, so an adverse event may or may not be considered "traumatic" in a child's viewpoint. While the experience, including displacement, may vary, refugees (like asylum seekers) have a well-founded fear of persecution by definition.[1] Psychologically, children who have experienced persecution or war-related trauma may have difficulty in knowing whom to trust, with understandable hesitancy about whether disclosure of mental health symptoms will affect their legal status or may have negative social consequences. Parents may worry about being judged unfavorably, that their child will be removed from the country, or that sensitive personal information could compromise future decisions on asylum status.

The effects of trauma can be mediated by the level of insecurity and violence youth have been exposed to, availability of a positive attachment figure/relationship to help buffer/mitigate the effects of the trauma, individual genetic or biological makeup of the youth, and community resources available to assist the youth in

---

[1] The 1951 Refugee Convention defines a refugee as "someone who is unable or unwilling to return to their country of origin owing to a well-founded fear of being persecuted for reasons of race, religion, nationality, membership of a particular social group, or political opinion."

returning to a normal developmental trajectory [5, 25]. For those with trauma-related symptoms and behaviors, executive functioning – the ability to organize, plan, strategize, and manage time – can be impaired [12]. Those who have suffered from traumatic events may have impaired memory, missing certain pieces of information or the ability to describe clearly dates and times of events.

Managing Silence and Disclosure

Caretakers and refugee children may have experienced "being silenced," which is a form of control and taking away power. "Being silent" is different than "being silenced" and can demonstrate personal agency and control. When interviewing refugee children and families, we should be mindful of the role of silence and respect people's preferences and needs to not disclose certain information [23]. Sometimes silence is a reflection of a cultural response to a situation where there is an asymmetry of power inherent in the interaction (such as the clinician and client roles). Clinicians can be mindful of nonverbal cues and aware that emotions and the expression of such are influenced by the social environment and culture in which youth are raised. How physically expressive or reserved or emotionally expressive or stoic one is may be shaped by one's culture. Clinicians should therefore be mindful of personal expectations of how one is supposed to react and can observe nonverbal communication and body language to complement any information already gathered.

Conclusion

While not comprehensive, this chapter provided a few key points to consider prior to conducting a mental health evaluation. This may be the first mental health evaluation for a refugee child. Therefore, the evaluation should be done with caution and care, in order to safely, effectively, and efficiently obtain the required information to inform a care plan. Underlying the mental health assessment is an understanding that an individual child's identity, values, ways of expressing him/herself, and experiencing the world is shaped and developed by the ecosocial environment. Family, community, and culture all influence the expression and perception of emotional and behavioral distress. Respect should be given to the child's developmental stage, sensitive to a child's functioning in relation to same age peers. Since many practitioners may not speak the same language as the child, consideration on how to work with persistent language barriers and how to use interpreters as cultural mediators can provide the practitioner with additional information to guide the assessment. We may tend to rely on verbal communication, but respect should be given to what is *not* discussed or held silent. This may be a response to exposure to potentially traumatic events or a reflection of culture. By considering the above before, during, and after a mental health evaluation, we can attempt to avoid any negative unintended consequences of engaging with a refugee child.

References

1. Bolton P, Bass J, Betancourt T, Speelman L, Onyango G, Clougherty KF, et al. Interventions for depression symptoms among adolescent survivors of war and displacement in northern Uganda: a randomized controlled trial. JAMA. 2007;298(5):519–27.
2. Bot H, Wadensjö C. The presence of a third party: a dialogical view on interpreter-assisted treatment. In: Wilson JP, Drozdek B, editors. Broken spirits: the treatment of traumatized asylum seekers, refugees, war and torture victims. New York: Brunner/Routledge; 2004. p. 355–78.
3. Bracken P, Tomas P, Timimi S. et al. Psychiatry beyond the current paradigm. Br J Psych. 2012;201(6):430–4.
4. Bronfenbrenner U. The ecology of human development: experiments by nature and design. Cambridge, MA: Harvard University Press; 1979.
5. Bronstein I, Montgomery P. Psychological distress in refugee children: a systematic review. Clin Child Fam Psychol Rev. 2011;14(1):44–56.
6. Cavallera V, Reggi M, Abdi S, Jinnah Z, Kivelenge J, Warsame AM, et al. Culture, context and mental health of Somali refugees: a primer for staff working in mental health and psychosocial support programmes. Geneva: United Nations High Commissioner for Refugees; 2016.
7. Cheung C, Swank J. Asian American identity development: a bicultural model for youth. J Child Adolesc Counsel. 2019;5(1):89–101.
8. Ehntholt KA, Yule W. Practitioner review: assessment and treatment of refugee children and adolescents who have experienced war-related trauma. J Child Psychol Psychiatry. 2006;47(12):1197–210.
9. Eruyar S, Huemer J, Vostanis P. How should refugee services respond to the refugee crisis? Child Adolesc Mental Health. 2017; https://doi.org/10.1111/camh.12252.
10. Flores G. The impact of medical interpreter services on the quality of health care: a systematic review. Med Care Res Rev. 2005;62(3):255–99.
11. Hassan G, Kirmayer LJ, Mekki Berrada A, Quosh C, el Chammay R, Deville-Stoetzel JB, et al. Context and the mental health and psychosocial wellbeing of syrians: a review for mental health and psychosocial support staff working with syrians affected by armed conflict. Geneva: UNHCR; 2015.
12. Herlihy J, Scragg P, Turner S. Discrepancies in autobiographical memories—implications for the assessment of asylum seekers: repeated interviews study. BMJ. 2002;324(7333):324–7.
13. Huemer J, Vostanis P. Child refugees and refugee families. Mental health of refugees and asylum-seekers. In: Bhugra D, Craig T, Bhui K, editors. Mental health of refugees and asylum-seekers. Oxford: Oxford University Press; 2010. p. 225–42.
14. Jordans M, Tol W, Komproe I, Susanty D, Vallipuram A, Ntamatumba P, de Jong J. Development of a multi-layered psychosocial care system for children in areas of political violence. Int J Ment Heal Syst. 2010;4:15. https://doi.org/10.1186/1752-4458-4-15.
15. Jordans MJ, van den Broek M, Brown F, Coetzee A, Ellermeijer R, Hartog K, et al. Supporting children affected by war: towards an evidence based care system. In: Morina N, Nickerson A, editors. Mental health of refugee and conflict-affected populations. Cham: Springer; 2018. p. 261–81.
16. Keselman O, Cederborg AC, Linell P. "That is not necessary for you to know!": negotiation of participation status of unaccompanied children in interpreter-mediated asylum hearings. Interpreting. 2010;12(1):83–104.
17. Kienzler H, Spence C, Wenzel T. A culture-sensitive and person-centred approach: understanding and evaluating cultural factors, social background and history when working with refugees. In: Wenzel T, Drožđek B, editors. An uncertain safety. Cham: Springer; 2019. p. 101–16.
18. Kirmayer LJ, Crafa D. What kind of science for psychiatry? Front Hum Neurosci. 2014;8:435.

19. Lewis-Fernández R, Aggarwal NK, Hinton L, Hinton DE, Kirmayer LJ, editors. DSM-5 handbook on the cultural formulation interview. Washington: American Psychiatric Publishing; 2015.

20. Patel V, Saxena S, Lund C, Thornicroft G, Baingana F, Bolton P, et al. The *Lancet* commission on global mental health and sustainable development. Lancet. 2018;392:1553–98.

21. Quintana SM, Kerr J. Relational needs in late adolescent separation-individuation. J Couns Dev. 1993;71(3):349–55.

22. Rohlof H, Knipscheer JW, Kleber RJ. Use of the cultural formulation with refugees. Transcult Psychiatry. 2009;46:487–505.

23. Song SJ, de Jong J. The role of silence in Burundian former child soldiers. Int J Adv Couns. 2013;36(1):84–95.

24. Tay AK, Islam R, Riley A, Welton-Mitchell C, Duchesne B, Waters V, Varner A, Silove D, Ventevogel P. Culture, context and mental health of Rohingya refugees: a review for staff in mental health and psychosocial support programmes for Rohingya refugees. Geneva: UNHCR; 2018.

25. Tol WA, Song SJ, Jordans M. Annual research review: resilience and mental health in children and adolescents living in areas of armed conflict – a systematic review of findings in low- and middle-income countries. J Child Psychol Psychiatry. 2013;54(4):445–60.

26. Tribe R, Morrisey J. Good practice issues in working with interpreters in mental health. Intervention. 2004;2:129–42.

27. Ventevogel P. Borderlands of mental health: explorations in medical anthropology, psychiatric epidemiology and health systems research in Afghanistan and Burundi. University of Amsterdam (PhD thesis). 2016.

28. Watters E. Crazy like us: the globalization of the American psyche. New York: Simon & Schuster; 2010.

Conducting the Mental Health Assessment for Child and Adolescent Refugees

6

Suzan J. Song and Julia Oakley

Introduction

Conducting a comprehensive mental health assessment of a child is critical before treatment or interventions are even considered. The child (defined here as 0–18 years old) should be viewed as an individual at a developmental stage, as part of a family, with an identity shaped by one or more cultures, within a social and environmental context. Oftentimes, helpers and clinicians may feel the pressing need to assist refugee children and rush to providing interventions or treatments before spending adequate time in the assessment. Jumping to interventions too soon places the child at risk of ineffective and potentially harmful interventions that only delay care. Understanding the potential root causes; meaning of symptoms to the child, family, and community; and cultural influence on the expression of symptoms is needed for an accurate assessment that will ultimately guide optimal interventions that are tailored for the child. Refer to Fig. 6.1 for the general outline of how to conduct a mental health assessment for refugee children. This assessment chapter is meant to be a general guideline for mental health clinicians working with refugee children and families. It is not meant to serve as a standard of care for all professionals working with youth.

S. J. Song (✉)
Department of Psychiatry, George Washington University, Washington, DC, USA

J. Oakley
Northern Virginia Family Services, Program for Survivors of Severe Torture and Trauma, Arlington, VA, USA

© Springer Nature Switzerland AG 2020

81

S. J. Song, P. Ventevogel (eds.), *Child, Adolescent and Family Refugee Mental Health*, https://doi.org/10.1007/978-3-030-45278-0_6

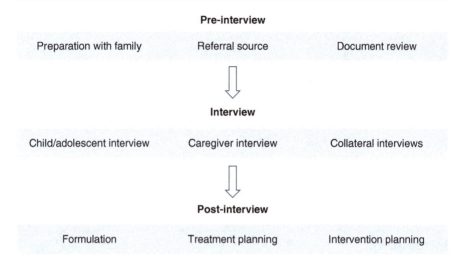

Pre-interview

Preparation with family   Referral source   Document review

Interview

Child/adolescent interview   Caregiver interview   Collateral interviews

Post-interview

Formulation   Treatment planning   Intervention planning

Fig. 6.1 Flowchart for the mental health assessment of refugee children

Practical Aspects Prior to the Assessment

Preparation

Preparing a child and his/her family for a mental health assessment is essential and should begin well before the assessment process. Clinicians should anticipate ambivalence to the mental health assessment due to legal, privacy, and stigma issues and then acknowledge and alleviate such ambivalence as soon as possible. The mental health assessment may possibly be the family's first contact with mental health care. Gathering information about the family's culture ahead of the assessment helps the clinician to set up the assessment in a culturally sensitive way. For many children, this will mean avoiding an overemphasis on the individual, instead placing the family in the context of their social, family, community, and political surroundings [13].

Clinicians should relay the practical and administrative aspects of an assessment at the beginning of session. This includes confidentiality, assessment process, length of interviews, clinician role, expectations from the assessment, and permission to gather information from other sources (e.g., school, resettlement agencies, case workers, physicians). Clinicians may also need to follow up with procedural reminders. One should be watchful for both verbal and nonverbal clues of unease, which could easily be missed through language and interpretation barriers.

Referral Source

First clarifying the purpose of the mental health assessment from the referral source, typically the caregiver, guardian, or a staff member, gives a sense of how a child's emotional or behavioral issues are understood, expressed, and managed. Caregivers may refer a child for evaluation of suicidal thoughts or a teacher may refer an adolescent for school truancy or substance abuse concerns. A pediatrician in the refugee camp may refer a child for suspected physical or sexual assault, or a case worker may report observing an adolescent with social difficulties with peers. The clinician must ensure that necessary consent is obtained to conduct the mental health interview, if the parent or caregiver is not the referral source. Understanding the main concerns that the referral source has, why the child is brought in now, as well as any questions they would like answered will help the clinician be focused and understand expectations for a mental health evaluation. The referral source will provide critical information about the family or social and environmental factors that could be causing or contributing to the presenting problems.

Review Documents

With the information provided in the referral, a clinician should be attentive to the child's immigration status and length of time in the current country. Such information will help to contextualize distress and protective factors. For example, the emotional wear that uncertainty and prolonged migration or waiting can have on a refugee. Documents can be useful in obtaining demographic information such as religion, country of origin, number and places of relocation, circumstances of persecution, age, and household composition. This information can be used to obtain general information about the cultural and socio-political background of their experience.

Any forms, such as consent for treatment or mental health questionnaires, should be given in the family's language of proficiency. Patience and understanding should be given to refugee children and their parents who may not be literate in their primary language, or who may have visual impairments to reading documents. While mental health questionnaires can be a quick way to gather information prior to an interview, clinicians should be mindful to use scales that are culturally and contextually validated. Many refugee children may feel uncomfortable and guarded about filling out such questionnaires that they are unaccustomed to using. Culture can play a role in the consent process, with some refugee children and referral sources looking to the interpreter for guidance on whether to sign or if the clinician can generally be trusted.

Clinical Mental Health Interview

Deciding Whom to Interview

Refugee children may be accompanied by extended family members or social supports. While it is important to help refugee children define who is in their family and acknowledge the importance of influential people in their lives, the interview itself should initially be limited to those most integral to the child's life. Other family members can be interviewed subsequently, as appropriate, so as not to disorganize the interview or become overwhelmed with simultaneous competing voices.

Logistics of the Mental Health Assessment

While mental health clinicians working with refugee children will each have their own time constraints, a 2-hour evaluation with all concerned persons – child, caregiver or referral source, and clinician – is ideal. This allows observation of the interaction between child and caregiver, which can provide information on the relational strengths and struggles. Observing the family as a whole can be informative to understanding how the family supports or hinders each member and how they perceive a problem. If the child is under 13 years old, an interview with the parents would be followed by an interview with the child. If the child is over 14 years old, typically the adolescent is interviewed first. Adolescents may have more to discuss and may have more developmental awareness about their own emotional health and capacity to maintain an alliance with the clinician. Interviewing the child independently from the caregiver can avoid exposure to criticism by an adult and allow an opportunity to learn about social or family issues that may not be appropriate for the child to hear. At the end, time is reserved for all parties to return to discuss the diagnostic formulation that includes the socio-cultural impact on a child's emotional and behavioral well-being as well as discuss potential interventions or a care plan for going forward.

Assessing the Impacts of the Humanitarian Setting

In humanitarian settings, such as refugee camps, staff may have difficulty finding a private area to conduct a proper interview for such a long period of time. Privacy is of paramount importance to minimizing stigma, making the client feel as comfortable as possible, and allowing disclosure of emotional experiences. These considerations (Box 6.1) can be considered in such settings.

Box 6.1 Considerations in Humanitarian Contexts
- If only tents/caravans are present, clinicians can try to walk in private with the child
- Children and their parents can be asked to choose a location where they feel safe and comfortable
- Best attempts should be made to allow adequate time to conduct a thorough assessment
- Parents should always be approached first, to obtain consent for a mental health assessment and describe the process, including risks (of eliciting stressful emotional responses) and benefits (developing a plan to ease emotional or behavioral distress)
- Parents and children should be told that they can share as much or little as they are comfortable with

Building an Alliance

The alliance, or relationship, between the child and clinician is of paramount importance, as is the alliance between clinician, family, and any collaborating agencies. Because the assessment is the beginning of the clinician's engagement with the child and family, it begins the clinician-client-family alliance and sets the tone for the efficacy of the intervention. An alliance incorporates building trust and negotiating to identify shared goals [5]. While an alliance can be built quickly, refugee children and their families may be guarded or protective of each other to give their recent history of persecution. A compassionate and professional demeanor may help the client feel more at ease to be able to share their true experience and emotions. Following a child's interest while maintaining structure and purpose to the interview is both intuitive and a learned skill. Different age groups may respond to different techniques for engagement (refer to Box 6.2).

Box 6.2 Example of Approaches to Build Alliance with Children

Younger children	Older children/adolescents
• Creative means such as play, drawing, use of stuffed animals • Gentle guidance and patience upon an initial meeting can show respect • Talk to children at their developmental level using language and expressions that a child at a certain age would understand, mindful that younger children may be more susceptible to suggestion	• Engaged directly, perhaps starting with "neutral" topics, such as their prior hobbies or music choice • Engage the child in asking their view point of their perspective and why they are seeing a mental health clinician

---

There is a balancing act between being able to obtain the information needed and staying present with the child and discussing what topics the child would like. If the child is focused on current problems, such as not having friends, the clinician should listen and re-direct if needed, but not impose his or her own order of pre-planned questions. When there is an appropriate moment, the clinician could ask their related question. For example, if the clinician wants to ask about the child's mood, but the client is focused on the boredom of school, the clinician could identify the connection between the two and first address the child's concerns. The clinician could say, "I wonder how school is different now than when you were at home…" Then link the child's concern to the clinician's inquiry, "How does it feel to be at school now?" and prompt if necessary: "Sad? Angry?" This allows the clinician to both hear and address the child's concerns while also obtaining information the clinician needs to complete an assessment. If the child becomes distressed when sharing emotional difficulties or sensitive topics, the interviewer should reassure the child and defer these unresolved questions to another contact.

Caregiver Interview

Engaging the Caregiver

The caregiver interview will inquire about the reasons for the referral, child's current difficulties as well as strengths, and impact of the child's difficulties on his/her social, academic, and family functioning. If multiple caregivers are present, they may have differing opinions on the youth's presenting problem as well as personal beliefs or stigma against seeking mental health care. Sensitivity, engagement, and multiple visits may be needed to adequately understand the family's perspective. Important in discerning the cause and manifestation of emotional and behavioral problems is identifying whether problems are evident at home, school, other settings, or all of the above. Asking direct, closed questions can be useful to obtain data on time-related events and details, and open-ended, exploratory questions may be helpful for relational and emotional information [10].

Practical Issues with the Caregiver Interview

The caregiver should be interviewed separately to discuss issues that may be uncomfortable or inappropriate to discuss in front of the child, including sexuality, substance abuse, or exposure to traumatic experiences. Oftentimes, caregivers will have differing opinions as to the child's behavior and social and academic functioning. Cultural values may dictate how parents and children communicate: some children may feel they are showing respect to elders by not responding to questions or speaking unless granted permission. Clinicians should consider how cultural etiquette may dictate who should be addressed first in the assessment as well as how family members should be addressed. Interviewing parents alone and children alone can help both more freely communicate. Caregivers can describe the impact of the child's symptoms on the family or home life and the response of influential people. Caregivers can also fill in historical information about a child, by asking about developmental milestones, early life experiences, past and present medical history, and the course or progression of mental health symptoms. Caregivers should be asked about family history of psychiatric or medical disorders that may be relevant. In the case of unaccompanied refugee minors, it may be that no adult has information on their previous developmental history.

Resilience Approach Toward the Child and Caregiver

Clinicians can inquire about what the family has already done to address the problem and how that strategy has been working. As well, clinicians should engage the caregivers in helping to understand what the child's life was like before displacement to help identify the contribution and influence of the child's environment on his/her current behaviors. Discussing the child's positive personal characteristics and behaviors before displacement and how they have/have not changed can help caregivers give a more longitudinal view of their child [17]. Clinicians should seek to understand a parental well-being and social supports during the interview, as both are strong protective factors for a child's resilience [11].

Assessment of Developmental History

Assessment of physical development is also critical, especially when working with children who may have neurological symptoms or intellectual/cognitive disabilities. An understanding of fine and gross motor development, puberty, illnesses, hospitalizations, and serious injuries can be related to mental health symptoms. Comparing a child's emotional, physical, social, cognitive, language (expressive and receptive), and learning capacity in the context of their chronological age will help identify areas of delay which could be targets for interventions, as well as to note strengths for resilience building.

Developmental history includes conception and pregnancy, birth, postnatal phases, and any major cognitive, social, or emotional issues of the youth, as well as any major life events or stressors during the first few years of life. If evaluating an adolescent, the history can also include the developmental assessment of social skills including prosocial behavior. For refugee children, understanding development in the context of the family system during war or persecution, migration, and post-migration processes can help obtain critical information of the impact of changes in the family (refer to Box 6.3).

Box 6.3 Example of Questions to Caregivers of Children About Developmental Histories

- What concerns do you have for your child?
- When did this [concern] begin, and what do you think is the cause?
- Has anyone else in the family had this problem? Has anyone in the family had any major emotional or behavioral problems?
- What does your child do well?
- What do you like about your child?

Medical/family history	Developmental history
Has your child had any surgeries? Hospitalizations? Illnesses or infections such as malaria?	Were there any main stressors on the mother when she was pregnant with the child?
Is your child on any medication? Has he/she ever taken any in the past? Does she have any allergies to medication?	Were there any complications during pregnancy, labor/delivery, or afterward?
How does your child play? Is your child able to play well with other children of the same age?	Were there any abnormal feeding, eating, or toileting issues in the first few years of life?
Do you know if your child is engaged in any substance abuse?	Did your child hit developmental milestones?
Do you think your child is engaged in any risky behavior or behavior you disapprove of?	Was the child separated from parents for a period of time? Under what circumstances?
	Have there been any major stressors in the child's life thus far?
	What has been the quality of your child's peer relationships since toddlerhood?

Mental Health Interview for the Refugee Child

Considerations for Refugee Children

While adults may be more verbally communicative about the presenting problem, it is important to also engage children in asking the children's viewpoint of why they are coming to see a mental health clinician and what is going on in their life. Initially, children may be guarded and hesitant to speak with a clinician. This is developmentally appropriate, and clinicians should be mindful that refugee youth may feel other adults have broken their trust or that they have been harmed by government or political officials (with whom they may be associating you). Therefore, clinicians should be clear about roles, purpose of the interview, confidentiality rules, and expectations from the assessment. Then, clinicians can begin the interview with neutral topics such as past hobbies, favorite games, or favorite songs/music.

> **Box 6.4 Considerations for the Mental Health Interview for Refugee Youth**
> - A child's ability, motivation, and eagerness to engage with a clinician may vary if in a new culture and context
> - Those who have experienced interpersonal traumatic events may not be forthcoming or feel at ease with a clinician whom they have never met before
> - Children may/may not describe or conceptualize well their emotions, associated causes and events, or what may help their distress
> - Children may have difficulty in adapting to multiple insecure environments
> - Managing with traumatic loss, cultural bereavement, and grief
> - Children of all ages may regress to developmentally younger behaviors, such as bed-wetting

Assessing for Mental Health Concerns

As many humanitarian staff may not be mental health clinicians, the purpose of the mental health evaluation is not necessarily diagnostic, but rather to develop an understanding of the child's presenting problems in order to inform a care plan. A mental health assessment tends to be one interview, though a cross-sectional evaluation of a child at a particular point in time may not accurately reveal overall level of functioning or distress. If possible, more than one interview with the child can give a more representative overview of the child's distress and strengths. The severity, timing, duration, associated factors, and help-seeking behavior around the symptom or problem should be assessed. Furthermore, the child's safety should be assessed via a risk assessment as part of the assessment process; for example, whether the child has past or present suicidal ideations, plan, or attempts and whether there is a risk that the client is a harm to himself/herself or others. Clinicians should further assess for self-injury and whether the child feels safe in his or her environment. Box 6.5 provides an overview of potential emotional or behavioral problems that may be seen in children.

Box 6.5 Broad Types of Mental Health Problems [26]

Category of mental health problem	Potential symptom/problem
Internalizing (emotional)	Sleep problems
	Avoidance of certain situations
	Physical presentations of distress
Externalizing (behavioral)	Acting out
	Aggression
	Defiance/yelling
Neurodevelopmental	Physical overactivity
	Attention impairment
	Language delay
	Repetitive behaviors
	Impaired social reciprocity
Somatic/body-brain	Sleep problems
	Feeding and eating disorders
	Somatoform and related disorders

Presentation of Mental Health Problems

The clinician must obtain an accurate picture of the youth's developmental functioning, nature and extent of the child's behavioral problems, any impairment of functioning, and subjective distress. Mental health problems may present similarly but have different causes and hence different intervention strategies. For example, aggression is a common concern, and when due to the experience of abuse or exposure to community violence such as war conflict, aggression may reflect the youth's difficulty with emotion regulation. However, if aggression is due to learned behavior from peers, this may be a sign of conduct problems. These two underlying conditions require different strategies – attachment-focused or trauma-focused interventions for abuse survivors and behavioral and social strategies for youth with conduct problems. These two types often co-occur, requiring both approaches, and a thorough assessment can give a detailed understanding of these patterns to match the youth's needs with intervention goals.

Somatic Concerns

Refugee children may present with somatic concerns (relating to the physical body) either due to cultural reasons or because they have difficulty articulating their emotional distress [1, 3, 12]. Any underlying physical cause of emotional distress or pain should be ruled out and youth and families can be asked what they believe the meaning, etiology, and treatment of the symptom to be. When physical investigations have been conducted and found negative, children and parents should not be challenged by emphasizing the lack of physical etiology. An approach that shows respect and curiosity about their symptoms can improve the alliance and help youth be open to engaging in interventions.

Unusual Beliefs or Sensory Experiences

Another difficulty in a mental health evaluation can be establishing the nature of unusual beliefs and sensory experiences, usually visual or auditory, that could indicate the onset of a psychotic illness. One needs to consider the cultural connotations of such thoughts and beliefs and children's potential expression of fear and distress through sensory perceptions. Children who experience trauma and abuse may describe sensory experiences that sound like psychotic hallucinations but are really disturbances consistent with trauma, for example, seeing illusions or hearing the voice of a perpetrator at night.

Ecosocial Assessment

As discussed throughout this book, each child is situated in a complex ecological system consisting of multiple levels (Benounna et al., in progress; Reis et al., in progress; Snider et al., in progress; Song et al., in progress). Each of these levels therefore requires an assessment of the influence they have on the child (refer to Box 6.6).

Box 6.6 Ecosocial Assessment

System	Example
The individual	Age
	Gender
Microsystem	Family
	Peers
	School
Mesosystem	Interactions between more than one microsystem
	Religious groups
	Home
Exosystem	Local government
	Social welfare system
	Friends of family
	Mass media
Macrosystem	Social and cultural context, such as ideologies,
	values, and attitudes

Cultural Environment

Acculturation

Acculturation is the process by which one becomes competent in navigating more than one culture [15]. Acculturative stress is the psychological impact of adapting to a new culture. When family members vary in their acculturation processes, refugee children can feel more or less supported, which can influence mental health symptoms and expression. Acculturative family stress can negatively impact child mental health and therefore be acknowledged and explored as a potential target for intervention (refer to Box 6.7). Potentially traumatic events may interfere with refugee children's acculturation processes, which may cause a fear of involvement with police or authority figures and forming new trusting relationships or avoidance of engaging in activities that may remind them of their trauma.

Box 6.7 Acculturation Considerations for Refugee Children
- Client and family's relative degree of comfort with aspects of mainstream culture
- Client and family's primary language spoken at home
- Exploration of potential bi-cultural stress
- Exploration of sources of support

Adapted from the Cultural Assessment Interview Protocol [6]

Culture and Expectations

The cultural environment the refugee child is in presently should be compared to the cultural environment from which the child is from. Cultural differences may account for child or family stigma around conceptualization of mental and physical health, seeking mental health services, and emotional expression. Exploration of cultural ideas around family roles, child-rearing practices, education, and communication is important to understand the issues present in the family. The child's religion and spirituality may also be culturally bound and may be inextricably linked to how the client views wellness, disease, healing, life, and loss. This discovery process will help the clinician not only to understand the context surrounding the child's presenting issues but also identify assets and protective factors as well as potential barriers to treatment adherence.

Family Environment

The family will be stressed by external forces such as exposure to violence, loss of loved ones or forced separation from their supports and community, as well as internal forces that change the roles, expectations, and ways of interacting between family members (refer to Box 6.5). The refugee child and his/her family may be struggling with cultural bereavement for the loss of homeland, culture, and associated memories left behind [4].

> **Box 6.8 Potential Changes in Family Dynamics for Refugee Children**
> - Changes during the refugee experience
> - Birth and loss of loved ones
> - Family exposure to violence
> - Ambiguous loss of loved ones
> - Long-term absence of a parent
> - Potential witnessed interpersonal or community violence
> - Forced separation from friends, family, community
> - Overall level of acculturative stress
> - Change of parental role
> - Marital conflicts about roles and responsibilities
> - Children assuming a parental role
> - Family conflicts about what constitutes acceptable behavior
> - Changes in social or economic status
> - Communication patterns among family members

Evaluating the Roles and Expectations of Family Members

The caregiver and child can be asked of the family's roles and expectation. Understanding the child's relationships to family members can help identify primary sources of nurturing and support, as well as who meets which of their needs. Children can be asked to draw their family or to map out who is in their family system and be asked about their relationships to everyone they draw or leave off the map. Clinicians should explore how family roles and expectations have changed with the migration and experiences the family has recently gone through.

Since refugees may arrive to a new country without family members, clinicians can ask whether all family members are present: Is anyone missing? Are all family members safe? If a family member is missing, clinicians can query how the family roles have changed: Is a primary caretaker or financial supporter missing? Who is filling that role presently? [22].

Historical Structure and Functioning of the Family

Understanding the historical structure and functioning of the family is useful to be able to identify available resources to promote well-being and prevent emotional distress. Families should be defined from the child's perspective, aware that non-blood relatives, extended family, or deceased loved ones may be perceived as critical family relationships. Clinicians may ask about how the family is organized and what the family's overall strengths are. It is important to inquire about the family beyond the presenting problem to obtain a sense of everyday life, which can give a lens into family norms and expectations. A clinician may explore family functioning, family roles, caregiver-child attachment, typical patterns of communication among family members, and methods of discipline employed by caregivers.

Assessing the Supportive Role of Families

The primary system in a child's life is family. Children may need support grieving for lost loved ones or their family system as they once knew it. Consideration of how the child and family members typically cope with adversity can give open communication about ways in which individual coping styles are helpful or stressful for other family members. For example, if a parent tends to cope by turning inward, finding solitude, and seeking silence, but the child copes by talking, engaging, and interacting, the child may feel his/her needs are not met, which can influence emotional and behavioral presentations.

Furthermore, ambiguous loss of family members may occur when it may be unknown whether a loved one is deceased or alive, or perhaps when a loved one is physically present but psychologically absent. The child may feel he/she has little support from a family member that is unavailable. In situations of ambiguous loss, the ambiguity of the loss itself needs to be validated and presence and tolerance for ambiguity should be enhanced [21]. Traumatic events experienced by parents or grandparents can also have a negative impact on the health and well-being of future generations, as evidenced by attachment style in relationships, family functioning and communication, and anxiety, depression, and post-traumatic stress levels of offspring [19], which can further the difficulty in children feeling supported.

Social Environment

The context in which the child is embedded should be evaluated, as discussed previously in this book (Chaps. 3, 7, and 12). Since the lack of basic needs like housing, poverty, school enrollment, available food, and safety have been linked to mental health (social determinants of health), identifying and prioritizing a response to the child's basic needs can be a critical step to understanding emotional and behavioral concerns. For refugee children, evaluation of the social environment also includes identifying past and ongoing potentially traumatic experiences, which are always external to a child. Such an evaluation would include the safety of the child and family (e.g., secure housing, safe neighborhood, potential of interpersonal violence); exposure to war-related events; community violence, and abuse; and the migration experience (if applicable). Moreover, sources of stress and support should be defined, as a lack of protective networks due to a breakdown of families and social systems can lead to greater risks of violence, exploitation, and abuse. Peer and community supports can be elicited and incorporated into care plans, to help restore a sense of belonging.

Involvement in school with educational attainment and social inclusion may be evaluated, since children typically spend the majority of their days in a school setting. Children may have experienced lack of access to schools or interrupted education, which can negatively impact education level and social development [11]. School challenges such as interrupted education, acculturation and language difficulties, and struggles with learning, coping, and adapting to a new environment should be discussed proactively and additional services provided such that a child always has a place to feel safe, to learn, to implement structure, and to belong.

Formulation

The case formulation is the integration of all previously described information from history, corroboration with other agencies, observations, and interview with the child and his/her parents into a coherent, distilled, and nuanced story that leads to the development of a hypothesized understanding of the child's presenting problem as well as a care plan. The formulation describes signs, symptoms, and areas of resilience where symptoms are not present and embeds these in family, social, educational, and cultural contexts (see Box 6.9). The formulation further makes diagnoses and provides hypotheses and justification, as well as describes intervention options based on all of these considerations [8]. This formulation can and should involve the family and, in a developmentally appropriate way, the child and is merely a hypothesis that can and should change with further understanding of the child and context.

Two models are used primarily as the structural basis for a formulation: the 4Ps and the biopsychosocial models. The Biopsychosocial Model incorporates biological, psychological, social, and even spiritual and cultural factors into the conceptualization of the client as a complete and complex person. The 4Ps Model for mental health formulation asks specifically about chronology and etiology based on predisposing factors, precipitating factors, perpetuating factors, and protective factors. It is also possible to mix both models together, or these models with other models, for an even more nuanced formulative approach [8].

Integrating the Biopsychosocial and 4Ps Models

The Biopsychosocial Model ensures that an evaluation of the client is informed by biological, psychological, ecosocial, and even spiritual and cultural factors so as to prevent reductionism. It includes a mental status exam, complete individual and family history, developmental history, social and environmental supports and challenges. These aspects are taken together to form the diagnoses, hypotheses, and case formulation, which then inform the care plan goals.

The 4Ps Model organizes a formulation by predisposing, precipitating, persisting, and protective factors. According to the 4Ps Model, some *Predisposing or vulnerability* factors will be obvious such as exposure to war trauma and migration, while others such as the impact of trauma on parenting can be missed. Doing so could exclude parents from an intervention that only focuses on the effects of trauma on the child. *Precipitating* factors can "push" a child's capacity over the threshold, for example, in the case of bullying. For refugee children, *perpetuating/maintaining* factors are likely to be related to current disadvantage such as protracted time spent in a humanitarian environment, poor housing conditions, unemployment, or a parent's own emotional distress. These also remind the assessor that focusing only on the child, particularly on past trauma, is unlikely to suffice. Finally, amidst all the concerns and anxieties that usually focus on problems, it is common to miss the identification of *resilience or protective* factors. These are particularly important in the face of multiple vulnerabilities, by pointing out at strengths within the child and their environment that could help break the cycle. A clinician should be attentive to personal characteristics and environmental supports that led the child to survive and participate in a mental health assessment in the first place.

Formulation for Refugee Children

In the context of a forced migration situation, negative emotions related to extremely difficult life circumstances and reactions to accumulative stress or past traumas or losses are often normal responses to abnormal events. Clinicians should avoid diagnoses for symptoms that can be better accounted for by normal adjustment to a new situation, typical human development, or usual adaptations following a traumatic event. We can take care to consider the particular circumstances and ongoing stressors related to the refugee experience while also seeking to understand the child's personality, symptoms, protective factors, and coping strategies before the forced migration.

The Influence of Attrition Stressors on Mental Health

A case formulation should seek to identify different manifestations, causes, and context behind the diagnosis (refer to Box 6.9). Unlike some types of clinical depression best targeted by pharmacology and brief psychotherapy, depression in refugees may be more related to situational, attrition symptoms. Attrition symptoms such as hopelessness, despair, demoralization, and helplessness are best targeted with distinct psychotherapy interventions, such as mobilizing hope, and resilience-focused psychotherapy, and identity transformation [7].

Box 6.9 Case Formulation as Informed by the 4Ps Model and Biopsychosocial Model

"P" characteristic	Biological	Psychological	Social
Predisposing "Why at risk?"	Compromised immune system	Temporary separation from attachment figure at early age	Fled home due to war and sectarian conflict
Precipitating "Why now?"	Malnourishment	Grieving loss of friend	Acculturation stress Starting new school
Perpetuating "Why still?"	Poor medical follow-up due to lack of resources	Coping skills breakdown due to several external stressors	Protracted stay in refugee camp
Protective "What to rely on?"	Now aware of accessible medical resources and personal motivation for medical follow-up	Quick improvement of adaptive coping skills	Extended family supports and faith community

Adapted from IACAPAP Textbook of Child and Adolescent Mental Health [8]

Culture and theFormulation

Particular attention in the formulation should also be paid to culture. If the child is experiencing distress related to racial, cultural, or physical relocation, consider at which stage the client is on the cultural identity development model: conformity, dissonance, resistance and immersion, introspection, or integrative awareness [23]. Clinicians can work to understand cultural concepts of distress, illness, and culture-bound syndromes and consider how the child is experiencing his distress and expressing using a cultural lens as a lens distinct from Western-oriented psychiatric symptoms [8, 18]. A clinician may want to consult, with the client and family's consent, with religious leaders or community leaders deemed important and trust-worthy so as to collaboratively create plan for care which is respectful of the client's beliefs and likely to succeed.

The Role of Family in the Formulation

Considering how the family can be part of the solution and including the family in psychoeducation sessions can help identify "sticking" points for client progress, make plans for accountability, and improve family communication. Care may include bringing lost family members into the room symbolically or enhancing the child's capacity to engage parents on questions of family secrets related to trauma or engaging parents and children together in discussions related to intergenerational acculturation difficulties.

Multimodal Care Planning

Once the case formulation is shared with the caregivers and the child, the clinician takes the next step of developing the care plan together with the caregivers and the child (if age appropriate). The clinician should work together with the family to prioritize issues to be worked on in the mental health-care process, transforming these issues into care goals to be worked on. The clinician should note symptoms or behaviors to target with care goals and propose recommended interventions for each goal. Questions from the child/adolescent and caregiver should be gently solicited and encouraged while also addressing concerns. A discussion of the risks and benefits of the proposed interventions should occur, to ensure children and families understand the impact of the intervention. Potential barriers to adherence could be brainstormed, with proactive ways to enable optimal efficacy of care.

Multimodal Approach to Care

Since refugee children and their families have a high risk of exposure to potentially traumatic events as well as complex daily life stressors, taking an approach that incorporates not only psychological functioning but also social and cultural adaptation and ongoing psychosocial functioning may be able to address some of the wide-ranging needs [14]. Such a multimodal approach would address the family, social, and individual psychological lives of children. A public health approach to refugee children may take a pyramidal interventional approach that targets mild distress or behaviors with social and family interventions and serious mental health symptoms with specialized treatment [2].

Ecosocial Targets for Care

The post-migration environment for a child is typically comprised of difficulties with language proficiency, unstable housing, lack of a sense of belonging, and lack of peer relationships when first arriving to a new country. Clinicians should consider how to leverage the child's access to community resources to reduce stressors in the child's current environment [20]. Addressing these daily life struggles through advocacy and support can help to ease the burden on the refugee child. Some social programs can foster a sense of connectedness and draw upon social networks integral to a collectivist culture such that they might be more appropriate than individual therapy. Since school is a critical environment for children, addressing school needs – both academic and social – can impact mental health [28]. A systematic review of community and school-based interventions for forcibly displaced children found interventions used both socio-ecological approaches and trauma-focused interventions [27].

Family-Centered Approaches

Family-centered interventions may be the most accepted intervention for refugee children, as parental support has been a consistent protective factor for children's mental health [25]. Children found to be experiencing minor emotional distress in congruence with their situation may best be aided by being connected to family support together with family psychoeducation, increasing community participation, and/or developing a sense of belonging in the current environment. A study among Afghan refugees in a Pakistani refugee camp showed that improvements in caregiver mental health via peace-building and violence prevention family programs were associated with improvements in child mental health [16]. Restoring social support networks for children and families [9] as well as cultural resources and extended family networks [24] are an important component of care for refugee youth.

Severe Mental Health Symptoms

When severe symptoms, such as suicidal plans or psychotic symptoms, have been identified, children will need to be referred to more specialized treatment. For example, children with psychotic symptoms not fully explained by a cultural perspective, with mood instability that significantly impairs daily functioning, will need to see a specialist. Children with psychosis in humanitarian settings are at risk of neglect, exploitation, and abuse [20]. Pharmacotherapy may be indicated for children whose symptoms significantly impair their daily functioning, who appear to have a biological predisposition to their psychiatric illness, or whose symptoms do not resolve using other evidence-based treatments. Children who may pose a danger to themselves or someone else should be evaluated for risk placed into emergency care if indicated.

Conclusion

This chapter has sought to provide a practical approach to the mental health assessment for children who are refugees. Often in humanitarian settings, or with children who have emotional or behavioral issues that are difficult to manage, clinicians and helpers may feel the urge to jump to treatment or interventions, without a comprehensive assessment. Doing so may be counterproductive and more time-consuming, as a quality mental health assessment aims to efficiently and effectively formulate a hypothesis of understanding the child's present experience to address through a care plan, which should incorporate a socio-ecological approach. From assessment to development of a care plan, a resilience lens that highlights current and past strengths to draw upon, both in the individual refugee child and his/her social and cultural resources, may serve to promote well-being and prevent worsening of mental health problems.

References

1. Batista Pinto Wiese E, Burhorst I. The mental health of asylum-seeking and refugee children and adolescents attending a clinic in the Netherlands. Transcult Psychiatry. 2007;44(4):596–613. Retrieved from https://journals.sagepub.com/doi/pdf/10.1177/1363461507083900.
2. De Jong J, Berckmoes L, Kohrt B, Song SJ, Tol W, Reis R. A public health approach to address the mental health burden of youth in situations of political violence and humanitarian emergencies. Curr Psychiatry Rep. 2015;17(7):60.
3. Betancourt TS, Newnham EA, Layne CM, Kim S, Steinberg AM, Ellis H, Berman D. Trauma history and psychopathology in war-affected refugee children referred for trauma-related mental health services in the United States. J Trauma Stress. 2012;25(6):682–90. Retrieved from https://onlinelibrary.wiley.com/doi/abs/10.1002/jts.21749.
4. Bhugra D, Becker MA. Migration, cultural bereavement and cultural identity. World Psychiatry. 2005;4(1):18–24. Retrieved from https://www.ncbi.nlm.nih.gov/pmc/articles/PMC1414713/.
5. Green J. Annotation: The therapeutic alliance - a significant but neglected variable in child mental health treatment studies. J Child Psychol Psychiatry. 2006;47(5):425–35.
6. Grieger I. A cultural assessment framework and interview protocol. In: Suzuki LA, Ponterotto JG, editors. Handbook of multicultural assessment: clinical, psychological, and educational applications. San Francisco: Jossey-Bass; 2008. p. 132–61.
7. Griffith JL. Mobilizing hope in the face of despair: Applying social neuroscience research at the bedside. Lecture. 2015.
8. Henderson SW, Martin A. Case formulation and integration of information in child and adolescent mental health. In: Rey JM, editor. IACAPAP e-textbook of child and adolescent mental health. Geneva: International Association for Child and Adolescent Psychiatry and Allied Professions; 2014.
9. Jordans M, et al. Development of a multi-layered psychosocial care system for children in areas of political violence. Int J Ment Heal Syst. 2010;4:15.
10. King R. Practice parameters for the psychiatric assessment of children and adolescents. J Am Acad Child Psychiatry. 1997;36(10):4S–20S.
11. Lustig SL, Kia-Keating M, Knight WG, Geltman P, Ellis H, Kinzie D, Keane T, Saxe G. Review of child and adolescent refugee mental health. J Am Acad Child Adolesc Psychiatry. 2004;43(1):24–36.
12. Mollica RF, Poole MARC, Son L, Murray C, Tor S. Effects of war trauma on Cambodian refugee adolescents' functional health and mental health status. J Am Acad Child Adolesc Psychiatry. 1997;36(8):1098–106.

13. National Child Traumatic Stress Network Refugee Trauma Task Force. Review of child and adolescent refugee mental health: White Paper. In: White Paper Committee with Lustig SL, Kia-Keating M, Grant-Knight W, Geltman P, Ellis H, Birman D, Kinzie JD, Keane T, Saxe GN. 2003. Retrieved from https://www.nctsn.org/sites/default/ files/resources//review_child_adolescent_refugee_mental_health.pdf.
14. Nickerson A, et al. A critical review of psychological treatments of posttraumatic stress disorder in refugees. Clin Psychol Rev. 2011;31:399–417.
15. Oppedal B, Røysamb E, Lackland Sam D. The effect of acculturation and social support on change in mental health among young immigrants. Int J Behav Dev. 2010;28(6):481–94.
16. Panter-Brick C, Grimon M-P, Eggerman M. Caregiver-child mental health: a prospective study in conflict and refugee settings. J Child Psychol Psychiatry. 2014;55(4):313–27. Retrieved from https://onlinelibrary.wiley.com/doi/full/10.1111/jcpp.12167.
17. Papadopoulos RK. Systemic challenges in a refugee camp. Context, the Journal of the Association of Family Therapy. 2008;99:16–9. Retrieved from http://repository.essex.ac.uk/2040/1/RKP_Context_paper_08.pdf.
18. Pumariega AJ, Rothe E, Pumariega JB. Mental health of immigrants and refugees. Community Ment Health J. 2005;41(5):81–597.
19. Sangalang CC, Vang C. Intergenerational trauma in refugee families: a systematic review. J Immigr Minor Health. 2017;19(3):745–54. Retrieved from https://www.ncbi.nlm.nih.gov/pmc/articles/PMC5362358/pdf/nihms-818645.pdf.
20. Silove D, Ventevogel P, Rees S. The contemporary refugee crisis: an overview of mental health challenges. World Psychiatry. 2017;16(2):130–9. Retrieved from https://onlinelibrary.wiley.com/doi/full/10.1002/wps.20438.
21. Utržan DS, Northwood AK. Broken promises and lost dreams: navigating asylum in the United States. J Marital Fam Ther. 2017;43(1):3–15.
22. Song SJ. Clinical strategies to address the mental health of forcibly displaced child (refugees, asylum seekers, and unaccompanied minors): the role of silence, family, and socio-ecological resilience. In: Parekh R. Culture and mental health. Arlington, VA (USA): APA Press; in press.
23. Sue DW, Sue D. Counseling the culturally diverse: Theory and practice (6th ed.). New York: John Wiley & Sons; 2013, p 297.
24. Tingold L, et al. Seeking balance between the past and the present: Vietnamese refugees parenting practices and adolescent Well-being. Int J Intercult Relat. 2012;36:260–70.
25. Tol WA, Song SJ, Jordans M. Annual research review: resilience and mental health in children and adolescents living in areas of armed conflict – a systematic review of findings in low- and middle-income countries. J Child Psychol Psychiatry. 2013;54:445–60.
26. Thapar A, Pine D, Leckman J, et al. Rutter's child and adolescent psychiatry, 6th ed. Hoboken: Wiley-Blackwell; 2015.
27. Tyrer R, Fazel M. School and community-based interventions for refugee and asylum seeking children: a systematic review. PLoS One. 2014;9:e89359.
28. Viner RM. Adolescence and the social determinants of health. Lancet. 2012;379:1641–52.

UNICEF Community-Based Mental Health and Psychosocial Support (MHPSS) Operational Guidelines

Leslie Snider and Zeinab Hijazi

The Importance of *Community* in MHPSS

Stable, secure, and positive environments are fundamental to supporting children and their caregivers to recover from stressful experiences and for children to learn, play, grow, and develop their full potential. Increasingly, however, contexts for children grow more threatening, due to conflict and displacement, as well as due to poverty, violence, and exploitation in many forms. The escalation and protracted nature of conflicts around the world, and the large-scale migration of families in search of safety and economic opportunity, have had significant impacts on the development and overall wellbeing of children. In such situations, vulnerable children and adolescents can also be targeted by violent extremist groups and may experience various forms of violence or recruitment into extremist ideologies. Combined with terrorism, disease outbreaks, intensifying natural disasters, and the impacts of climate change, the changing dynamic of threats has led to a child protection crisis presenting the humanitarian and development community with acute challenges.

Children and their caregivers in these contexts may lack adequate security, access to dignified basic services and livelihood opportunities, and school for months and sometimes years. They also often lack access to mental health and psychosocial support (MHPSS) services to address their varying and complex needs and to help them to cope in the face of challenging circumstances. These threats also damage community resources, structures, systems, and social cohesion – the "social ecological" fabric of community life that provides critical safety and support to its members, including families, teachers, and other child caregivers. Children's

L. Snider (✉)
The MHPSS Collaborative, Save the Children, Copenhagen, Denmark
e-mail: les@redbarnet.dk; http://www.mhpsscollaborative.org

Z. Hijazi
Mental Health and Psychosocial Support Specialist, Child Protection in Emergencies, Programme Division, New York, NY, USA

© Springer Nature Switzerland AG 2020

S. J. Song, P. Ventevogel (eds.), *Child, Adolescent and Family Refugee Mental Health*, https://doi.org/10.1007/978-3-030-45278-0_7

development benefits from positive attachment to caregivers [1], with the presence of a stable, caring adult mediating children's responses and coping in crisis situations. Emerging findings presented during the symposium "Growing Up in Conflict: The impact on children's mental health and psychosocial wellbeing," convened by UNICEF, the government of the Netherlands, and a wide range of humanitarian and academic partners [2], reinforce the importance of the social environment of children and families in reducing risk and promoting wellbeing through factors such as cultural adherence, social cohesion, material resources, and identity. Participants described MHPSS interventions as helping to "promote resilience by aiming to strengthen protective factors in children's lives so that they are able to develop attachments and rebuild hope and agency" (UNICEF 2015, p 15).

To strengthen these protective factors in children's lives in humanitarian settings, there is renewed focus on ensuring MHPSS interventions are grounded in *communities*. UNICEF and members of the Inter-Agency Standing Committee (IASC) Reference Group for MHPSS in Emergencies promote a holistic, community-based approach to child programming as a quality standard of practice. Still, there is a need to reaffirm and better operationalize this commitment in evolving humanitarian contexts and crises, due to:

1. *The protracted nature of conflict and displacement*: The number of people fleeing their homes in search of safety worldwide increased from 43.3 million in 2009 to 70.8 million people by the end of 2018, about half of whom are children, and 78% are in protracted displacement situations [3]. As the average duration of displacement for refugees is 20 years [4], many refugee children spend their entire childhoods "in displacement" and are thus at risk of disrupted access to education and its promotive effects for their safety and development [5]. Also, 61% of refugees in 2018 were living in urban areas [3], with important implications for host communities and local service systems and resources. Traditional humanitarian aid systems geared toward short-term aid and camp environments have had to adapt to this new reality, and there is a greater need to assess and strengthen community resources and care systems to meet the long-term and complex needs of evolving humanitarian crises.

2. *Emerging evidence on standard interventions for children in emergencies*: Establishing child-friendly spaces (CFS) is an important first-line intervention to ensure children have a protected space in emergencies to gather for supervised and structured psychosocial support activities. They are intended to be embedded in and implemented together with local communities. However, models centered on CFS have demonstrated certain limitations in engaging families and communities, necessary for transitioning CFS from early emergency response to recovery and regular programming. Evaluations of CFS approaches also emphasize the need to improve both the scale and quality of MHPSS interventions in these spaces to improve children's wellbeing [6].

3. *The need to better contextualize programming*: Interventions with a single focus on treatment of psychological symptoms demonstrate similar limitations. There is a need to shift to "contextually appropriate, multi-layered systems of support that build on existing resources" [7] – including strengthening refugee communities' own capacities for protection and psychosocial wellbeing. While approaches may have many similarities across contexts, caution is needed, and adaptation or modifications may be critical to the success of MHPSS programs.

These findings and lessons learned from decades of MHPSS programming in humanitarian settings inform the UNICEF Community-Based MHPSS Operational Guidelines [8] that serve as the main source material for the content in this chapter. The guidelines offer practical information and tools (see information about accompanying Compendium of Resources in text box below) to implement a range of MHPSS interventions to rapidly address the protection, mental health, and psychosocial support needs of children and families, in parallel with specialized MHPSS interventions and referral for those most in need. The guidelines present an operational framework that emphasizes engaging actors at all levels (children and caregivers, community service providers, humanitarian workers across sectors, and governmental actors) to design and implement MHPSS strategies that are locally relevant, comprehensive, and sustainable. Restoring, strengthening, and mobilizing family and community supports and systems ultimately aims to support child and family wellbeing by:

1. Reducing and preventing harm and enhancing coordination of quality, culturally relevant interventions.
2. Strengthening the resilience of children, families, and communities to recover from adversity and promoting their full participation.
3. Improving the care conditions that enable children and families to survive and thrive and to receive referral to ensure MHPSS needs are met.

Developed through a wide consultative process and evidence review, the UNICEF Community-Based Operational Guidelines include an online Compendium of Resources available through the open-access platform MHPSS.net. The various resources, guidelines, training manuals, and tools in the compendium can be used as references in designing and implementing MHPSS approaches in different contexts. It will be continually updated with new resources and evidence-based approaches as they become available, including the *IASC MHPSS guidance note on community-based approaches to MHPSS*, World Health Organization's *Scalable Interventions*, and others.

What Does it Mean to Design and Implement *Community-Based* MHPSS?

As part of a strategic psychosocial and mental health approach, community-based MHPSS aims to build on existing individual and community resources, capacities, and resilience. See the box below for key elements in designing and implementing community-based MHPSS.

> A community-based MHPSS approach:
> - Strengthens natural supports and systems.
> - Makes use of community knowledge and capacities.
> - Requires skills and a thorough analysis of local practices and resources to ensure the principle of "do no harm".
> - Engages the community in all phases of programming.
> - Addresses interventions at all layers of the IASC MHPSS pyramid.
> - Includes both non-specialist and professional services and psychological and social supports.

Skills Needed to Strengthen Natural Community Supports and Systems

At the heart of community-based MHPSS is the meaningful engagement and participation of the community through all phases of the program management cycle, working in ways that enhance, rather than damage, natural family and community supports to children. This requires skills and knowledge, time, commitment, and flexibility. Working through a community's natural supports and systems can strengthen the overall care environment for children and families – including more effectively identifying those most vulnerable, reducing stigma and discrimination, and ensuring their inclusion in interventions and relief efforts. It also recognizes the resilience, capacities, skills, and resources for coping that all people have, even if those may be weakened by the emergency. Community-based approaches further ensure interventions are relevant to local realities, cultural values, and understandings; strengthen childcare systems for broad impact; and promote ownership of programs for long-term sustainability.

It is important to remember that a *community* is diverse and dynamic, constantly changing to adapt to new realities, environments, challenges, and resources – particularly when familiar ways of life are disrupted by an emergency. For example, people displaced by an emergency may or may not be identified as part of the same community. Subgroups may or may not feel included, safe, or respected. Host communities must also be engaged, and their relationship with displaced communities examined. There may also be harmful practices in communities, and some groups may historically have been marginalized or excluded. Community-based MHPSS programmers must be able to critically examine and effectively and respectfully address these issues to ensure interventions align with international human rights standards. They must also learn the nuances of the community, including appropriate entry points, power structures, and other political, social, and cultural dynamics that influence who is included and who participates in decision-making. As stated in the IASC MHPSS Guidelines (IASC, 2007, p. 100),

> Communities often include diverse and competing subgroups with different agendas and levels of power. It is essential to avoid strengthening particular subgroups while marginalizing others, and to promote the inclusion of people who are usually invisible or left out of group activities.

Box 7.1 outlines the principles for inclusion and participation of communities, and the case study below underscores the importance of deep understanding of and engagement with communities.

Box 7.1 Inclusion and Participation
Inclusion and participation of all community members in MHPSS is based upon certain principles:
- A rights-based approach that incorporates an age, gender, and diversity analysis to ensure broad participation of community members.
- The value of empowering individuals to understand their situation, make informed decisions, and assume ownership of solutions for sustained impact.
- Transparency and accountability of all stakeholders.

Case Study. Importance of Community Engagement in Ebola Response in the Democratic Republic of Congo
In the midst of the tenth Ebola outbreak in the Democratic Republic of Congo, UNICEF and its partners integrated MHPSS into all areas of the public health response, acting on lessons learned from previous Ebola outbreaks. Locally led psychosocial commissions were set up in various Ebola affected areas, staffed with non-specialist MHPSS providers identified and trained from within the communities. MHPSS workers were able to use existing social networks and in-depth understanding of cultural norms to reach children and families that might have otherwise been hesitant to seek assistance. Services provided included family tracing; temporary care and durable solutions for orphans and unaccompanied children; daily individualized household visits to mitigate the discrimination, stigma, and isolation associated with Ebola; and addressing psychosocial problems that may result following an Ebola case. This model of engaging communities aimed to reduce child and family distress and promote healthy behaviors and recovery.

However, following community attacks on Ebola treatment centers, community-based needs assessments among Ebola-affected communities revealed pressing social, humanitarian, and infrastructure needs beyond the Ebola public health response.

UNICEF and partners then called for mainstreaming MHPSS throughout the response to better strengthen community ownership and engagement in addressing the complex needs and continued mistrust toward the (inter) national Ebola response. This included:

- Developing MHPSS capacities of local staff to provide psychoeducation and support community engagement, accountability, and mobilization.
- Strengthening MHPSS support to (suspected) and recovered patients, their families, and the wider community in dealing not only with Ebola virus disease, its stigma and sequelae, but also the wider concerns and needs of the communities (e.g., socioeconomic and conflict/violence-related concerns).
- Reinforcing coordination and referral mechanisms to improve both intra-agency collaboration and closer engagement and active participation of the communities, creating a co-owned localized Ebola response.
- Including community sensitization at the heart of the response, through prevention and control messages by teachers in schools, by religious leaders in sermons and other religious teachings, and by community volunteers through house-to-house visits and community meetings.

Involving the Community in All Phases of Programming

Community engagement and participation involves the following six steps:

1. *Learn about the context* – beginning with a desk review, a situation analysis can elucidate the sociocultural context for children and families and maps the risks, resources, and priority areas for intervention in the emergency context.
2. *Identify and meet community stakeholders* – a stakeholder analysis undertaken with the community helps to ensure inclusive representation in community engagement activities including government and civil society actors, childcare organizations (e.g., school boards), religious organizations, youth and women's groups, women leaders, people with disabilities, and others.
3. *Conduct an inclusive, participatory assessment of needs and resources* – this requires bringing diverse voices to an understanding of the community, how the emergency has affected coping capacities, and how different communities see their own risks and resources. Care should be taken to safely and appropriately engage boys and girls, women and men, and vulnerable or marginalized children and families.

4. *Facilitate inclusive participatory planning of solutions and interventions* – ensure the stakeholder analysis and participatory assessment findings are shared with stakeholders (such as a planning committee representative of diverse voices) to plan the way forward together. Ensure children, youth, and families have the opportunity to input into the design of programs relevant to their needs. It is often necessary to support members of planning committees to be able to participate effectively, particularly if they are unaccustomed to speaking up and having their opinions regarded seriously.

5. *Support program implementation by community actors* – the role of external agencies is usually to support program implementation with technical and financial assistance. Wherever possible, this means maximizing community and governmental resources for sustainability, supporting existing community initiatives, and building capacity of the community to sustain their own solutions (see text box below on capacity building).

6. *Monitor and evaluate interventions together* – ensuring a wide range of voices (including boys and girls and marginalized children and families) in feedback about program outcomes and effectiveness gives a comprehensive and clear view of the impact and shortcomings of interventions and is critical for transparency and accountability.

Non-specialist and Professional Supports

There is a close relationship between the social and psychological aspects of children's wellbeing and development, and MHPSS approaches therefore cover both social and psychological interventions. These utilize both non-specialist and professional staff to meet the needs of children and families within the community. Both non-specialist and professional staff must have relevant competencies for their tasks, and setting minimum standards and qualifications for all providers is important in a successful community-based MHPSS program. For example, professional staff such as doctors and nurses may provide clinical psychological or psychiatric services (e.g., medication for treatment of neurological or mental disorders, counseling), and social service professionals may provide specialized protection and social services (e.g., case management). With training and supervision, non-specialist providers can provide nonclinical support to children and families, such as peer support, psychological first aid[1] [9], and identification and referral of those in need of specialized help.

---

[1] Psychological first aid involves assessing needs and concerns; helping people address basic needs; listening to and comforting people and helping them feel calm; helping connect to information, services, and social support; and protecting people from further harm – as described in Psychological First Aid: Guide for Field Workers, World Health Organization (WHO), War Trauma Foundation and World Vision International, WHO: 2011.

Take the following steps to ensure program implementers have the skills, knowledge, and systems to implement community-based MHPSS interventions and track their quality and progress over time (see Box 7.2).

Box 7.2 Steps for Implementing Community-Based MHPSS

1. *Recruit* staff or volunteers locally, being careful to ensure cultural and gender appropriateness; to screen for child protection concerns; and not to weaken existing structures by pulling away skilled staff members.
2. *Train and supervise* local staff and volunteers through participatory, skills-based training and ongoing, regular supervision. Set minimum qualifications for various roles and ensure they are equipped for their tasks. It is absolutely essential to include staff care strategies in addition to regular supervision – this is fundamental to both quality programming and preventing burnout.
3. *Establish information management systems and standard operating procedures (SOPs)* as an essential part of any program. Ensure these systems meet ethical requirements (e.g., confidentiality), are user-friendly, and that local program implementers are trained in them.

How Was the Content Structured and Developed?

The UNICEF operational guidelines were constructed upon two frameworks: (a) the social ecological model [10] which illustrates the importance of networks of people and structures that surround children, safeguarding their wellbeing and supporting their optimal development, and (b) the intervention pyramid within the IASC guidelines on MHPSS in emergency settings (IASC, 2007). The operational guidelines combine these two frameworks demonstrating how MHPSS interventions, designed across layers of the pyramid, with referrals between layers according to the needs of children and families, can best protect and support children by strengthening and enhancing connections between the personal, family, and community resources in each context. A multilayered, community-based MHPSS system helps to create the conditions for child and family wellbeing and protection.

The Social Ecological Model of Children's Development

Children's development is inextricably connected to the social and cultural influences that surround them, particularly the families and communities that are children's 'life support systems' [11].

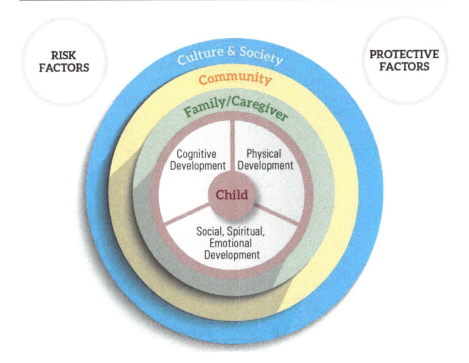

Fig. 7.1 The social ecological model of children's development

The social ecological model is a framework that examines the multiple effects and connections between social elements in an environment, recognizing the relationships between the child and their environment at multiple levels at which risk and protective factors operate. The model explores how the environment and child continually interact at various levels of the social ecology to influence human development and life transitions, and how children develop and cope with change. Interactions between the child and their context influence growth not only in obvious domains such as physical development but also in cognitive, psychological, and social areas [12].

The model (see Fig. 7.1 below) illustrates the child nested within networks of people and structures that safeguard children and promote their wellbeing and optimal development. The relationships and networks that exist within and between the circles provide for children's social and practical needs, protection, learning, belonging, and identity as well as their recovery from critical events. Children are active agents in this rich social ecological dynamic, being influenced by and, in turn, influencing their environment. Their "wellbeing" and "resilience" (see definitions in the text box below) are similarly influenced by personal factors, such as the presence or absence of a disability, genetic factors, and the child's personality, and their capacities depend upon their age and developmental stage.

Definitions of Wellbeing and Resilience

In MHPSS work, *wellbeing* is commonly understood in terms of three domains:

1. Personal wellbeing: positive thoughts and emotions such as hopefulness, calm, self-esteem, and self-confidence.
2. Interpersonal wellbeing: nurturing relationships, a sense of belonging, and the ability to be close to others.
3. Skills and knowledge: the capacity to learn, make positive decisions, effectively respond to life challenges, and express oneself.

Resilience is the capacity to overcome adversity and adapt after difficult experiences.

For more information, see Chap. 4, by Videvogel., S., and Verelst, A. Supporting mental health in young refugees, a resilience perspective.

As stated in the IASC Guidelines for MHPSS in Emergencies (IASC, 2007), "Emergencies create a wide range of problems experienced at the individual, family, community and societal levels. At every level, emergencies erode normally protective supports, increase the risk of diverse problems and tend to amplify pre-existing problems of social injustice and inequality." The resilience of children in emergencies results from their innate strengths and capacity for coping, and the risk and protective factors in their social and cultural environments (e.g., positive or negative family environments, supportive teachers, access to essential services and protection).

MHPSS interventions work to reduce risks and strengthen protective factors for children – building capacities both within the child (e.g., problem-solving abilities) and within their care environments. Caregivers are also directly affected in emergencies, and attention to caregiver wellbeing is essential to their ability to provide the necessary safety, stability, and nurturance that help children maintain optimal development in the face of adversity.

Key Terms: Multilayered Interventions, Integrated Services and Mainstreaming

Several terms are used to describe how community-based MHPSS programs can best be implemented: multilayered interventions, integrated services, and mainstreaming across sectors.

Multilayered: The term *multilayered interventions* refers to the complementary, multiple layers of MHPSS approaches that are needed to meet the continuum of needs of all children and families in emergencies – from those with needs for general support to those with more specialized needs including mental, neurologic, or substance abuse (MNS) disorders or serious protection needs (*see the section below for an elaboration of multilayered supports*).

Integrated services: Community-based MHPSS services are most effective when *integrated* within community structures, such as local health centers, schools, community centers, or youth clubs. In this way, community-based MHPSS approaches support and strengthen existing structures and ensure services are accessible to all children and families. Integrating within existing supports also helps to reduce the stigma of children and families who may seek MHPSS services.

Mainstreaming: Mainstreaming MHPSS interventions across different sectors of humanitarian response – such as education, health, protection, camp management, and water and sanitation – improves the way in which other sectoral services are delivered in support of children and families who have experienced very distressing events. This can enhance the protective qualities of humanitarian interventions and reduce their potential risks. It also improves the reach of MHPSS interventions and the access of children and families to dignified, humane, and supportive humanitarian services.

Community-Based MHPSS Activities Across the IASC Pyramid Layers

In emergencies, children are affected in different ways and require different kinds of supports. A key to organizing MHPSS approaches is to develop a multilayered system of complementary supports that meets their needs, as described above. The pyramid demonstrates how mental health specialists, protection actors, social service staff, community members, and other actors and systems operate together to support child and family wellbeing. It is essential to view the layers of the pyramid as connected, with functional referrals up and down the layers (see Fig. 7.2 below).

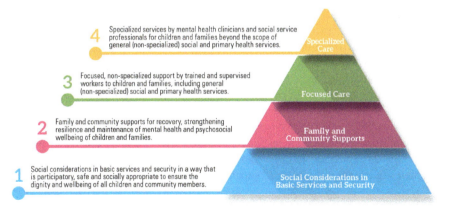

Fig. 7.2 The IASC MHPSS pyramid (adaptation) (This is an adaptation of the IASC MHPSS intervention pyramid that continues to benefit from application in the field and further discussion among experts. Original source: IASC MHPSS Guidelines in Emergencies, IASC (2007).)

All layers of the pyramid are important and should ideally be implemented concurrently. The layers include the following:

Layer 1: Once basic survival needs (food, shelter, water, basic health care, controlling communicable diseases) are met in supportive and socially appropriate ways and safety and security have returned, most children and families will go back to functioning normally without professional support.

Layer 2: Some children and families will need specific support to restore the protective factors within family and community systems. Useful responses in this layer include family tracing and reunification, supportive parenting programs, formal and non-formal educational activities, livelihood activities, and the activation of social networks, such as through women's groups and youth clubs.

Layer 3: The third layer represents the support needed for the still smaller number of children (e.g., survivors of gender-based violence or recruitment) who also need more focused individual, family, or group interventions. These interventions are delivered by workers who are trained and supervised but who may not have had years of training in specialized care.

Layer 4: The top layer of the pyramid represents the additional support required for the small percentage of the population whose suffering, despite the supports already mentioned, is intolerable and who may have significant difficulties in basic daily functioning. These children may have pre-existing mental disorders not related to the disaster but worsened by it, or they may have been exposed to traumatic events or serious protection risks [13].

UNICEF Operational Guidelines: A Framework for Implementation

The UNICEF Community-Based MHPSS Operational Guidelines join the Social Ecological Model and the IASC MHPSS intervention pyramid into one framework. MHPSS approaches and specific activities are suggested at each of the IASC pyramid layers and across child, family/caregiver, and community tiers. They include tables and intervention examples elaborated at each layer, offering ideas for MHPSS intervention strategies that can have sustained beneficial impacts. Users of the guidelines can select from among the approaches to develop implementation strategies for particular programs. In each program, different intervention strategies may be prioritized depending on needs, resources, and contextual realities. An accompanying Compendium of Resources further provides useful resources at each layer of the pyramid, including training manuals, toolkits, and guidance documents. Examples of resources from the Compendium are indicated throughout the text.

Layer 1 Interventions

Layer 1 interventions are aimed at advocating for service delivery that fosters inclusive and participatory community engagement; gives special attention to the sociocultural context in how aid is delivered, and security is achieved; and ensures appropriate services reach the most vulnerable children and families. Examples from the guidelines include:

IASC Pyramid Layer 1: Social considerations in basic services and security: fulfilment of basic needs and security in dignified, safe, and culturally appropriate ways

Tier of intervention		
Child	Family/caregivers	Community
• Work with the community and other sectors to ensure children's access to safe living, playing, and learning areas (e.g., communal areas, formal/ non-formal school structures) • Work with health and nutrition actors to identify and include vulnerable children in basic health care and to promote a psychosocial perspective in nutrition programs and feeding practices for infants and children	• Raise awareness and promote access for vulnerable families to basic services (e.g., shelter, infant, and/or school feeding programs) • Work with other sector actors to ensure appropriate shelter accommodation for the privacy and comfort of families	• Make sure age, diversity, and gender are reflected in the design and delivery of basic services and security for children and families • Advocate across sectors for safe spaces for children, women and families • Include children and parents/caregivers with MNS disorders or disabilities in basic service delivery and security

Layer 1 field example. Terre des Hommes Sports Clubs in Sri Lanka engage children and youth participation in sports activities. They aim to develop children and youth's active role in the development of sports in their communities, and to rebuild relationships based on trust, peer support, mutual respect, and an appreciation of the value of rules and fair play. By emphasizing rights and inclusion, the project contributes to gender and minority equality and to a greater participation in sports and community life of disadvantaged groups such as widows and low-caste communities.

Layer 2 Interventions

Family and community supports are the foundation of enabling environments for children's safety, wellbeing, and optimal development. When these foundations are disrupted due to displacement, poverty, and loss of or separation from key family and community members in emergencies, strengthening the ability of families and communities to reestablish routines and normalcy and supportive connections can greatly enhance the capacity for coping and recovery. Examples from the guidelines for layer 2 interventions include:

IASC Pyramid Layer 2: Strengthening family and community supports: enabling environments for children's optimal development, including positive social relationships and learning

Tier of intervention

Child	Family/caregivers	Community
• Support identification, family tracing, and reunification and appropriate care, for separated children • Support children's access to quality, psychosocial structured activities (e.g., creative and expressive activities) within the community (e.g., in child friendly spaces) • Support the inclusion and meaningful participation of vulnerable children (e.g., children with disabilities, marginalized children) in community activities and services	• Strengthen family care and nurturing family environments through positive parenting training (e.g., how to help children of different ages and developmental stages cope with emergencies) • Help to strengthen networks of support for parents and other child caregivers in the community (e.g., support groups for mothers, safe spaces for women, self-care strategies) • Build capacity and self-care of teachers to create positive, safe classroom environments	• Support integration of child and family MHPSS services in other sectors (e.g., health care, social services, education, and protection) • Work with schools to strengthen safe, positive school environments for children's protection, recovery, wellbeing, and social and emotional learning • Develop community awareness campaigns to promote awareness of appropriate coping and recovery strategies and support child protection messaging to reduce risks to children's safety

Layer 2 field example. International Rescue Committee's Parenting Skills Training in Liberia [14] aims at decreasing violence in the home and improving parenting practices and parent-child relationships. Through behavioral skills training, parents learn child development concepts, negative effects of punishments, and positive parenting skills. *The training supports parents in managing the challenges of raising children in the midst of crisis and helping their children to cope with the severely distressing events and displacement they have witnessed or experienced. Through the parenting skills training, Syrian parents gain a better understanding of their own stress, and learn ways to support their coping and healing. The also learn to enhance the role that they play in their children's wellbeing, including through communication, nurturing practices, empathy and positive behavior, and understanding and providing support to children with psychosocial needs.*

Layer 3 Interventions

Although most children and families can cope and recover well if their basic needs are appropriately met (layer 1) and with strengthened family and community supports (layer 2), focused care may be needed for a smaller number whose coping capacity has been overwhelmed. This may include children and families in acute distress due to exposure to serious stressors such as violence or abuse; who have been exposed to protection risks and require psychological, health, and legal support; who are survivors of severe human rights violations such as trafficking; or who are unable to make use of existing services and support networks to meet their basic needs (e.g., children or caregivers with specific health or mental health problems or disabilities). Layer 3 interventions are delivered by trained and supervised nonclinical staff, and examples include:

IASC Pyramid Layer 3: Focused care: person-to-person support to address psychosocial distress and protection challenges

Tier of intervention		
Child	Family/caregivers	Community
• Ensure access of children to age- and gender-appropriate individual and group psychosocial interventions by trained, non-specialized staff • Build capacity of children of different ages in self-care and appropriate support to their peers (e.g., adolescent peer support) • Build capacity among community MHPSS workers in identification, referral, and case management for children in need of specialized care (layer 4 services)	• Provide focused psychosocial care for distressed parents and caregivers – including psychological first aid [9] and WHO scalable interventions[a] • Support outreach services to vulnerable families for psychosocial support, protection services, and referral to specialized care and other sector services as needed • Train and supervise non-specialist staff to provide individual and group psychosocial interventions for vulnerable caregivers/families (e.g., support to mothers with postpartum depression, interpersonal group therapy)	• Strengthen social service systems for coordinated care, case management, and referral for children and families with MHPSS and protection needs • Raise awareness and build capacity in school systems to support children with distress, MNS disorders, or intellectual disabilities, including identification and referral of at-risk children • Promote mental health and community awareness campaigns about available, focused care and supports for children, caregivers, and families in need

[a]Evidence-based individual and group interventions developed by a range of agencies (including WHO) that show promising results in helping parents and caregivers in emergencies. Scalable interventions can be delivered by non-specialized providers with proper training and regular supervision by mental health clinicians.

> *Layer 3 field example. Save the Children's Psychological First Aid (PFA) for Child Practitioners (2013)* [15] is a defined set of skills and competencies that any staff working with children in crisis should have, to be able to reduce the initial distress of children caused by accidents, natural disasters, conflicts, or other critical incidents. The approach developed by Save the Children is fully in line with the WHO's orientation manual in PFA and adapted to the specific needs of children according to child development theories. *PFA for Child Practitioners* is for anyone working with children in distress, particularly social workers, volunteers, aid workers, and other staff. The tool is relevant for colleagues across sectors and not limited to those working in child protection or psychosocial programming.

Layer 4 Interventions

In any emergency, a small percentage of children and caregivers will require specialized care, such as clinical mental health care by mental health and social service professionals. This includes care for children and caregivers with pre-existing MNS disorders and disabilities that can worsen in crisis situations; child survivors of serious protection violations or traumatic events; and parents and caregivers who have experienced serious stressors and require specialized care for their own coping and recovery and to be able to meet the needs of their children. It is important that children and families can access specialized services without the risk of stigma, isolation, or additional harm. Examples of layer 4 interventions from the guidelines include:

IASC Pyramid Layer 4: Specialized care: clinical mental health care and professional social services for MNS disorders, developmental disabilities, serious distress, or serious protection violations

Tier of intervention		
Child	Family/caregivers	Community
• Ensure referral and access to appropriate clinical MHPSS care and professional social services for children with MNS disorders or exposed to serious protection risks • Facilitate the management and support of children with MNS disorders or serious protection risks (e.g., assisting their access to medications and follow-up appointments)	• Assist referral and access of vulnerable families to therapeutic interventions (e.g., psychotherapy) and specialized social services • Build capacity and support the work of mental health and social service professionals (e.g., school psychologists, clinical social workers) in working with at-risk children and families	• Work with health and mental health professionals to support and strengthen available, accessible, high-quality clinical MHPSS care for children and families within health and mental health systems (e.g., hospitals, child and adolescent mental health units, community mental health systems) • Promote quality standards for clinical care of MNS disorders (e.g., mhGAP[a] training for mental health care providers)

[a]The WHO Mental Health Gap Action Programme (mhGAP) aims at scaling up services for mental, neurological, and substance use disorders in countries especially those with low and middle incomes. The program asserts that with proper care, psychosocial assistance, and medication, tens of millions could be treated for depression, schizophrenia, and epilepsy, prevented from suicide, and begin to lead normal lives – even where resources are scarce.

> *Layer 3 and 4 field example.* Key program description and examples of focused, non-specialized, and specialized supports for children include *International Medical Corps MHPSS and child protection case management services* set up throughout the Middle East in response to the Syria crisis. A multidisciplinary team of social and para-social workers are trained and supervised to work within the primary healthcare system and IDP shelters. They ensure a continuum of effective services for affected populations that have

multiple and complex needs and require a comprehensive mental health and psychosocial case management approach. In Syria, International Medical Corps has also developed psychosocial support and child protection training packages and has developed the capacity of volunteer frontline and childcare workers supporting IDP families in inaccessible areas outside of Damascus.

Summary and Next Steps: Scaling up and Scaling Deep

Existing resources and capacities are not sufficient to meet the significant MHPSS challenges posed by protracted, large-scale conflicts, such as those seen from the Syria crisis and other countries hosting displaced populations. Displaced populations tend to reside in the most deprived areas where locals are already struggling with inadequate services, few support systems, and few mental health professionals available to meet demand. Scaling up in these contexts is needed, and there is willingness and drive to do so within the international MHPSS community. At times, however, providing MHPSS to a more significant number of people *AND* ensuring quality and effectiveness of approaches – scaling "deeply" – can be considered a trade-off. Nonetheless, there have been valuable experiences in scaling up community-based MHPSS interventions and lessons learned that can inform future implementation and sustainability.

The UNICEF-Community Based Operational Guidelines recommend approaches that emphasize the need to improve both the scale and quality of community-based MHPSS in humanitarian settings, promoting interventions for prospective scale-up based on implementation science research that contributes to the evidence base of those interventions. The guidelines include a monitoring and evaluation framework to assess facilitators and barriers to quality implementation at scale – limiting the risks of compromising effectiveness while improving reach. Furthermore, UNICEF launched the guidelines in a field test version in 2018 [16] and will continue to collect feedback from users and pilot agencies through 2020, incorporating lessons from the field in the final version and maximizing their utility and relevance among various humanitarian actors in complex contexts.

The benefits of community-engaged MHPSS programming are myriad. As described in the UNICEF operational guidelines (UNICEF 2018, page 41), community engagement ensures programs:
- Are relevant to local realities, cultural values, and understandings.
- Make the best use of local resources.
- Effectively identify children and families who are vulnerable or have special needs and actively promote their inclusion in interventions and relief efforts.
- Strengthen the natural supports in families and communities to care for children.
- Strengthen the capacities of childcare systems for broad impact.
- Promote local ownership of programs for long-term sustainability.

Quality, community-based MHPSS programming is a worthwhile investment, but it requires sufficient time, skills, and resources. Longer-term funding across the emergency-development nexus is necessary to develop the capacities needed on the ground to meet the demands of the current child protection and developmental crisis. Community-engaged work requires particular skills and knowledge in traversing social, cultural, economic, and political particularities in each context, reducing threats of various kinds to positive mental health and psychosocial wellbeing of children and families (e.g., stigma, marginalization, violence) and maximizing the potential resources that already exist among caregivers, communities, and within children and adolescents themselves. This foundational work in capacity building is a starting point to "build back better" [17] protection and care systems for children, and to strengthen systems that ensure solid safety nets and seamless MHPSS care for children and families in the short term. It is also essential to the work of addressing the global disparities in adequate mental health care and social service financing and structures within national healthcare systems in the longer term [18].

References

1. Bowlby J. Attachment and loss, vol. 1 Attachment. New York: Basic Books; 1969.
2. United Nations Children's Fund (UNICEF). Growing up in conflict: the impact on children's mental health and psychosocial well-being, report on the symposium, 26–28 May 2015, New Babylon Meeting Center, The Hague. New York: UNICEF; 2015. http://www.unicefinemergencies.com/downloads/eresource/docs/MHPSS/Growing%20up%20in%20conflict-20160104112554.pdf.
3. United Nations High Commissioner for Refugees (UNHCR). Global trends forced displacement 2018. 2019. https://www.unhcr.org/globaltrends2018/.
4. European Civil Protection and Humanitarian Aid Operations (ECHO). Fact Sheet: Forced displacement: refugees, asylum seekers and internally displaced people (IDPs). 2019. Last updated 19/06/2019. https://ec.europa.eu/echo/what-we-do/humanitarian-aid/refugees-and-internally-displaced-persons_en.
5. Overseas Development Institute (ODI). Education cannot wait: proposing a fund for education in emergencies. 2015.
6. Hermosilla S, Metzler J, Savage K, Musa M, Ager A. Child friendly spaces impact across five humanitarian settings: a meta-analysis. BMC Public Health. 2019;19:576.
7. Jordans M, Pigott H, Tol W. Interventions for children affected by armed conflict: a systematic review of mental health and psychosocial support in low and middle income countries. Curr Psychiatry Rep. 2016;18(9):2016. https://doi.org/10.1007/s11920-015-0648-z.
8. United Nations Children's Fund. Operational guidelines on community based mental health and psychosocial support in humanitarian settings: three-tiered support for children and families (field test version). New York: UNICEF; 2018a.
9. World Health Organization, War Trauma Foundation and World Vision International. Psychological first aid: guide for field workers. Geneva: WHO; 2011.
10. Duncan J, Arntson L. Children in crisis: good practices in evaluating psychosocial programming. International Psychosocial Evaluation Committee and Save the Children Federation, Inc. 2004. p. 16.
11. Save the Children. Children in crisis: good practices in evaluating psychosocial programming. Save the Children Federation; 2004. p. 6.

12. Lippman LH, Moore KA, McIntosh H. Positive indicators of child Well-being: a conceptual framework, measures and methodological issues. Working paper no. 2009-21. UNICEF research Centre, Florence; 2009.
13. Baron N. Global tool kit of orientation and training materials. Inter-Agency Standing Committee (IASC); 2009.
14. Sim A, Puffer E, Green E, Chase R, Zayzay J, Garcia-Rolland E, Boone L. Parents make the difference: findings from a randomized impact evaluation of a parenting program in rural Liberia. International Rescue Committee; 2014.
15. Save the Children. Psychological first aid for child practitioners. Denmark: Save the Children; 2013.
16. United Nations Children's Fund. Humanitarian Annual Report. New York: UNICEF; 2018b.
17. World Health Organization (WHO). Building Back better: sustainable mental health care after emergencies. Geneva: WHO; 2014. https://apps.who.int/iris/bitstream/handle/10665/85377/9789241564571_eng.pdf?sequence=1.
18. Patel, V., Saxena, S., Lund, C., et al. (2018) The Lancet Commission on global mental health and sustainable development, Lancet 392 (10157), P1553–1598.

Part III

Mental Health Symptom Clusters in Refugee Children and Adolescents

Grief and Loss in Displaced and Refugee Families

8

Lynne Jones

Introduction

Why do we grieve? Wouldn't life be much simpler if we did not experience all those painful emotions that occur when someone we love dies? Perhaps so: no weeping and wailing, no stoical silence, no anger and irritation, no smiling and carrying on as usual, no sudden flood of pain and memories to overwhelm and paralyse, or the rush of tears when you hear a familiar tune. That sounds much easier. The trouble is that grief is actually the price tag on another emotional experience without which human life would be quite unbearable. We grieve because we love. Love is the essential emotion that keeps us connected and attached to family and friends and allows us to survive as rather puny animals in a hostile world. If we did not love, we could not suffer loss, but neither could we survive in selfish isolation.

This chapter provides a brief introduction to understanding grief and loss in families who have been displaced by disaster and conflict and provides some guidance as to how to support them. It will address the following questions:

- What losses are experienced by displaced and refugee individuals and groups?
- How is grief related to attachment and do we grieve in stages?
- Is grief an illness?
- How does bereavement affect our health?
- When is grief abnormal?

This is an adapted and updated version of the chapter that appeared in: Maternal and Childhealth Advocacy International (2014). *International Maternal & Child Health Care: A practical manual for hospitals worldwide.* London, Radcliffe

L. Jones (✉)
FXB Center for Health and Human Rights, Harvard University, Cambridge, MA, USA

© Springer Nature Switzerland AG 2020   123
S. J. Song, P. Ventevogel (eds.), *Child, Adolescent and Family Refugee Mental Health*, https://doi.org/10.1007/978-3-030-45278-0_8

- What is mourning and why does it matter?
- What happens when large numbers die at one time?
- What happens when it is not clear if someone has died or not (ambiguous loss)?
- How do we distinguish between the effects of traumatic events and the effects of loss?
- What is 'cultural bereavement'?
- How does bereavement affect children?
- What can we do to help grieving families and children?
- Should we tell children the truth about death?
- Some guidelines for grieving children.

Most children will be seen in the company of their surviving adult relatives whose own mental state will have a profound effect on the child. A health worker must therefore be responsive to, and able to assess and support, the whole family. For this reason, this chapter looks at grief in both adults and children. It outlines a general approach to supporting families and children but does not give detailed management advice on the wide variety of specific symptomatic problems that can occur in grief (e.g. bedwetting or sleep disturbance). Readers interested in specific management guidance on this topic can consult existing manuals [6, 29].

Some notes on terms and definitions: The terms grief and bereavement are often used interchangeably. In this chapter I use the term bereavement to mean the experience of loss and the term grief to mean the emotions, thoughts and behaviours that occur in response to the experience of bereavement.

What Losses Are Experienced by Individuals and Groups in Conflict and Disaster Settings?

The central experience for almost all those displaced by conflict or disaster is loss. Even if no one in your family dies, something will be lost. You may be injured or lose your health. Your home or your school may be destroyed, the neighbourhood swept away. Your friends or workmates may be killed or flee. When you flee, you lose everything that made up your world and kept you rooted and connected. As well as the external losses just mentioned, you may lose aspects that are internal to your sense of self: feelings of being safe and in control and your sense of identity as a mother, father, schoolchild, farmer or shopkeeper. Some possibilities are illustrated in Table 8.1. Their effect can be overwhelming. Understanding how people react to such losses, how to distinguish between normal and abnormal grief and how to assist in appropriate mourning will be one of the key tasks for health workers in these contexts. It is also essential to understanding other psychological reactions such as PTSD and set them in context.

Table 8.1 Some of the losses experienced by those exposed to conflict, disaster or life as refugees. Can you think of others?

Internal	External
Control	Family members
Autonomy	Friends
Security	Home
Identity	Community/country
Self-respect	Work/school
Belief in future	Money and other material possessions
Sense of belonging	Physical health
Trust	Religion
Past	Language
Meaning of life	Familiar life

How Is Grief Related to Attachment and Do We Grieve in Stages?

The ability to form strong relationships with others is necessary for our survival as human beings. We call this ability *attachment.* The sense of loss we feel when a loved one is absent results in us searching them out. Attachment is the glue that keeps families and groups connected and together. Human beings could not have survived in previous eras if they did not live in groups which would enable them to cooperate, feed and shelter themselves. *Loss* is the sense of sadness, fear and insecurity we feel when a loved person is absent. It can also be felt for things and places.

In the 1950s the British psychiatrist and psychoanalyst John Bowlby became interested in what happened to small children when they were separated from their mothers. In Britain in those days, if a child went to hospital for an operation, the parent was not allowed to remain with them. John Bowlby and his colleague James Robertson observed the infant to see how they reacted, how they adapted to the separation and how they behaved when the parent returned [5]. Bowlby described behaviours which might be observed in any infant separated from its mother and then reunited with her [4].

There would first be a period of loud and angry *protest*. The child would hope that its cries would bring mother running back. When this did not happen, a period of *despair and withdrawal* followed in which the child would cry, not wish to engage with others, and not eat or play. Later the child might appear to 'adapt'. She would start eating again, play with other children, make friends with the nurses and appear *detached* and indifferent to her loss. Indeed, if the parent reappeared in this stage, the first response might be to ignore them and then if they did engage to be naughty and *angry*. Only after some time would the original relationship reform and *re-engagement* occur. Bowlby noted that this *attachment/separation behaviour* is most visible in children of 6 months to 3 years old. However, these behaviours might reappear in any of us throughout the life cycle when faced with separation from someone we love:

Attachment behaviour is any form of behaviour that results in a person attaining or maintaining proximity to some clearly identified individual who is conceived as better able to cope with the world. It is most obvious whenever a person is frightened, fatigued or sick, and is assuaged by comforting and care-giving. At other times the behaviour is less in evidence. Nevertheless, for a person to know that an attachment figure is available and responsive gives him a strong and pervasive feeling of security and so encourages him to value and continue the relationship. Whilst attachment behaviour is at its most obvious early in childhood, it can be observed throughout the lifecycle, especially in emergencies. Since it is seen in virtually all human beings (though in varying patterns), it is regarded as an integral part of human nature and one we share (to a varying extent) with members of other species. The biological function attributed to it is protection. To remain within easy access of a familiar individual known to be ready and willing to come to our aid in an emergency is clearly a good insurance policy - whatever our age. (Bowlby [4], p. 27).

Many writers, including Bowlby himself, noted the similarity between a child's behaviour after separation from a parent and our reactions to the loss of a loved person who has died. Death reactivates attachment behaviour. Faced with the permanent loss that death represents, we may find ourselves angrily protesting, searching and yearning, trying our best to maintain and hang onto the connection. Or we may experience periods of indifference and denial as a way of avoiding the pain. Many people move between periods of acute grieving and yearning and periods of avoidance/detachment. In the past some have argued that these feelings occur in stages. Elisabeth Kubler-Ross constructed a stage model of grief in which the individual was said to progress through periods of (1) denial, (2) anger, (3) bargaining, (4) depression and (5) acceptance [17].

It was suggested that people could become stuck at different stages and that 'grief work' was necessary to progress through all the stages to recovery. However, although this approach continues to be popular and widely taught, some decades of research have failed to show scientific foundation for this theory. What has become clear is that 'most people do not grieve in stages. Using stages as a guide in work with the bereaved is unhelpful and may even cause harm' [24].

How people grieve and how they cope will depend on multiple factors interacting with one another. What were their experiences as a child? Were they loved and securely attached to those who cared for them or abused or insecure? This will affect the way they form relationships with other people and the way they experience loss; so will their age, sex and the experience of previous losses. It will also depend on the nature of the loss and how it occurred: was it sudden or expected? Was it violent, unjust, part of a massive loss or after a prolonged illness? What did the loss mean to the person? Were they thrust into isolation and poverty or, possibly, liberated from an abusive relationship? In all cases social factors such as cultural and religious beliefs and community and family dynamics will play a role in determining how grief is experienced and expressed. As will the current social situation: is the family in flight, still in danger or settled in a camp? If in a camp, are their familiar neighbours close by, or do they live next to strangers? Does anyone speak their language? Is there social support or are they isolated? What material resources are there? Do they face legal difficulties because of the loss? The case examples below all illustrate these variations.

Table 8.2   Reactions to bereavement

Affective	Cognitive	Behavioural	Physiological-somatic
Depression, despair, dejection, distress	Preoccupation with thoughts of deceased, intrusive ruminations	Agitation, tenseness, restlessness	Loss of appetite Sleep disturbances
Anxiety, fears, dreads	Vivid memories Sense of presence of deceased	Fatigue, apathy Overactivity	Energy loss, exhaustion
Guilt, self-blame, self-accusation	Lowered self-esteem, self-reproach	Searching Weeping, sobbing, crying	Somatic complaints Physical complaints similar to deceased
Anger, hostility, irritability	Helplessness, hopelessness, pessimism about future	Social withdrawal Normal behaviour and continuation of normal activities	*Endocrine and immunological changes*
Anhedonia – Loss of pleasure	Suicidal ideation Sense of unreality	Agitation, tenseness, restlessness	Susceptibility to illness, disease, mortality
Loneliness	Memory, concentration difficulties	*In children:*	
Yearning, longing, pining	Suppression, avoidance, disbelief	Acting out Regressive behaviour	
Shock, numbness	Fantasies	School difficulties Rapid maturing	
No reaction		Bedwetting	

Source: Stroebe et al. [22]

Table 8.2 illustrates the wide variety of emotional, cognitive, behavioural and physiological changes that can occur in reaction to bereavement. An individual may have some, all or none of these. The reactions may occur in many patterns and combinations depending on the factors above. Some individuals experience few, others more. In some people reactions change over time or come in varying combinations.

People may feel anger and sadness at the same time. An anniversary or a particular place may trigger a memory, which reactivates the feelings of grief again, years after the event, perhaps interrupting a long period of acceptance. Some have described grief as a 'relapsing illness'. Stroebe and her colleagues have created a model to show how many people may fluctuate between a 'loss orientation' of yearning and sadness and a 'restoration orientation' of more avoidant states of denial and getting on with things [22, 23] (see Fig. 8.1).

Which feelings and behaviours occur, which state dominates and what is regarded as normal for both children and adults will depend very much on how grief is expressed in that culture, by that family and in that individual as well as the religious values, temperament and personality of the individual. For example, in Bosnia, it is regarded as appropriate for Serbian women to attend the funeral and to display their emotions visibly, keening and weeping. Many Muslim cultures value a more stoical approach and see the vivid display of emotions as inappropriate. In some cultures, for example, in parts of Southeast Asia, vivid dreams may be regarded as appropriate messages from the dead. In Western culture, dreams may be seen as an upsetting form of sleep disturbance. In Kosovar families with whom I have worked, there was often one individual (usually an older adolescent girl), who might

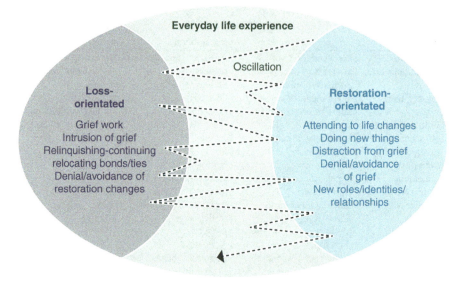

Fig. 8.1 The dual process model of coping with bereavement. (Source: Stroebe et al. [22])

cry a great deal, hyperventilate and faint, while the rest of the family remained stoical. The fainting girl might cause concern but also seemed to play a role in vividly expressing grief for the rest of the family, whose concern for her also acts as a form of distraction from the loss.

Is Grief an Illness?

> Near the end of his life Sigmund Freud was consulted by a woman who had become depressed following the death of her husband. After listening to her, Freud quietly stated, "Madam you do not have a neurosis, you have a misfortune". (Wahl [26], p. 104)

Acute grief may be painful and feel like an illness, but it should be understood, in all its variety, as a normal reaction to loss. Some combinations of reactions do appear to mimic some acute mental illnesses. For example, loss of appetite, combined with sleep disturbance, sadness, ruminations and various somatic complaints, appears similar to clinical depression. But the diagnosis should not be made if someone has suffered an acute loss [29, 30]. Some individuals may adopt the behaviours of the deceased, dress in their clothes, act strangely or hear their voice, see them and talk to them. Again, this should not be regarded as psychotic behaviour but as a possible manifestation of acute grief. Or there may be flashbacks, vivid intrusive thoughts and dreams of the deceased, and the individual may be anxious and aroused, similar to those with post-traumatic stress disorder (PTSD). None of these reactions are necessarily pathological.

How Does Bereavement Affect our Health?

That is not to say that bereavement does not have physical and mental health consequences that require attention, understanding and support [25]. Bereaved people experience more physical complaints, make more health consultations, use more medication and experience more hospitalisations. Paradoxically, those grieving intensely actually make less health consultations than the normal population, and high-intensity grief is a predictor for more severe physical disorders a year later. Perhaps this is because early warning signs are missed. Regarding the impact of bereavement on mental health, the majority of people recover, but there is a greater vulnerability to depression, anxiety and PTSD [22].

Bereavement is associated with increased mortality from many causes. People who have suffered a recent bereavement are more likely to die of alcohol-related disorders, coronary artery disease, unnatural deaths and suicide. It is thought that the additional risk may be due to a variety of factors: loneliness, changes in social circumstances, less material resources and lack of care. The risks are higher in the earliest months and greater in specific groups: particularly those who have lost a child, spouse or sibling [22, 31]. So it is not nonsensical to say that you can die of a 'broken heart'.

When Is Grief Abnormal?

The decision as to what is abnormal and inappropriate grief will depend on an understanding of the individual, the family, the culture and the context from which they come. You cannot decide what is abnormal without this cultural and personal knowledge. The community and family may be able to tell you when they feel the grief is too intense or too long or unusual in its manifestations. In the newly released ICD-11, the definition for prolonged grief disorder is as follows:

> Prolonged grief disorder is a disturbance in which, following the death of a partner, parent, child, or other person close to the bereaved, there is persistent and pervasive grief response characterized by longing for the deceased or persistent preoccupation with the deceased accompanied by intense emotional pain (e.g. sadness, guilt, anger, denial, blame, difficulty accepting the death, feeling one has lost a part of one's self, an inability to experience positive mood, emotional numbness, difficulty in engaging with social or other activities). The grief response has persisted for an atypically long period of time following the loss (more than 6 months at a minimum) and clearly exceeds expected social, cultural or religious norms for the individual's culture and context. Grief reactions that have persisted for longer periods that are within a normative period of grieving given the person's cultural and religious context are viewed as normal bereavement responses and are not assigned a diagnosis. The disturbance causes significant impairment in personal, family, social, educational, occupational or other important areas of functioning (World Health Organization [28]).

Epidemiological research around this concept is still in the early days. In normal circumstances it is thought that approximately one in ten bereaved persons suffer from prolonged grief disorder although the variations in definition and different methodologies used in research mean that specific risk factors have yet to be agreed [19]. However, recent studies of PGD in refugee and displaced populations show that they may be particularly vulnerable. Among Iraqi Mandaean refugees in Australia, 17% experienced prolonged grief disorder, while 16% suffered from a combination of PGD and PTSD [20]. A study of 308 internally displaced victims of conflict in Colombia found that 25% suffered from PGD alone and 27% from combined PGD and PTSD [11]. This research suggests that prolonged grief disorder is a relevant and distinct condition in refugee and displaced populations, characterized by particular risk factors: traumatic loss, experiencing more abusive and assaultive events, being older and/or female, the loss of a close relative and experiencing difficulties in adapting to the new environment. PGD was characterized by distinctive symptoms: separation distress, longing and yearning, difficulties in accepting the death and bitterness. Knowledge of these risk factors and symptoms may assist health workers in identifying those at risk of PGD.

What Is Mourning and Why Does It Matter?

Mourning is the name for those processes which help people to cope with bereavement. All societies and cultures mourn but in different ways. Mourning processes usually include methods for acknowledgement and acceptance of the death, saying farewell, time periods for grieving, processes to continue attention towards the dead and to move beyond it and make new attachments. It might be helpful to take a moment and jot down on a piece of paper the ways that you mourn the dead in your own society. Try answering the questions in Box 8.1:

Box 8.1 Questions to Reflect on Mourning in your Own Society
- How do other people know that someone has died or that you are bereaved?
- What happens at the funeral?
  - What are the burial customs?
  - What happens to the body?
  - Who visits the bereaved?
- What are the different roles, if any, for men and women?
- What do younger and older children do?
- Are there different ceremonies at different time periods after the death to mark different stages of mourning?
- What ways do you use to remember the dead?
- What is the role of dead person in continuing family life?

Different societies have different time periods set aside for mourning, and different ideas about what is appropriate behaviour for different family members. They may also have different views on the appropriate role of children in these rituals. Sometimes families may be in conflict over what is appropriate to communicate to children and what is the appropriate way to mourn. This is particularly the case in communities in flight or whom have been displaced (see Vignette 1).

What Happens in Situations of Massive Loss?

As we noted above, all displaced people have experienced losses, even if not the loss of a person. The loss of culture and familiar landscape may be overwhelming, but there are no formal mourning rituals for such losses, which may contribute to prolonged feelings of yearning and distress that are not recognised. When it comes to the loss of people, conflicts, disaster and displacement all disrupt the possibilities of appropriate mourning. There may be uncertainty over missing relatives (see the section on ambiguous loss below). The body may have been lost, abandoned, treated inappropriately or buried in a mass grave. The normal mourning rituals are impossible to carry out during flight. Other processes also occur in large-scale upheavals. For example, in Aceh after the 2004 tsunami, displaced people found themselves living in a landscape swept completely clean by the wave, where every familiar marker had disappeared along with their communities, families and livelihoods. There were no bodies and no places to go to remember the dead. In Haiti, after the earthquake, people camped out among crushed houses that entombed their families. Massive losses that affect whole communities may remove entire social networks of support and the resources needed to make grief endurable and mourning possible.

Even in functioning communities, massive losses have the effect of depriving each individual of the normal support that they would have received if their loss had been singular occurrence. Because everyone is affected, few are in the position to play the role of visitor and comforter. There is no one to come round, help the bereaved widow with the child care and household tasks, arrange the funeral and cook a meal, because everyone who survived is in the same situation. Everyone struggles alone. And the bereaved may become more reticent than usual about their own feelings, not wishing to burden similarly affected neighbours. At the same time, the pain of the loss is amplified by the knowledge that the bereaved person's loss is one of many in a community. The outside world is focussed on the scale of the event: '300,000 dead, half a million killed'. Lost within these figures, the individual bereavement may seem insignificant – just one of many thousands. This lack of significance adds to the pain of the survivor.

Case Example: The Dead Mother

Giving significance to loss: In early 2005 I was working on the East Coast of Sri Lanka after the tsunami. On one occasion, walking along a completely deserted, devastated street, a man came running up to me. I was holding my camera and assumed I might have offended him by taking pictures. 'No, no', he said, 'please take a picture of THIS HOUSE'. I looked at the gutted empty building and did as he requested and then turned back. He was near to tears. 'My mother died here'. We sat on the ground and he talked for some time about his mother. I suddenly realised that for this man I was more than just a sympathetic ear, I was the outside world witnessing and memorialising his individual loss. Not just 10,000 dead, but his mother. I was making her significant.

What Happens When It Is Not Clear if Someone Has Died or Not (Ambiguous Loss)?

Imagine that you had to flee your home abruptly. Bombs were falling on the city, or a flood threatened. In the chaos loved ones were left behind and you have no idea what happened to them. You sit with other survivors who tell you everyone in that place died. That is what the news reports say as well. And yet there is no list of the dead, no body, no clear information as to what actually happened – maybe they escaped as well, maybe they are in another camp somewhere, maybe they are trapped, maybe they were forcibly recruited or abducted. The months and years pass and still there is no information. Grieving and mourning would mean giving up hope for the person and in some sense betraying them, letting them down, abandoning them. But continuing to hope means continual preoccupation, searching, anxiety. It roots you in the past, may fill you with longing and yearning and prevents you starting life anew. You do not know where to settle in case they cannot find you. Should you save money to spend on someone you may never see again? Should you look for employment that will take time from searching? This is ambiguous loss, unfortunately a common experience for many displaced by war and disaster. Some have argued that this continuing preoccupation with the missing person should be treated as prolonged grief disorder, as many exhibit the same symptoms. In a qualitative study of parents in Northern Uganda whose children had disappeared between 8 and 28 years earlier, the majority described persistent yearning, continuing emotional pain, anger and bitterness on a daily basis. The combination of hope and despair created a constant state of anxiety and restlessness ([13], p. 298). One of the Ugandan families explained:

> It is very important to have someone confirmed dead and buried in the compound. It is better than the thought that the person is still alive, this feeling is accompanied with the feeling that the person is dead. This is so painful. So we are never settled. We are always living in unrest. There is the hope, but the hope is always accompanied by the worries and the sad feeling that the person is dead. There is no closure. (Hollander [13], p. 298)

Ambiguous loss may generate additional stresses. Families may break up because of differing views on what has happened to the missing person. The survivors may find themselves isolated from their community because 'culturally condoned grief has an expiration date'. People no longer know what to say to them. Or they may be stigmatised because of questions over the role a missing person is playing in continuing conflict. There may be cultural and spiritual stress because the family cannot carry out the normal mourning rituals. For all these reasons, many argue that ambiguous grief should not be regarded as a pathological disorder, because in spite of its similarities to PGD, the problems are caused by these external stressors and pathologising does not help. To date the most useful therapeutic approaches have been those that offer group support, address isolation, restore relationships and focus on normalising the ambiguity, so that people can learn to live with it while looking forward and finding enjoyment and meaning in life once more [13].

Traumatic Experiences, Grief and Mourning

Exposure to traumatic events can interfere with mourning. Avoidance that may be protective in coping with the memories of a traumatic event may make it difficult for the bereaved to mourn their loss because the memories of the lost person are always accompanied by painful memories of the circumstances of the loss, so 'remembering' is too painful. In such circumstances, the traumatic symptoms may need treatment before the bereaved person is able to mourn. Table 8.3 illustrates the differences in emotional cognitive and behavioural reactions that may occur.

Table. 8.3 Distinguishing the impact of traumatic events and loss

Reactions to Loss	Reactions to Traumatic Event
Separation anxiety	Anxiety about threat posed by recurrence of traumatic event
Sadness more than anxiety	Anxiety more than sadness
Yearning and preoccupation with loss	Fearful, anxious and preoccupied with traumatic event
Sense of security intact	Personal sense of safety challenged
Primary relationships disrupted	Primary relationships intact
Intrusive memories are images and thoughts of the deceased	Intrusive memories of traumatic event plus re-experiencing accompanying emotions
Memories sought after positive and comforting	Uncontrollable intrusions: Negative and distressing
Dream of dead person is comforting	Nightmares of event are terrifying
Seek out reminders of loved ones	Hypervigilant, scanning environment for threat
Avoidance of reminders of absence of loved one	Avoidance of reminders of threat
Anger at loss	Irritable, diffuse unfocussed anger and rage
Guilt at not doing enough	Guilt at surviving
Mourning as a tribute to dead	
Sleep EEG normal	Increased REM sleep intensity
Coping involves reconstructing life without loved one	Coping involves re-establishing sense of safety
Recovery: Resolve attachment issues	*Recovery*: Habituate to fearful responses

Source: Hendricks [12]

Cultural Bereavement

When working with displaced or refugee populations, you may find the concept of 'cultural bereavement' more useful than trying to decide whether or not someone is suffering from a 'disorder'. The term was coined by the Australian anthropologist and child psychiatrist Maurice Eisenbruch to encompass the experiences of massive losses and uprooting suffered by refugees.

> Cultural bereavement is the experience of the uprooted person - or group - resulting from loss of social structures, cultural values and self identity: the person - or group - continues to live in the past, is visited by supernatural forces from the past while asleep or awake, suffers feelings of guilt over abandoning culture or homeland, feels pain if memories of the past begin to fade, but finds constant images of the past (including traumatic images) intruding into daily life, yearns to complete obligations to the dead and feels stricken by anxieties, morbid thoughts and anger that mar the ability to get on with daily life. It is not in itself a disease but an understandable response to catastrophic loss of social structure and culture. (Eisenbruch [8])

In his work with Cambodian adolescents, Eisenbruch found that those refugee children, who had been encouraged to assimilate rapidly into a new culture, suffered more cultural bereavement than those encouraged to participate in traditional ceremonies and cultural practices. He believes that the concept allows for a more integrated and culturally sensitive approach to the experience of loss, than attempting to classify any disabling symptoms only in terms of pathological categories according to Western diagnostic criteria such as PTSD or traumatic bereavement. Disabling symptoms may be best addressed by a combination of restoring appropriate cultural practices and, if necessary, symptomatic relief.

How Does Bereavement Affect Children?

These are some frequently asked questions about children who have suffered a bereavement:

- Do children grieve?
- Are they too young to understand?
- Should we protect them from unpleasantness and distress?
- Will loss in childhood cause later mental or physical illness?

Children's Understanding of and Reactions to Death

Children's reactions to death are as variable as those of adults, and any or all of the reactions listed above in Table 8.2 may occur. The most important point to note is that their understanding of death changes according to their development and life experiences. The following notes are based on Western experiences and should be taken as a guide only. For example, working with displaced and refugee children in many low-resource settings has taught me that in many societies, particularly rural ones, children understand death at an earlier age.

Under 5 Years

There is little understanding that death is final. For example, a 4-year-old child in England, having helped to formally bury his dead pet rabbit in the garden, then asked if he could now dig it up so that he could have the rabbit back. He had not yet understood that death is forever. Magical thinking results in misconceptions about causes and effects. An egocentric view of the world can lead to feelings of responsibility. 'Mummy won't come back because I was naughty'. Reactions are similar to those following any separation: The longer the absence, the greater the distress. It may be followed by detachment, so that the surviving family may think the child does not care. Clinginess and reluctance to be separated from the surviving carer is very common, as is regressive behaviour. Soiling, wetting, sleeplessness and minor illnesses can all occur.

Over 5 Years

Children begin to understand that death is irreversible, that certain physical changes occur and that there is permanent separation. They may still not regard it as something that can affect them. They may continue to have some magical, concrete and egocentric thinking. At this age, children more commonly use concepts of good and bad, they are curious about cause and effect, and they are able to articulate concern for others.

There is a desire to stay connected to the dead parent. Many children dream about and talk with the dead parent frequently; feel the dead parent is watching them; and keep physical objects associated with them. One study found that 43% of children in a large community sample thought about the dead parent on a daily basis 1 year after death. The reactions are variable. Boys are already learning to suppress feelings. 91% of the children in the same study cried on the first day; 50% had transient emotional and behavioural problems. Concentration and school work are affected. Repetitive play is very common [21].

Ten to Adolescence

There is a growing understanding of abstract concepts: that death is universal and inevitable and can affect them personally. There is a growing concern with justice and injustice, and an awareness of inconsistencies. The conflict between the desire for autonomy and need for closeness can be resolved by 'indifference and detachment', or by identification and nostalgia. In a group of adolescent refugee boys 'ethnically cleansed' from Northern Bosnia (all had lost their homes; some had lost their family), all spoke passionately and with great longing about their home towns, describing them as the 'most beautiful place to live' [14]. Revenge fantasies are not unusual. There are less somatic and behavioural problems, and a depressed mood is common. Poor concentration and lack of interest occur at school. The oldest child who has lost a same-sex parent is at greatest risk.

Case Example: The Surviving Brother

G is a 13-year-old boy. During a long and brutal war, his elder brother was killed on the front line. G was always very close to his brother. Three years later he continued to think about him on a daily basis. He visited the grave frequently and watched the video of the funeral once a week. He did not like to sleep alone and felt sad much of the time, although he was doing well at school. He talked about his brother a great deal. He wanted to be as much like his brother as possible, whom he believed was one of the bravest and most incorruptible people. He was angry about the peace agreement. He felt it was unjust and made a mockery of the aims for which his brother fought.

Source: Jones [15], p 64–65.

As in adults, the reactions to bereavement at all ages are enormously variable: age, personality, closeness to the deceased, culture and family values, especially the way the parents or surviving caretakers react, will all affect the expression of grief. There is an increased vulnerability to psychiatric disorder. Sudden death in particular is associated with higher rates of PTSD and depression, particularly if it is accompanied by disruption in the child's social networks and their sense of security. These risk factors are of obvious relevance to refugee children [10, 16].

Children within one family exposed to the same losses may all handle grief in different ways. (See 'Case example: Telling the story'.) Children need to understand that the experience of grief may wax and wane. When discussing grief feelings with children, I sometimes use the image of a wave.[1]

I ask them to imagine they are standing at the edge of the sea and a big wave comes along and knocks them over. They feel terrible, overwhelmed. There may be a whole mix of emotions, anger, tears, bewilderment, despair, but somehow, they manage to struggle to their feet. Then there is a period of calm water before the next wave. Perhaps it is a significant date – a birthday – or they hear a favourite tune which acts as a reminder. But this time they are more prepared, so that when the next wave – and all those painful feelings – comes along, it does not knock them over because they saw it coming and braced. What will happen over time is that, although the waves never go away completely, the periods of calm sea grow longer, the waves get smaller, and the child grows stronger and more able to cope.

Long-Term Effects

Unfortunately, if children experience the loss of someone significant early in life, it may have long-term health effects. A large three-country cohort study of more than seven million young adults in Scandinavia showed that those who had lost a parent between 6 months and 18 years of age had a 50% greater chance of dying from any

---

[1] This is only appropriate for children familiar with the sea and obviously not in the context of loss caused by a tsunami or flood.

cause (natural or unnatural) in young adulthood than those who had not. The authors argue that genetic susceptibility only accounts for a small part of the risk and that a number of other causes should be considered including biological responses in the immune system to early life adversity; changes in behaviour including increasing risk behaviours; and more social and economic adversity, all of which are relevant to refugee populations [18]. Research evidence also suggests that children who suffer an early bereavement do have an increased risk of psychiatric disorder and poorer psychological wellbeing in the long term, particularly if the loss is associated with other disruptions in the child's life [1, 9, 15].

Life events research shows that the following events are the most likely to be associated with later mental illness:

- Those that require people to undertake a major revision of assumptions about the world
- Those that are lasting in their implications
- Those that take place over a short period of time without preparation

The intangible losses of displacement after conflict and disasters as well as traumatic bereavement can have all these features. However, there are significant factors that can mediate the impact of both the innumerable losses experienced by a refugee and bereavement. The child's long-term mental health also depends on:

- The response and wellbeing of the surviving parent or relatives
- The availability of other support
- Subsequent life circumstances
- The degree of continuity in the child's life
- How the loss is viewed by others
- What resources are available

This list provides an immediate guide as to what needs to be done to enhance a child's resilience and coping in the face of loss. The 'Case example: Different girls' from Pakistan illustrates how important these aspects are and how much difference the behaviour of surviving relatives can make: Such behaviour will in part depend on the resources and support given to them.

Case Example: Different Girls, Different Ways to Grieve
After the Pakistan earthquake in December 2005, I worked with children who had lost their parents. Contrast the experiences of two young teenage girls from the same rural, Islamic society, affected by the same terrible event but living in somewhat different settings with quite different responses from those caring for them and the support systems around them. Samira was 14 and living with her aunt and uncle and her six younger brothers and sisters in one tent in a displaced persons camp. Her village had been completely destroyed and her mother and father killed. Samira acted as mother

to her sibs and helped her aunt care for her cousins. The aunt and uncle had told the children 'your mother is in the village and will come soon'. Samira and her smaller sisters looked ill-kempt and neglected. They cried constantly, which suggested the comforting lie was not working. They knew their house had been turned to rubble, so where was their mother now? When I asked Samira what she thought, she told me in a whisper that her mother was dead. The aunt and uncle gave me permission to explain to all the children what had actually happened. Their calm reaction suggested I was confirming something they already knew. Samira also told me she would like to get out of the tent. As Samira was the eldest girl, she carried the burden of household tasks and childcare, and her aunt was very reluctant to let her go the camp school or any other of the activities arranged for children. However, she let the younger children attend and their improved mood was obvious. Samira continued to weep and neglect herself. Finally, when the Aunt herself was engaged in a livelihood programme with other camp women, she became more cheerful and gave Samira permission to go to school. This had the immediate effect of alleviating some of Samira's sadness.

In contrast, 12-year-old Aisha still lived in her village higher up in the mountains above the town. She too lost her mother when the house was destroyed. She moved in with her grandmother but stayed in her village. I met her laughing and playing with other village children. She had just had her hands hennaed in beautiful flower patterns. She had been told her mother was dead and said she still felt very sad. But she liked living with her grandmother and she did not cry all the time. When playing with other village children, she was able to be happy, and she told me she had many relatives and friends that cared about her.

These two stories illustrate the vital role of continuity in a child's life and the importance of the wellbeing and support for the carer as well as the benefits of honest communication. It is harder to achieve these things with displaced families under stress, but the Samira's story illustrates that it is possible.

What Can We Do to Help Grieving Families and Children?

Not all grieving families require a health worker's intervention. But in situations of conflict, disaster and displacement, the natural sources of social support are absent for the reasons listed above. In this case, the health worker is the supportive community. Some key activities are listed in Table 8.4.

Your role may be to accompany, support and advocate for the bereaved as any neighbour might do in normal times. Obviously if a family lacks basic resources

Table 8.4 Key actions to support grieving families	Attend to basic needs
	Access resources
	Assist mourning in culturally appropriate manner
	Answer questions; provide information
	Accompanying
	Available
	Attention to individual loss: Give significance
	Altruism opportunities
	Avoidance as required
	Advice as needed

or is not safe, helping to address these basic needs is a priority. Help may be needed to connect to agencies like the International Committee of the Red Cross, to trace missing relatives or identify them. Outsiders may have a significant role to play simply by encouraging and partaking in the normal processes of mourning. This may be through assisting an individual to organise a funeral or it may be helping a community. If any individual has symptoms of distress that are so great they cannot function or carry out necessary tasks, providing symptomatic relief will help.

Regarding discussion of the loss, you should follow the lead of the bereaved. With both adults and children, this means being able and available to listen without forcing talking. There is no evidence that 'grief work', that is the experiencing, confronting and working through of negative emotions, is helpful. There is some evidence that it may have long-term negative consequences. Contrary to some popular Western stereotypes, positive emotions in the early period after loss are indicative of good outcomes, not pathology. Individuals who choose the more avoidant orientation (see Fig. 8.1) are not in harmful denial, and this does not have to be challenged [7, 24, 27].

Nor is it necessary to 'break down' continuing attachment to the deceased. Good memories assist mourning and give pleasure and comfort. This connection may be maintained throughout a bereaved person's life without pathological effect. Depending on the culture, it may involve regular visits to the grave, talking actively or praying to the dead, frequent dreams or visions. Indeed, ritualised celebrations of connection with the dead in some societies actually strengthen living family bonds as they bring families together [2, 3]. A continuing connection should only cause concern if continuing yearning, searching and longing causes misery and dysfunction, dominates life in the long term and prevents the bereaved from forming any new attachments.

If the loss has occurred as a result of some form of political injustice or abuse, unresolved issues of reparations and justice may prolong grief and make mourning difficult. Helping victims to access justice may be another part of your role. See *Case example: When to tell the story.*

Case Example: When to Tell the Story

The family consisted of 3 surviving children (2 girls and a boy) who had witnessed the death of their mother and aunt and 15 other members of their extended family. They had been physically injured in the attack and spent some time in hospital. At our first meeting 4 months after the event, two of the children did not believe their mother was dead. They hoped she had survived as they had. We sat together with the children's father who told them gently that he thought that in all probability she was dead. The children cried and we did not discuss it further that day. The following week the bodies had been identified, funeral notices posted and the funeral arranged. The family had returned to the house where the massacre had occurred and appeared to be functioning well. The boy had no symptoms, although the younger girl was sad and quiet. When asked if they wanted to talk about what happened, she said no. Her brother said that he had already talked with journalists and did not feel a need to go over it again. The elder girl (14) had some intrusive thoughts and memories, and poor sleep and appetite. She wanted to walk me around the site and retell the events in detail.

The other children did not wish to join in. During the walk the elder girl told me that she now knew her mother was dead. All the children then wanted to show me all their old photographs, and all the children participated in identifying their dead relatives and telling me stories about their life before the war. After the funeral (which only the elder girl attended at her own request), the children appeared more cheerful, and all were looking forward to school. The surviving family provided an extremely loving and supportive network, and although the father was extremely sad, he allowed the children to talk about their mother whenever they wanted. Later the whole family was sent to another country for medical treatment for the children. They attended local schools where they learnt English and appeared to be adjusting well.

A year after the events, the International Criminal Tribunal wished to interview them regarding the massacre, and the three children insisted that they would like to give their accounts. All the children made statements recorded on video and gave similar detailed stories about the events surrounding the massacre. Although they found it distressing, each obviously regarded it as significant and important and was pleased to have had the chance. This example illustrates that children in the same family will not all deal with their grief in the same way. If given the opportunity, they will find the most appropriate time to tell their own stories in the way that will give it significance and meaning for themselves.

Long-term follow-up of these children 16 years after the massacre showed that all are doing well.

Should We Tell Children the Truth?

Many families present to health workers because they have concerns about the long-term impact of events on the child and want advice on how to talk about such abnormal events with their children. The health worker's role should be to facilitate the process of normal grieving, help to sustain and support the protective aspects mentioned in this chapter. While treating pathology where it is evident, you should take care to avoid pathologising where it is not. A particularly important role may be facilitating clear communication between family members. As some of the case studies and the vignette illustrate, many families are concerned that telling the child what happened will cause unnecessary distress and that as the child is 'too young to understand', it is better to lie or avoid the subject when it comes up. Children are very protective of surviving parents and quick to sense when a question causes distress. They may avoid asking for information because the questions make the parent cry. False information leads to confusion and a lack of trust. There is research evidence to suggest that this lack of trust may have an enduring effect in adult life [9]. The following case, *Case example: Telling the truth*, illustrates the benefits of telling the truth.

> **Case Example: Telling the Truth**
> The father was a member of a 'Liberation Army' and killed in the fighting. His 32-year-old wife had two surviving children of 8 and 9 and continued to live with her husband's relatives. She told the children their father was working in another country. The children would frequently ask her why he did not phone and if he would bring them presents. They were confused because other children in the village told them their father was dead. When they questioned their mother, she would start to cry, so they became nervous of asking her. Mother and brother-in-law asked for advice as to what to do and accepted my suggestion of sitting with the children and explaining in simple terms what had happened, answering all the children's questions as they came up and sharing the experience of grief. Mother told me that the relief of not having to lie to the children had slightly eased her own distress and made it easier to respond to them. Moreover, rather than being bewildered by their father's silent absence, the children now talked about him in the village with pride.

Guidelines for Grieving Children

1. Provide consistent, enduring, appropriate care.
   - Reunite children with their families or extended families as soon as possible.
   - In the absence of family, create enduring family-type networks with a low ratio of caretaker to children.
   - Consistent caregiving by one or two caretakers, not multiple different volunteers (however well intentioned), is essential to prevent attachment problems particularly in younger children.

2. The more continuity with the child's previous life the better.

   This is difficult to achieve with bereaved refugee children who may be griev-
   ing over both the loss of a parent or close relative and the loss of all that is
   familiar: home school, normal routines, familiar food, and pets. The following
   are examples of steps that can help:
   - Re-establish familiar routines including school in their own language.
   - Allow families that have fled together to live close to one another.
   - Provide facilities and support for families; allow them to cook their own food.
   - Provide culturally appropriate space for religious worship.
3. Support the carers by attending to basic needs and their own mental states.

   Help them to access the appropriate agencies to solve the practical problems
   they will encounter. Attending to basic needs is essential. Engaging in the process of rebuilding their lives helps families to come to terms with their losses.
4. Facilitate normal grieving and mourning.

   This can be done with memorials and rituals for absent bodies, and appropri-
   ate religious ceremonies
5. Don't hide the truth.
   - Children need clear, honest, consistent explanations appropriate to their
     level of development.
   - Answer the child's questions about the dead relative honestly in an age-
     appropriate way.
   - They need to accept the reality of the loss, not be protected from it.
   - Magical thinking should be explored and corrected. What is imagined may
     be worse than reality, and children may be blaming themselves for events
     beyond their control.
6. Grief work and debriefing may not be therapeutic or appropriate.

   The insistence on getting a child to 'debrief' or tell the story of their loss
   may not be therapeutic or appropriate. Not all cultures put a high value on the
   ventilation of individual feelings, as Western culture does. The therapist's goal
   should be to encourage a supportive atmosphere for the children, where open
   communication is possible, difficult questions answered, and distressing feelings tolerated. This means that the child will be free to express their grief in the
   manner they find appropriate to the person they most trust, and at a time of their
   own choosing.
7. Provide symptomatic relief.

   Help the family to cope with traumatic symptoms such as bedwetting, nightmares, and regressive behaviour, if they exist. Give the parents information as
   to what to expect and straightforward management advice.
8. Restart normal educational and play activities as soon as possible.

   Encourage communities and families to create or rebuild structured, safe
   opportunities for children to play and restart their education. This might be in
   the form of child friendly spaces or school classes.
9. Help the child maintain connection with the lost parent.

   Encourage the carer/surviving parent to allow the child to choose a memento
   to keep, access to photographs, or let the child draw a picture, make objects,
   create a memory box.

10. Help the child access justice.

The question of justice will be important for families in situations of political violence. Many will state that they cannot come to terms with their losses while the fate of loved ones is unknown, bodies unidentified, or perpetrators at large. These issues will affect the children, and older children may bring them up spontaneously and wish to discuss them. Health workers may be asked their own views. Stating a willingness to learn and understand, along with an awareness of one's own biases and subjectivity is the most helpful position. Political and cultural literacy are essential. The family should be put in touch with the appropriate human rights or justice agencies if they wish to give formal evidence, so that the therapeutic and confidential nature of your own work remains clear and the family are not confused as to the purpose of the interview. Giving testimony to such agencies should always be at their own request. In this case it may prove therapeutic (see *Case example: When to tell the story*).

Vignette 1: Complex Needs in a Displaced, Grieving Family

Alba was a high school student of 18, living in a rural area in the heart of a conflict region, the second eldest of seven children (four girls and three boys). She wanted to study medicine. Her life and health were normal, until the shelling began and her family fled to the forest, where they spent 3 months. The local police of a different ethnic origin found them and separated men from women and elderly men and sent the latter home. They got home to find their village full of army and police and themselves under siege at their home, where they were harassed and sometimes beaten. Meanwhile their invalid, pensioner father was shot in a massacre of ten men from the village. He was buried while they were under siege. I first met Alba one month after these events, living with seven family members in one room of their fire-damaged house. She was extremely sad and frightened. She was crying all the time, ruminating about her father being captured. She found everywhere frightening, and was too frightened to go to sleep, but when she did fall asleep, she woke early. She had no appetite, and a diurnal mood swing.

However, when I visited her a week later to my surprise, Alba was a great deal better, her sleep and appetite having returned to normal over the week. She informed me that she felt this was because of feeling she had someone to talk to, and who 'wanted to come and visit'. However, all the female members of the family were preoccupied with father's death, tearful in discussion of it, and in conflict over how to manage the grief. The mother and one sister no longer wanted to wear the symbolic mourning clothes and to move on. The other three sisters were wearing black mourning bands in their hair and wanted to do so for the appropriate period of a year. One of these sisters complained she was having some panic attacks. They also all felt angry and concerned about their material circumstances. They had no access to father's pension as this would have meant going to a police station run by the ethnic group in power to get new identity papers (all burnt) and identifying themselves as from a conflict area, and as members of a family that had lost a relative in a massacre. Anxiety made sleep difficult. Interestingly, the boys in the family (14, 8 and 7) appeared cheerful, busy and well, insisting they were symptom-free, although they missed their father. All the boys attended school regularly. The girls did not go, as there was no money for books. They therefore sat around at home with little to do.

We agreed to have family meetings to help them resolve their conflict about how to grieve, and relaxation therapy to provide some symptomatic relief. We did this as a group, and they practised themselves on a daily basis, mother running the group. Over the weeks there was a marked improvement in the whole family. The three girls continued to wear their mourning bands and the mother was more tolerant of this. Alba began to press me to help her get an ID card so that she could go to a nearby town, get a job and earn some money. However, the security situation deteriorated too much for this to be possible. My last visit before evacuation was distressing, as there was fighting on the nearest main road and the sound of shelling of nearby villages. We all knew that they might have to flee again in the near future.

I returned to the family 3 months later. They had spent these months internally displaced pushed from one village to another, with very little to eat. During this time the 14-year-old son, who had separated himself from the family believing he endangered them, had been killed along with another male relative. The family had returned to their home to find it completely burnt to the ground except for an outhouse. They had nothing left and were using an ammunition box as a table and sleeping under a small piece of plastic in the garden, because the outhouse attracted snakes. As previously, the healthiest members of the family appeared to be the smallest boys, who denied any symptoms except some tearfulness now and then. They appeared active and cheerful except when witnessing their mother's distress. The mother was devastated and could not stop crying. She could not sleep or eat or function and expressed suicidal ideas. Alba had moved to an aunt in a nearby town and had a number of somatic symptoms. We provided clothes and basic material equipment for the house. The mother was started on antidepressant therapy.

The family then lost contact with our service for 6 months. They had been provided with materials to build a warm room, but the aid agency had failed to realise that with no adult males left, there was no one to build it. The family therefore moved into a grim damp refugee flat in town. The mother had found the antidepressants helpful but had run out of medication. Two daughters had escaped the situation by marriage. The boys were well and attending school. The other daughters remain trapped within the prison of their mother's unremitting grief. They spent all day in the flat with their mother talking and crying. She did not wish to be left alone. They wanted to show her how much they cared for her and insisted on doing every household task, which added to her feeling of being a useless burden. We began 'family work' again: encouraging the girls to join the free local youth club and to allow the mother to re-establish her maternal role in the family, supporting her by restarting the antidepressant medication at her request, and getting in touch with the aid agency about their house.

Some Reflections on this Case.

For most families of this particular ethnic group, the immediate and respectful burial of the dead is crucial. This is followed by 7 days of visiting by friends and family, who sit all day with the bereaved and discuss the dead. These normal mourning processes had not been possible either for the father or son. It seems likely that the surprisingly sudden symptomatic relief Alba gained from my initial intervention was through my contribution to some of this normal mourning by being an outsider who visited and listened. A family approach meant that differences could be brought out in the open in a respectful way. The family also formed a natural group that could encourage and support each other in doing relaxation work. Attending to human rights concerns such as identity papers and security was also important. However, all this was undone by the second round of conflict and loss. There is something particularly devastating about loss coming again immediately after having begun to work one's way to recovery. Being made homeless and not being given support to rebuild their house has contributed to their sense of bereavement and powerlessness and prolonged the period of grief. The mother told me repeatedly that if she could start rebuilding her house, she would feel better.

Some families are strongly patriarchal. There are different coping strategies available to boys and girls. All the women in this family came across as strong and capable, but all felt that the loss, first of an invalid father, and then of the eldest boy, had destroyed the family's capacity to function at all. Much of the work with grieving female survivors has to address their insecurity and lack of confidence in their own self-worth. This family required a complex approach: participation in normal mourning; attention to basic needs; help with family communication; symptomatic relief; and help in re-establishing normal family roles and adapting to new ones in the absence of male support.

Additional Notes on Approaches to Assessing Grieving Children

I am often asked how I approach conducting an assessment with a grieving child. The following notes are drawn from 25 years of clinical experience with war-affected and displaced children:

Basic Principles

1. The assessment should be therapeutic.
2. Work with children within their surviving families if possible.
3. Give children the opportunity to talk to you on their own if they would like to do so.
4. Be well-informed – always get the 'story of what happened' from a surviving carer. If the child is unaccompanied and no one knows, go to 5.
5. *Do not* force talking but be able to listen.
6. Create situations where it is comfortable and possible to talk if desired.
7. Ask about distressing symptoms.

8. Ask about daily life problems.
9. Offer symptomatic relief.
10. Explain what you are going to do next:
    (a) See the child again – when and where.
    (b) Explain how you plan to address any problems they have raised.
11. All communication should aim to foster children's natural resilience and the resilience of the communities in which they live.

Initiating discussion with a grieving child can be very difficult. Below I describe two approaches that have worked well for me:

Family Trees: An Interviewing Approach

When dealing with familial loss, I have found the joint construction of a family tree/family network is helpful particularly when there have been multiple losses. I meet with the child (or children) and their surviving family together and ask the child to help me draw the family tree. The pace of the activity is set by the child. I start with whoever is present in the room and ask the child to tell me what their relationship to the child is. Even children as young as 3 quickly understand how the diagram works with circles for women and squares for men and how connecting lines between them work. If working with smaller children, we made add faces and decoration to enhance it.

I then ask the child: *Is anyone missing from the picture?* This allows the child to name absent family members and say as much or as little as they wish about them. I do not ask why they are not there, or what happened. On most occasions children have spontaneously identified and named dead or missing relatives (see case example below), often to the surprise of the observing surviving adults. Any further discussion is up to the child. The advantages of this systemic approach are:

1. It is a collective act: everyone joins in; everyone introduces themselves and explains their connection to others.
2. It is interesting for the children. I usually place a large piece of paper on the floor in the centre of the room and use coloured crayons.
3. Asking the children to include those who are missing or dead allows the whole family to learn what the children already know and facilitates truth telling.
4. Naming the dead allows the person to be identified and honoured. Symbolically putting a black simple line through the names gives ritual significance.
5. How much that is said about that person or what happened is up to the family. The naming opens up the possibility for story telling but does not force the issue.
6. Whatever is said about the dead is said in front of the whole family so that there is a collective narrative from which the children are not excluded.
7. The picture allows for children to identify who is the network of support around them. They can add in lines to other people, friends, and neighbours who matter to them. We then colour and strengthen these lines.
8. The picture can be kept as a basis for discussion in other sessions.

Case Example: Using Family trees to Explore Loss

Family B had lost more than 20 members – mostly female and children – in a massacre. I was asked to visit because of concerns for the mental health of the surviving children who had witnessed the attack and were all under 6. At the first session, most of the remaining extended family, including the children, had gathered to meet me in the only intact room of a house where they had taken shelter.

I already knew the outline of what had happened and used this first meeting to draw a family tree. This is particularly useful in cultures where extended family is of central importance. On this occasion the children all pointed out when I had missed a dead person, but we did not discuss the massacre. Once the genogram was done, the family told me their concerns about the children and their own fears about letting the children talk as it seemed to upset them. At this meeting I gave the simple advice about communication outlined above and arranged to meet the family regularly and to do non-directive play therapy with the children.

I continued with family meetings and play therapy over the next 6 months. During this time the oldest child (5 years) of the section of the family in which the mother had died began to tell his father fragments of what he had seen and to ask questions about his mother. The father had taken out photographs of her to show to all the children. At no point did the children tell the story to me, nor did I insist upon it, seeing my role as facilitating and supporting communication within the family. Over the following year, the children changed from tearful and withdrawn to outgoing, cheerful, communicative and energetic. They all attended the formal reburial of their family. Their father remarried and their new step-mother was well accepted. He began on the process of rebuilding his house. They remained well at follow-up, and when I visited 15 years later, all the children were in productive employment and doing well.

Using Puppets to Open Discussion with Younger Children

Puppets are a particularly useful tool with younger children as they provide an external object onto which they can project their feelings. They may not want to talk about themselves, but they may be happy to talk about the puppet. I usually carry a glove puppet in the form of a familiar non-threatening animal and hold the animal up in a gesture that can be interpreted in multiple ways.

For example, my cat puppet can cover both its eyes with its paws. I then ask:
What is the cat doing?
Crying. (I have also had children say, *playing hide-and-seek* which would suggest less distress on their part and can also be followed up with the question below).
How is she/he feeling? (I will give the cat the same gender as the child).
Very sad.

I am sorry to hear that.

Her mummy died (children often provide concrete information).

I am so sorry, poor cat; that is terrible; no wonder she is crying. (Pause to see if child wants to say more. If not continue with concrete questions.)

Is cat sleeping/does cat eat breakfast/go to school, etc.?

Note: I only *ask what and how* concrete questions focussed on the present to learn how she is feeling at present and how she is functioning. I *avoid why* questions and questions about the past as I do not want to push the child to discuss anything she does not wish too, even indirectly, although the child may spontaneously provide information as above. At the end I will ask if the cat is worried about anything or has any questions. I will make clear that anytime the cat wants to talk more about how she is feeling now, any difficulties she is having or what happened, she can do so.

References

1. Akerman R, Statham J. Childhood bereavement: a rapid literature review. London: Child Wellbeing Research Centre; 2011.
2. Bonanno GA, Brewin CR, Kaniasty K, Greca AML. Weighing the costs of disaster: consequences, risks, and resilience in individuals, families, and communities. Psychol Sci Public Interest. 2010;11(1):1–49.
3. Bonanno GA, Papa A, O'Neill K. Loss and human resilience. Appl Prev Psychol. 2001;10(3):193–206.
4. Bowlby J. The origins of attachment theory. In: A secure base. Clinical applications of attachment theory. London: Routledge; 1988. p. 20–38.
5. Bowlby J, Robertson J. A two-year old goes to hospital. Proceedings of the Royal Society of Medicine, 1953;46(6):425–27.
6. Cavallera V, Jones L, Weisbecker I, Ventevogel P. Mental health in complex emergencies. In: Kravitz A, editor. Oxford handbook of humanitarian medicine. Oxford: Oxford University Press; 2019. p. 101–32.
7. Currier JM, Neimeyer RA, Berman JS. The effectiveness of psychotherapeutic interventions for bereaved persons: a comprehensive quantitative review. Psychol Bull. 2008;134(5):648.
8. Eisenbruch M. From post-traumatic stress disorder to cultural bereavement: diagnosis of southeast Asian refugees. Soc Sci Med. 1991;33(6):673–80.
9. Ellis J, Dowrick C, Lloyd-Williams M. The long-term impact of early parental death: lessons from a narrative study. J R Soc Med. 2013;106(2):57–67.
10. Gormez V, Kılıç HN, Orengul AC, Demir MN, Demirlikan Ş, Demirbaş S, et al. Psychopathology and associated risk factors among forcibly displaced Syrian children and adolescents. J Immigr Minor Health. 2018;20(3):529–35.
11. Heeke C, Stammel N, Heinrich M, Knaevelsrud C. Conflict-related trauma and bereavement: exploring differential symptom profiles of prolonged grief and posttraumatic stress disorder. BMC Psychiatry. 2017;17(1):118.
12. Hendricks, J. H., Black, D., Kaplan, T. (2000). When father killed mother: guiding children through trauma and grief. London: Routledge.
13. Hollander T. Ambiguous loss and complicated grief: understanding the grief of parents of the disappeared in northern Uganda. J Fam Theory Rev. 2016;8(3):294–307.
14. Jones L. Adolescent groups for encamped Bosnian refugees: some problems and solutions. Clin Child Psychol Psychiatry. 1998;3(4):541–51.

15. Jones L. Then they started shooting: children of the Bosnian war and the adults they become. New York: Bellevue Literary Press; 2013.
16. Jones L, Kafetsios K. Exposure to political violence and psychological Well-being in Bosnian adolescents: a mixed method approach. Clin Child Psychol Psychiatry. 2005;10(2):157–76.
17. Kübler-Ross E. On death and dying. London: Routledge; 1973.
18. Li J, Vestergaard M, Cnattingius S, Gissler M, Bech BH, Obel C, Olsen J. Mortality after parental death in childhood: a nationwide cohort study from three Nordic countries. PLoS Med. 2014;11(7):e1001679.
19. Lundorff M, Holmgren H, Zachariae R, Farver-Vestergaard I, O'Connor M. Prevalence of prolonged grief disorder in adult bereavement: a systematic review and meta-analysis. J Affect Disord. 2017;212:138–49.
20. Nickerson A, Liddell BJ, Maccallum F, Steel Z, Silove D, Bryant RA. Posttraumatic stress disorder and prolonged grief in refugees exposed to trauma and loss. BMC Psychiatry. 2014;14:106. https://doi.org/10.1186/1471-244X-14-106.
21. Silverman PR, Worden JW. Children's reactions to the death of a parent. In Stroebe MS, Stroebe W, Hansson RO (Ed.), Handbook of bereavement: theory, research, and intervention (pp. 300–316): Cambridge: Cambridge University Press; 1993.
22. Stroebe M, Schut H, Stroebe W. Health outcomes of bereavement. Lancet. 2007;370(9603):1960–73.
23. Stroebe MS, Schut H. The dual process model of coping with bereavement: rationale and description. Death Studies. 1999;23:197–24.
24. Stroebe M, Schut H, Boerner K. Cautioning health-care professionals: bereaved persons are misguided through the stages of grief. OMEGA. 2017;74(4):455–73.
25. Stroebe M, Stroebe W, Schut H, Boerner K. Grief is not a disease but bereavement merits medical awareness. Lancet. 2017;389(10067):347–9.
26. Wahl CW. The differential diagnosis of normal and neurotic grief following bereavement. Psychosomatics. 1970;11(2):104–6.
27. World Health Organization. Guidelines for the management of conditions specifically related to stress. Geneva: WHO; 2013. http://apps.who.int/iris/bitstream/10665/85119/1/9789241505406_eng.pdf.
28. World Health Organization. International classification of diseases for mortality and morbidity statistics. 11th ed. Geneva: Author; 2018. https://icd.who.int/browse11/l-m/en#/http://id.who.int/icd/entity/1183832314.
29. World Health Organization, & United Nations High Commissioner for Refugees. Assessment and management of conditions specifically related to stress: mhGAP intervention guide module. Geneva: WHO; 2013.
30. World Health Organization, & United Nations High Commissioner for Refugees. mhGAP humanitarian intervention guide (mhGAP-HIG): clinical management of mental, neurological and substance use conditions in humanitarian emergencies. Geneva: WHO; 2015.
31. Zisook S, Iglewicz A, Avanzino J, Maglione J, Glorioso D, Zetumer S, Vahiam I, Young I, Lebowitz B, Pies R, Reynolds C, Simon NM, Shear K. Bereavement: course, consequences, and care. Curr Psychiatry Rep. 2014;16(10):482.

Intervening to Address the Impact of Stress and Trauma on Refugee Children and Adolescents Resettled in High-Income Countries

9

Cécile Rousseau and Melanie M. Gagnon

Introduction

War and displacement have always been associated with high exposure to stress and potentially traumatic events for children, youth, and their families. The characteristics of war and organized violence in the countries of origin and of transit and the multiple forms of structural violence in host societies considerably influence the refugee predicament. In the last two decades, the receiving country contexts in North America and Europe have been rapidly changing with an upsurge in xenophobia and the emergence of anti-refugee discourses [34]. This has major consequences for refugee families but also for the clinicians or community workers caring for them.

The process of legitimization or de-legitimization of refugees and migrants is not a new issue. It has always been a socio-politico-historical phenomenon, product of a specific time and space, which directly influences the ways in which refugee families and their children are represented. In the last two decades, and certainly after 9/11, as migrants and refugees were increasingly perceived as potential criminals, refugee children have become the object of growing ambivalence, as if the threatening other was overlaying the vulnerable child [21]. In the present international context, discourses of criminality and vulnerability are associated with representation of both helpless and irresponsible children, unable to have a voice of their own [24].

Negative perceptions and negative mirroring of migrants and refugees have progressively eroded the access to health, education, and other services in high-income host societies. Rights which have a universal valence are slowly replaced by ideas

C. Rousseau (✉)
Division of Social and Cultural Psychiatry, McGill University, Montreal, QC, Canada
e-mail: cecile.rousseau@mcgill.ca

M. M. Gagnon
CIUSSS West-Central Montreal, Montreal, Qc Canada, Montreal, QC, Canada
e-mail: melanie.gagnon.ccomtl@ssss.gouv.qc.ca

© Springer Nature Switzerland AG 2020
S. J. Song, P. Ventevogel (eds.), *Child, Adolescent and Family Refugee Mental Health*, https://doi.org/10.1007/978-3-030-45278-0_9

of deservingness and entitlement, which are relative and vary with time and subjects [52, 56]. Even more important than the erosion of available resources, the increase in direct and structural discrimination against refugees and the associated public representations contributes to a very insecure environment, which hinders both healing and resettlement processes [17].

In this ambivalent, and at time toxic, social environment, what can we do to protect refugee children and their families from further stress, buffer the ongoing stressors, and favor a healing environment from past trauma? This chapter addresses the exposure to stress and direct and indirect trauma of refugee children, describes the main consequences for their mental health, and delineates some perspectives to propose contextually and culturally adapted interventions.

Being Overwhelmed and Deprived: Child Exposure to Direct and Indirect Social Adversity

Armed conflicts, flight, and resettlement experiences inevitably expose refugee families to multiple forms of adversity which have a range of consequences for children. When these form of stress clearly exceeds the adaptation capacities of the child or his or her family, these may lead to the development of mental health problems and be considered as traumatic. However, what is considered traumatic vary across cultures and contexts, with some events being universally considered as potentially traumatic (rape, torture, executions), although often associated with different meanings [11]. Thus it may be more pertinent for clinicians to consider a continuum of stressful events and conditions which may have additive effects than to establish an arbitrary cutoff between diverse stressors and traumatic events. Because children are highly dependent on their families, particularly when they are very young, the assessment of stress and trauma exposure should not only consider whether they directly experienced adversity but also if they were indirectly exposed to it through their family, a process often referred to as intergenerational transmission.

Direct Exposure to Stress and Traumatic Events

Disruption of their daily environment may have a significant impact on children and youth. Partial or total interruption of schooling may be associated with under stimulation but also with the loss of a protective and child-friendly space. During armed conflict and flight, play and exploration, which are key to development, often resume in unsafe spaces in which children are at increased risk of being hurt and abused. Food deprivation is also common and can also interfere with normal physical and cognitive development [50]. For example, iron deficiency, which is frequent in refugee children and may manifest through sleepiness and learning difficulties, is often missed because the child difficulties are attributed to linguistic or familial problems.

Many children are witnesses of war and violent events in their proximal environment and the media. Witnessing family members being hurt, humiliated, or killed is very painful for children who experience not only impotence because they cannot prevent these events from happening but also a loss of trust in adults who they before considered as being able to protect them [48]. Some children are physically hurt, assaulted, or abused, although this does not always have more consequences than witnessing other loved ones being hurt.

Age and gender are major determinants of exposure to direct stress and trauma (cite). Prenatal exposure is often forgotten or minimized despite vast literature emphasizing the evidence of harm to the future child [45]. Food deprivation during pregnancy and a stressful maternal environment may affect the fetus. Extreme trauma (rape, torture) during pregnancy is relatively common, with children of rape being at higher risk since they may be seen as embodying the aggressor and may experience rejection from their mother, family, and community [22]. Other high-risk groups are adolescents and preadolescents who get affiliated with armed forces and armed groups and may be exposed to and involved in high levels or violence and sexual abuse and unaccompanied minors who travel alone and resettle without the support of their family [13].

Finally, exposure to stress and trauma is often prolonged and cumulative [15] making it difficult to disentangle the effects of trauma from the loss of a protective environment.

Intergenerational Transmission of Trauma

If the family plays a key role in enhancing or undermining the child's capacity to face stress and recover from trauma, these events may also shatter the capacity of the family to provide an optimal environment for the child. Importantly, family trauma is not automatically associated with children psychopathology [46, 51] and may actually endowing children with a mission [38]. Intergenerational transmission of trauma should thus be conceptualized as a multilevel process related to intrafamilial communication about trauma, the ways in which parent-child relation and family functioning are affected by trauma and the transformation of the family environment (Fig. 9.1).

How a family communicates about trauma can impact children. Unfiltered discourse, a situation in which parents speak in front of the child without acknowledging that (s)he can understand or be affected, has been associated with more distress in children [10]. Modulated disclosure, in which the explanations given by the parents vary with the child's age and needs, may be more protective for a child's mental health [23]. While the literature centers mainly on within family disclosure of trauma and meaning-making processes, certain authors have insisted on the idea of validation, which acknowledges that children often have more experiential knowledge than what adults think and that they require a confirmation of their intuitions and experiences [2, 4].

Trauma-related parental psychopathology (usually post-traumatic stress disorder or depression) may affect child well-being because they are distressed by their parent's anxiety, sadness, or fear of their anger [14]. Parental trauma may also affect

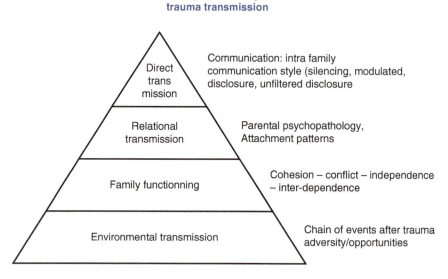

Fig. 9.1 The multiple layers of intergenerational trauma transmission

parent-child attachment since parents may be psychologically unavailable [47] or have emotional regulation problems associated with insecurity and ambivalence toward the parent.

The systemic family adaptation to trauma is not the sum of individuals consequences. Stresses and trauma may transform family functioning in different ways. Sometimes the family may internalize environmental adversity, which can exacerbate pre-existing couple and parent-child tensions [30]. In other cases, traumatic experiences may improve family relations, and family cohesion may increase to better confront to external adversities [3]. These dynamics have important consequences for children who may suffer from the conflict but also sometimes feel overprotected by parents who perceive the external world as uniformly dangerous.

Finally, the chain of negative events following trauma and exile may profoundly transform the family environment. This change may become more important for children than the traumatic events themselves. Parental changes in social status, loss of family social networks, difficulties with employment, and direct and structural discrimination may have cumulative effects to shatter the protective nature of a family [12, 16, 17].

Stress and Trauma Consequences for Children and Youth Mental Health and Development

Although the literature emphasizes the importance of the post-traumatic stress disorder (PTSD) diagnosis for refugee children [59], an approach considering the continuum of stress-related disorders and their relation to time both in the exile trajectory, and with relation to child development, may be more appropriate to guide action.

Different clinical issues are related to three moments of the resettlement process of refugee children: arrival, the first 2 years after resettlement, and long term. The NICE guidelines (2005) and subsequently the guidelines for PTSD in migrants and refugees of the Canadian Medical Association [40] emphasize a phased approach to treatment. Settlement and social issues should be at the forefront of intervention in the first phase after arrival of the refugees in a host country. All international guidelines emphasize the importance of (1) including social considerations in addressing basic needs and providing essential services and security and (2) the importance to support to families and communities in providing protective and supportive environments for children [1, 18, 54]. Specialized therapeutic intervention, if required, becomes a focus of the second phase.

Around Arrival

When arriving from refugee camps or armed conflict settings, refugee children may exhibit symptoms of acute stress (with a whole range of internalizing and externalizing symptoms) which will quite rapidly decrease in the first month if a warm and reassuring environment prevails. Normal mourning processes may also be very disruptive in the first months after arrival.

During this period, disturbing behaviors may stem from traumatic experiences or losses, but they can also reflect survival behavior.

Schools often have mixed feelings about these new students, expecting both catastrophic trauma symptoms and adaptation difficulties. In addition, the wide tendency to ignore or minimize the cognitive consequences of trauma exposure [31] frequently leads to a misinterpretation of learning difficulties. Refugee children can be diagnosed with attention deficit hyperactivity disorder (ADHD), oppositional defiant disorder (ODD), and autism spectrum disorder (ASD) and quickly prescribed psychotropic medication. During the arrival period, formal education testing may constitute a form of humiliation for children who have been under-schooled and whose cognitive capacities may still be affected by traumatic symptomatology and deprivation [58].

Because of the high risk of stigma associated with early intervention, schools and primary care health services may choose to withhold specialized mental health and education evaluations during the early resettlement period until a strong alliance with the child and his or her family is established. School teams can be trained to emphasize the restoration of safety and focus on the establishment of routines and daily rules of peaceful interactions. In the first months, academic performance should not be a priority. The focus should be on encouraging broad forms of learning and socialization. Teachers and school staff have not all chosen to work with refugee children. Influenced by media anti-refugee portrayal, they may see them as damaged children, as fraud, and/or as dangerous. Holding and appeasing their beliefs around refugee children and reframing their sense of urgency to intervene and to mobilize specialized resources may be useful steps to empower school teams, help to restore a sense of normalcy in the school environment, and decrease the risk of stigma for refugee families.

The First 2 Years: A Key Period?

A few months after arrival, the distinction between children who are re-engaging in life and learning and those who remain with difficulties is much clearer. Distinguishing stress-related symptoms from pre-existing difficulties becomes an important issue.

Both the DSM5 and the ICD11 emphasize the specificity of PTSD in children and the associated challenges in diagnosis. The DSM-5 revision of the PTSD diagnosis has incorporated a number of recommendations to draw the clinician's attention to maturational processes and their associated age-related PTSD manifestations [32]. They specify the form that the adult PTSD criteria can take in children (reenactment, nightmares without specific themes). Reckless or self-destructive behavior, frequent in adolescents, has been added as an example of the possible alterations in arousal and reactivity. Studies have shown that identifying PTSD in children aged 6 or under was difficult and that there was a need to modify the diagnosis process [44]. The alternative age-related criteria proposed in DSM5 is meant to be used only for children under 6 even if it has been shown to identify PTSD in the 7 to 10 age group better than the previous criteria [44]. This has important clinical consequences for these age groups for which the most disturbing comorbidity manifestations (concentration problems, agitation and aggressivity, acting-out behaviors) often lead to erroneous diagnosis like ADHD, ODD, or conduct disorder if the traumatic exposure is not given enough attention.

Because of the relative nonspecificity of externalizing, symptoms, when a history of traumatic events and attachment disruption is present, stress-related disorder assessment and treatment should be prioritized. Only after ruling out a stress-related disorder and/or treating them adequately, if other problems interfere with the child adaptation, should a co-morbidity be considered.

With respect to cognitive difficulties, the first 2 years constitute a key period to distinguish possible intellectual disability and language difficulties from the cognitive effects of the war context [31]. Too often, cognitive evaluation may be delayed year after year due to language proficiency, resulting in persisting impairment and eventually a chronic course of problems.

Because stress-related disorders are associated with a favorable prognosis, it is important that they can be recognized and treated in a timely fashion, in a culturally safe environment. Paying attention to the multiple manifestations of stress-related disorders (particularly externalizing symptoms) is important because they may confirm in the adult of the child new environment the circulations social representations about the dangerous/criminal refugees, and this may result in stigmatising interventions (very commonly assigning the child to a behavior and learning difficulty class). Attention to persisting problems during these 2 first years requires a prolonged joint mobilization of education and health professionals, a mobilization which may be challenging in a context of scarce health and education resources [34].

Long-Term Intervention

As life goes on, previous experiences tend to be forgotten by the school and clinical milieu. But the reactivation of trauma, separation, and other difficult relational experiences may happen at any time and can be associated with external or family triggers, or with more internal processes, like the transformations of adolescence. The literature emphasizes that the host-country practitioner has to be culturally competent [19]. Beyond cultural competence, as sensitivity to cultural and contextual differences, they also need to be aware that the families may have good historical and social reasons not to trust that country institution and thus lack cultural safety. Because of this frequent lack of cultural safety for the youth and families, and of their subsequent distrust of health personnel, the role of external social stressors, like discrimination or ostracism, tends to be missed or minimized, resulting in serious alliance problem between the families and the practitioners. Furthermore, after a few years, some persistent symptoms may not well be represented by the PTSD diagnosis. Often associated with cumulative trauma and deprivation, some children present challenges acting-out and risk-taking behaviors which may lead to a diagnosis of conduct disorder, personality disorder, or delinquency. A more applicable diagnosis for those youth may be complex post-traumatic stress disorder (CPTSD), which describes the consequences of exposure to stressors of an extreme or prolonged nature, from which escape is difficult or impossible. The symptom pattern of CPTSD is defined by re-experiencing, avoidance, emotional dysregulation, self-concept changes, and disturbances in relational functioning. Although not child-specific, this diagnosis is particularly important for refugee children and adolescents because they are very commonly exposed to chronic interpersonal trauma and deprivation, and may not have the capacity and resources needed to escape, given their situation of dependence associated with normal development. Services are often ill-equipped to respond to the need of these children who tend to receive multiple unrelated diagnoses with an emphasis on behavioral control [7, 42]. In countries with high resources, specific treatment for CPTSD may benefit children [5]. A sequenced therapy, with interventions tailored to specific symptoms set, appear to be most promising [6]. This includes emotion regulation strategies, narration of traumatic events memory, cognitive restructuring, anxiety and stress management, and interpersonal skills as first-line interventions. Importantly, this diagnostic category may play a role in promoting understanding and social support for many children who have endured chronic adversity, relational problems, or social rejection. Presently, the behaviors (and anger) of youth with CPTSD can easily be misinterpreted or seen as criminal tendencies to confirm the negative representations of refugees. These children will need firm limits, warmth, and empathy.

Assessment and Intervention

A few general principles should structure interventions to address the consequences of stress and trauma for refugee children:

- Systematic screening of children for PTSD should be avoided as there is no evidence of added benefits. Intrusive questioning may instead cause some harm. However, clinicians should remain alert if behavioral, emotional, or cognitive difficulties or unexplained medical symptoms are present and consider potential exposure to traumatic events [40].
- Family and community strategies and resources need to be identified, valued, and incorporated in the intervention plan.
- Power dynamics in the clinical context can be a significant barrier for refugee children and families. Approaches which are too directive must be used cautiously since they could suggest that families and children do not have the capacity to help or to "heal" themselves which in turn may fuel feelings of helplessness.
- An eco-systemic model which considers the whole environment of the child from the assessment to the intervention plan is to be favored [25]. In this perspective, reestablishing a protective environment and enhancing family and community resources may be more important than addressing directly symptoms.

In terms of assessment, it is important to remember that exposure to traumatic events from wars is variable. Prematurely pushing disclosure about traumatic experiences may cause harm and severe potential alliance with the child or his or her parents (Song & Ventevogel, in process). Assessment can be viewed as a process unfolding through time rather than a discrete encounter. For acute stress and cognitive difficulties, evolution of the symptoms and response to the intervention may confirm the initial hypothesis and complete the assessment.

A first level of intervention is aimed at reestablishing safety and normalcy in the child's environment. Different psychological first-aid guidelines such as the World Health Organization (WHO) psychological first-aid toolkit [55], the Save the Children Guidelines [43], or the Structure, Talking and time, Rituals, Organized play, Parents support (STROP) guidelines elaborated by the Rehabilitation and Research Centre for Torture Victims (RCT) [33] may be helpful to organize these nonspecific interventions with the community and the schools.

During this initial phase, the aim is to reestablish socialization processes, provide positive reinforcement for acquired skills, propose verbal and nonverbal expression spaces, and buffer anxiety and aggressive impulses through physical activities.

Schools are a privileged environment to support the shift from a survival predicament to normal life and should be the key actor during this first phase. Schools are highly valued by parents and children, who do not feel stigmatized by general population interventions but may resent being singled out and targeted by special interventions.

If after this first phase of resettlement symptoms or impairment persists, more specialized treatment may be warranted. Presently, there is limited evidence that medication is helpful to treat children with PTSD, and WHO clearly discourages the use of antidepressants in children with PTSD [53, 57]. It should thus not be a first choice for treatment and may be used only exceptionally if clinically justified for targeted symptoms. Different forms of psychotherapy can help children to heal

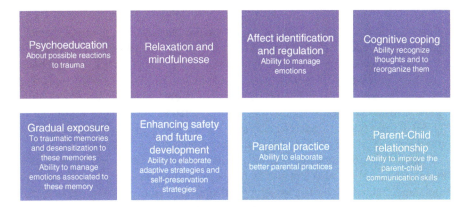

Fig. 9.2 Trauma-focused behavioral therapy main components

from trauma [20]. The choice among then should be guided by availability, cultural appropriateness, and of course parents and children preferences.

Therapeutic approaches with a focus on trauma typically focus on pre-migratory traumatic experiences. Some researchers and clinicians who advocate for these approaches suggest that post-traumatic symptoms may be addressed sooner, even if resettlement issues are not resolved [28].

Trauma-focused cognitive behavioral therapy is the most common evidence-based approach for children who display symptoms of post-traumatic stress disorder following a traumatic event (TF-CBT) [8, 9]. This approach's main components are shown below in Fig. 9.2:

Empirical findings in young refugees have confirmed its potential usefulness for this group [26, 49] as well as for children from diverse ethnocultural background who were exposed to multiple complex traumas [9].

The narrative exposure therapeutic approach [27] has been specifically designed for persons who have experienced war and torture and is also adapted to children [27]. This therapeutic approach implies the creation of a timeline representing the child's life from birth to the present, which comprises a detailed narration of traumatic events. The narrative aspect can help refugee children "heal" from the trauma by providing a collective interpretation of their experiences, by reinforcing their cultural and historical identity, by diminishing their feelings of personal responsibility, and by providing them a perspective for the future. Studies with young survivors of armed conflict and refugee children have shown significant improvement in post-traumatic stress symptoms [41]. The approach can also be used with a family focus, to support family meaning-making and overcome intergenerational transmission of trauma.

> Lin is a 7 years old boy of Chinese origin referred by the school to child-psychiatry because of isolated symptoms of elective mutism in an otherwise well-adjusted child. Family interview reveal that both parents had survived Pol Pot death camps because their parents instructed them to stop talking, in order to hide their identity. The disclosure of the family story in front of Lin, and the invitation to the parents to share some of their past with their son resulted in a rapid resolution of the symptoms.

Integrative interventions have been applied in school contexts for children and refugee youth, which combine creative therapeutic techniques (e.g., music therapy, creative games, and theater) and verbal treatment of past traumatic experiences. The school can provide an informal and non-stigmatizing context which can convince refugee children engage in therapy [49]. Art-based therapy [39] can offer a viewpoint which transcends cultural and language barriers and are nonthreatening because they do not push disclosure and are usually not considered stigmatizing expression [35–37]. All of these interventions are not to be used exclusively by psychologists and can be adapted so that other professionals from the school context can use them.

Confronted with stories of horror, it is however important to remember that a focus on trauma can also sometimes be harmful and not culturally appropriate. When undertaking supportive or structured therapies with children and families, consideration should be given to the potentially protective elements, and so working "around the trauma" rather than an approach that focuses directly on the traumatic experience can be more culturally sensitive [29]. Evidence is there to provide tools, not to replace clinical judgment.

Conclusion

In summary, the shift of our collective representations of refugee children interacts with our clinical and educational approaches. These polarized representations of the children as victims or aggressors are weaved in with our expectations about the temporal evolution and resolution of the problems. Decreasing our sense urgency around arrival, preserving an awareness of the long-term effects of their experiences on these children and youth, while being alert to the multiple impacts of the host society and international context on the safety of the resettlement process, may be helpful to balance the impact of these extreme representations.

With the increased number of displaced children and families in recent years, clinicians and community workers will meet more and more refugees. The root causes of refugee suffering are multiple and most closely related to social adversity, both in their home countries and in host societies. In addressing the mental health of refugee children and adolescents, clinicians and community workers should take an eco-systemic approach that contextualizes child distress into wider family, social, and global perspectives.

References

1. Alliance for Child Protection in Humanitarian Action. Standard 10: mental health and psychosocial distress, child protection minimum standards in humanitarian action. 3rd ed; 2019. Retrieved from Geneva.
2. Almqvist K, Källström Å, Appell P, Anderzen-Carlsson A. Mothers' opinions on being asked about exposure to intimate partner violence in child healthcare centres in Sweden. J Child Health Care. 2018;22(2):228–37.

3. Beiser M, Hou F. Mental health effects of premigration trauma and postmigration discrimination on refugee youth in Canada. J Nerv Ment Dis. 2016;204(6):464–70.
4. Björn GJ, Bodén C, Sydsjö G, Gustafsson PA. Brief family therapy for refugee children. Fam J. 2013;21(3):272–8.
5. Cloitre M, Cohen LR, Koenen KC. Treating survivors of childhood abuse: Psychotherapy for the interrupted life. New York, London: Guilford Press; 2011.
6. Cloitre M, Courtois CA, Charuvastra A, Carapezza R, Stolbach BC, Green BL. Treatment of complex PTSD: results of the ISTSS expert clinician survey on best practices. J Trauma Stress. 2011;24(6):615–27.
7. Cloitre M, Stolbach BC, Herman JL, van der Kolk B, Pynoos R, Wang J, Petkova E. A developmental approach to complex PTSD: childhood and adult cumulative trauma as predictors of symptom complexity. J Trauma Stress. 2009;22(5):399–408.
8. Cohen JA, Mannarino AP, Deblinger E. Treating trauma and traumatic grief in children and adolescents. New York, United States: Guilford; 2016.
9. Cohen JA, Mannarino AP, Kliethermes M, Murray LA. Trauma-focused CBT for youth with complex trauma. Child Abuse Negl. 2012;36(6):528–41.
10. Dalgaard NT, Montgomery E. Disclosure and silencing: a systematic review of the literature on patterns of trauma communication in refugee families. Transcult Psychiatry. 2015;52(5):579–93.
11. De Haene L, Rousseau C, Kevers R, Deruddere N, Rober P. Stories of trauma in family therapy with refugees: supporting safe relational spaces of narration and silence. Clin Child Psychol Psychiatry. 2018;23(2):258–78.
12. DeJong J, Sbeity F, Schlecht J, Harfouche M, Yamout R, Fouad FM, et al. Young lives disrupted: gender and well-being among adolescent Syrian refugees in Lebanon. Confl Heal. 2017;11(1):23.
13. Derluyn I, Vandenhole W, Parmentier S, Mels C. Victims and/or perpetrators? Towards an interdisciplinary dialogue on child soldiers. BMC Int Health Hum Rights. 2015;15(1):28.
14. Eruyar S, Maltby J, Vostanis P. Mental health problems of Syrian refugee children: the role of parental factors. Eur Child Adolesc Psychiatry. 2018;27(4):401–9.
15. Fazel M, Reed RV, Panter-Brick C, Stein A. Mental health of displaced and refugee children resettled in high-income countries: risk and protective factors. Lancet. 2012;379(9812):266–82.
16. Goosen S, Stronks K, Kunst AE. Frequent relocations between asylum-seeker centres are associated with mental distress in asylum-seeking children: a longitudinal medical record study. Int J Epidemiol. 2013;43(1):94–104.
17. Hynie M. The social determinants of refugee mental health in the post-migration context: a critical review. Can J Psychiatry. 2017;63:297–303.
18. Inter-Agency Standing Committee. IASC guidelines on mental health and psychosocial support in emergency settings. IASC: Geneva; 2007.
19. Kirmayer LJ, Guzder J, Rousseau C. In: Rousseau KG, editor. Cultural consultation encountering the other in mental health care. New York: Springer; 2014.
20. Kronick R. Mental health of refugees and asylum seekers: assessment and intervention. Can J Psychiatry. 2018;63(5):290–6.
21. Kronick R, Rousseau C. Rights, compassion and invisible children: a critical discourse analysis of the parliamentary debates on the mandatory detention of migrant children in Canada. J Refug Stud. 2015;28(4):544–69. https://doi.org/10.1093/jrs/fev005.
22. Marotte C, Rousseau C. Éclaboussures traumatiques et regards sur la filiation: les enfants nés du viol. In: Baubet T, Lachal C, Moro M-R, editors. *Bébés et traumas*: Éd. La pensée sauvage; 2006.
23. Measham T, Rousseau C. Family disclosure of war trauma to children. Traumatology. 2010;16(2):14–25.
24. Meloni F, Rousseau C, Montgomery C, Measham T. Children of exception: redefining categories of illegality and citizenship in Canada. Child Soc. 2013;28:305–15. https://doi.org/10.1111/chso.12006.

25. Miller KE, Rasmussen A. War exposure, daily stressors, and mental health in conflict and post-conflict settings: bridging the divide between trauma-focused and psychosocial frameworks. Soc Sci Med. 2010;70(1):7–16.

26. Murray LK, Cohen JA, Ellis BH, Mannarino AP. Cognitive behavioral therapy for symptoms of trauma and traumatic grief in refugee youth. Child Adolesc Psychiatr Clin N Am. 2008;17:585–604.

27. Neuner F, Catani C, Ruf M, Schauer E, Schauer M, Elbert T. Narrative exposure therapy for the treatment of traumatized children and adolescents (KidNET): from neurocognitive theory to field intervention. Child Adolesc Psychiatr Clin N Am. 2008;17:641–64.

28. Nickerson A, Steel Z, Bryant R, Brooks R, Silove D. Change in visa status amongst Mandaean refugees: relationship to psychological symptoms and living difficulties. J Psychiatry Res. 2011;187(1–2):267–74. https://doi.org/10.1016/j.psychres.2010.12.015.

29. Pacione L, Measham T, Rousseau C. Refugee children: mental health and effective interventions. Curr Psychiatry Rep. 2013;15(2):1–9.

30. Panter-Brick C, Grimon MP, Eggerman M. Caregiver—child mental health: a prospective study in conflict and refugee settings. J Child Psychol Psychiatry. 2014;55(4):313–27.

31. Pechtel P, Pizzagalli DA. Effects of early life stress on cognitive and affective function: an integrated review of human literature. Psychopharmacology. 2011;214(1):55–70.

32. Pynoos RS, Steinberg AM, Layne CM, Briggs EC, Ostrowski SA, Fairbank JA. DSM-V PTSD diagnostic criteria for children and adolescents: a developmental perspective and recommendations. J Trauma Stress. 2009;22(5):391–8.

33. Rehabilitation and Research Centre for Torture Victims (RCT). RCT field manual on rehabilitation. Copenhagen: Rehabilitation and Research Centre for Torture Victims; 2007.

34. Rousseau C. Addressing mental health needs of refugees. Can J Psychiatry. 2018;63(5):287–9.

35. Rousseau C, Beauregard C, Daignault K, Petrakos H, Thombs BD, Steele R, et al. A cluster randomized-controlled trial of a classroom-based drama workshop program to improve mental health outcomes among immigrant and refugee youth in special classes. PLoS One. 2014;9(8):e104704.

36. Rousseau C, Benoit M, Lacroix L, Gauthier M-F. Evaluation of a sandplay program for preschoolers in a multiethnic neighborhood. J Child Psychol Psychiatry. 2009;50(6):743–50. https://doi.org/10.1111/j.1469-7610.2008.02003x.

37. Rousseau C, Drapeau A, Lacroix L, Bagilishya D, Heusch N. Evaluation of a classroom program of creative expression workshops for refugee and immigrant children. J Child Psychol Psychiatry. 2005;46(2):180–5.

38. Rousseau C, Drapeau A, Rahimi S. The complexity of trauma response: a 4-year follow-up of adolescent Cambodian refugees. Child Abuse Negl. 2003;27(11):1277–90. https://doi.org/10.1016/j.chiabu.2003.07.001.

39. Rousseau C, Guzder J. School-based prevention programs for refugee children. Child Adolesc Psychiatr Clin N Am. 2008;17(3):533–49.

40. Rousseau C, Pottie K, Thombs B, Munoz M, Jurcki T. Post traumatic stress disorder: evidence review for newly arriving immigrants and refugees. Can Med Assoc J. 2011; www.cmaj.ca/lookup/suppl/doi:10.1503/cmaj.090313/-/DC1.

41. Ruf M, Schauer M, Neuner F, Catani C, Schauer E, Elbert T. Narrative exposure therapy for 7-to 16-year-olds: a randomized controlled trial with traumatized refugee children. J Trauma Stress. 2010;23(4):437–45.

42. Sar V. Developmental trauma, complex PTSD, and the current proposal of DSM-5. Eur J Psychotraumatol. 2011;2

43. Save the Children. (2013). Psychological first aid training - manual for child practitioners. Retrieved from https://resourcecentre.savethechildren.net/node/7838/pdf/final_pfa.pdf

44. Scheeringa MS, Zeanah CH, Cohen JA. PTSD in children and adolescents: toward an empirically based algorithm. Depress Anxiety. 2011;28(9):770–82.

45. Schwerdtfeger KL, Goff BSN. Intergenerational transmission of trauma: exploring mother–infant prenatal attachment. J Trauma Stress. 2007;20(1):39–51.

46. Sigal JJ. Long-term effects of the holocaust: empirical evidence for resilience in the first, second, and third generation. Psychoanal Rev. 1998;85(4):579–85.
47. Sigal JJ, Perry C, Robbins JM, Gagné M-A, Nassif E. Maternal preoccupation and parenting as predictors of emotional and behavioral problems in children of women with breast cancer. J Clin Oncol. 2003;21(6):1155–60.
48. Terr LC. Childhood traumas: an outline and overview. Am J Psychiatr. 1991;148:10–21.
49. Tyrer RA, Fazel M. School and community-based interventions for refugee and asylum seeking children: a systematic review. PLoS One. 2014;9(2):e89359.
50. UNHCR. Global Report 2016. Retrieved from Genev. 2017.
51. van Ee E, Kleber RJ, Jongmans MJ, Mooren TT, Out D. Parental PTSD, adverse parenting and child attachment in a refugee sample. Attach Hum Dev. 2016;18(3):273–91.
52. Vanthuyne K, Meloni F, Ruiz-Casares M, Rousseau C, Ricard-Guay A. Health workers perceptions of access to care for children and pregnant women with precarious immigration status: health as a right or privilege? Soc Sci Med. 2013;93:78–85. https://doi.org/10.1016/j.socscimed.2013.1006.1008.
53. Ventevogel, P., & de Jong, J. T. V. M. Depression and anxiety in refugee children. In S. Song & P. Ventevogel (Eds.), *Child, Adolescent and Family Refugee Mental Health. A Global Perspective*. 2020; Cham: springer. (this volume).
54. Ventevogel, P., Schinina, G., Strang, A., Gagliato, M., & Hansen, L. J. *Mental Health and Psychosocial Support for Refugees, Asylum Seekers and Migrants on the Move in Europe: a multi-agency guidance note*. www.mhpss.net: Antares Foundation, Care International. Church of Sweden, Psychosocial Centre of the International Federation of the Red Cross and Red Crescent Societies, International Medical Corps. International Organisation for Migration, Medecins du Monde, MHPSS.net, Psychosocial Services and Training Institute Cairo, Save the Children, Destinatin Unknown, Terre des Hommes, United nations High Commissioner for Refugees, UNICEF, Un Ponte Per., War Child Holland, War Trauma Foundation, World Health Organisation Regional Office for Europe, International Rescue Committee, World Vision International. 2015.
55. WHO. Risks to mental health: an overview of vulnerabilities and risks factors. Background paper by WHO secretariat for the development of a comprehensive mental health action plan. Retrieved from Geneva, Switzerland. 2012.
56. Willen SS. Do "illegal" Im/migrants have a right to health? Engaging ethical theory as social practice at a Tel Aviv open clinic. Med Anthropol Q. 2011;25(3):303–30.
57. World Health Organization. Guidelines for the Management of Conditions Specifically Related to stress. Geneva: WHO; 2013. http://apps.who.int/iris/bitstream/10665/85119/1/9789241505406_eng.pdf
58. Yasik AE, Saigh PA, Oberfield RA, Halamandaris PV. Posttraumatic stress disorder: memory and learning performance in children and adolescents. Biol Psychiatry. 2007;61(3):382–8.
59. Yule W, Williams RM. Post-traumatic stress reactions in children. J Trauma Stress. 1990;3(2):279–95.

Depression and Anxiety in Refugee Children

10

Peter Ventevogel and Joop T. V. M. de Jong

Introduction

Depression and anxiety disorders are characterized by persistent emotional disturbances such as worrying, fear, anxiety, and unhappiness. In adults, the hallmark of
depression is a pattern of excessive and persistent inner sadness paired with an
inability to experience pleasure that is not or only partially responsive to changes in
the immediate context, such as involvement in activities that are usually pleasurable, attention from loved ones, or finishing tasks. In younger children, however,
depression may manifest primarily through somatic symptoms and irritability [56].
Anxiety disorders are characterized by a pattern of anxious emotions that are excessive in intensity, duration, or appropriateness to context. The term "emotional disorders" is often used in children because of the overlap in symptoms. The most
commonly seen emotional problems in refugee children are depression, separation
anxiety, social phobia, and generalized anxiety. Emotional disorders are often
accompanied by avoidance and behavioral withdrawal. It is not the intention of this
chapter to give an extensive overview of the diagnostic criteria for emotional disorders as these can be found in the International Classification of Diseases [73] or the
Diagnostic and Statistical Manual [1]. Neither will we exhaustively discuss extant
treatment protocols [15, 48, 71, 74]. Rather, the chapter focuses on salient aspects
of emotional disorders in refugee children, particularly those aspects that have relevance for the identification and management of such conditions in refugee

P. Ventevogel (✉)
Public Health Section (Division of Resilience and Solutions), United Nations High
Commissioner for Refugees, Geneva, Switzerland
e-mail: ventevog@unhcr.org

J. T. V. M. de Jong
Cultural Psychiatry and Global Mental Health, Amsterdam UMC,
Amsterdam, The Netherlands

Boston University School of Medicine, Boston, MA, USA

© Springer Nature Switzerland AG 2020
S. J. Song, P. Ventevogel (eds.), *Child, Adolescent and Family Refugee Mental
Health*, https://doi.org/10.1007/978-3-030-45278-0_10

children. The main reason to discuss conditions related to depression and anxiety in one chapter is the large overlap in symptoms, leading to high level of "comorbidity" [24] particularly in children seen in primary care [37]. Moreover, the subdivision of syndromes may be artificial, with the concept of separate disorder categories potentially being flawed [10]. In child psychiatry, depressive and anxious symptoms are often grouped together as "internalizing symptoms," more common among girls. Boys may more often display externalizing symptoms, reflected in reckless, risk-taking, or antisocial behavior. Examples of problems on the internalizing spectrum include anxiety, depression, avoidance, separation anxiety, and enuresis. In preadolescent children, anxiety may be more commonly recognized than depression. This pattern reverses in adolescents where sizeable numbers of children develop depressive symptoms, which fuels the hypothesis that anxiety problems in younger children can develop into depressive disorders during adolescence.

Types of Emotional Disorders in Children

Depression

Most children have short periods of feeling sad and unhappy This is norrmal, but when these states become prolonged or are very intense, it may be appropriate to consider the diagnosis of depressive disorder [19]. The core signs of depressive disorder include persistent feelings of sadness or hopelessness and the inability to enjoy things that were previously pleasurable (anhedonia). However, in children, depression symptoms may be expressed differently than in adults. Younger children may not have anhedonia, and do not necessarily have sadness all the time. Additional symptoms may include a lack of energy, wish to be dead, sleep problems, feeling constantly bored, and diminished appetite. Younger children are often not able to verbalize their feelings, and diagnosis will be informed by behavioral observations and collateral information. In children, depressive states may manifest primarily through irritability, anger, aggressive behavior, being easily upset, and have a reluctance to go to school or social situations [56]. In adolescents, depression may be characterized by hopelessness, social withdrawal, and thoughts about death and suicide, which can lead to abuse of alcohol and drugs, involvement in self-destructive behavior, truancy, and running away from home. Many children may, at one period or another, have transient symptoms, often related to changes in their life situation or as part of their development. It is therefore important to assess if there is a *persistent pattern* of such symptoms and to weigh in whether the symptoms can be directly attributed to an identifiable stressor such as the death, absence, or sickness of a caregiver or sibling, or in the context of major changes in life circumstances such as going to a new school, migration, or other stress factors. It may also be relevant to ask caregivers about the child's prior level of functioning and symptoms. Bedwetting or speech problems may be related to a child's regression to an earlier developmental level.

Separation Anxiety

Normal childhood development includes a phase in which the young child (usually between 18 months and 4 years) experiences significant anxiety when the primary caretaker leaves temporarily. There are significant cultural differences here, based on the way child care/parenting is organized – in extended families where elder siblings, aunts, grandmothers, and others play major roles in child rearing, separation of the mother or father will often be less manifest, while it may be stronger in children who are raised by single parents or in nuclear families without much social support. In general, separation anxiety in children under 4 years is considered normal unless the child is seriously and consistently troubled when the primary caretaker leaves. If strong separation anxiety occurs in children older than 4 years, there may be a reason for clinical concern, particularly when the child refuses to go to school, develops persistent worries about danger that may happen to the absent caretaker, or refuses to sleep without the mother. Children may not always be able to verbalize their feelings but may develop stomachaches, headaches, or other physical symptoms. Separation anxiety disorder is the most common childhood anxiety disorder.

Social Phobia and Excessive Shyness

One speaks of social phobia when children are extremely uncomfortable in social situations, such as in school, or when the child has the feeling of being looked at or been asked to talk. This could lead to being "socially mute" ("selective mutism") in more extreme cases when a child talks normally within the household but not in other social situations.

Generalized Anxiety Disorder

The key feature of generalized anxiety is excessive and uncontrollable worry. This could include worry about personal safety and that of family members, things that may go wrong, and in particular, worry that the child may be doing things wrong. These are the same concerns that any child may worry about, but children with generalized anxiety disorder do so in excess, leading to problems in social functioning and/or great intrapersonal suffering. Generalized anxiety disorder has many commonalities with depression. Often, children present physical symptoms such as muscular tension, headaches, palpitations, tears, and stomach upset. Generalized anxiety disorder is relatively common particularly among school children and adolescents. It often starts gradually with symptoms worsening in stressful periods.

Prevalence

Globally, the point prevalence of depressive disorders in children is thought to be around 1–2% in preadolescent children and 3–8% in adolescents [7]. Globally, the 6–12-month prevalence of anxiety disorders in children ranges from 2% to 24%, with the caveat that the distinction between normal and pathological anxiety is often not clear cut [53] and shows major variations across cultural contexts [3]. In the normal emotional development of children, fears and anxieties are typical age-bound phenomena that do not necessarily represent psychopathology. Infants and toddlers are fearful of immediate, concrete environmental threats, but when children become older, their fears will incorporate potential future events and stimuli of a more imaginary or abstract kind [5]. Symptoms may become full-blown anxiety disorders if they become persistent, are exaggerated given the context, or occur beyond normal developmental trends. While there are universalities across cultural contexts, there is also significant cross-cultural variability in the expression of anxiety symptoms with individuals from "non-Western" societies often presenting more or less cultural specific constellations of somatic symptoms as a key aspects of pathological worry and depressed emotional states [35, 38].

Research with refugee children finds the prevalence of emotional disorders to be generally higher than in non-refugee children with up to 30% of resettled children suffering from depression [8]. The higher prevalence of emotional disorders in refugee children is linked to increased occurrence of risk factors for these disorders such as adverse experiences (including loss of or separation from parents and violent experiences) and to anxiety/depression in parents [5, 7]. Frequently occurring risk factors for refugee children include experience of extreme stress during the flight and re-exposure to stressful events after the flight. However, predictors of depressive and anxiety or other internalizing problems go far beyond the traumatic events of the past and are significantly influenced by factors in the current or more recent social context, such as having a stressful life in exile, low family cohesion, low parental support, absence of parents, feeling discriminated or marginalized, loss of supportive social structures in the community, financial hardships, repeated migration in the host country, poor accommodation, and challenges in accessing legal, health, and social services [23, 43, 55]. The detrimental effects of parental mental health problems on the mental health of their children has not been well researched, but there is growing evidence that these effects are significant [21, 41, 49].

Cultural Aspects of Emotional Disorders

Terms related to emotions can be confusing in psychiatric assessment with refugee children and adolescents, even when using interpreters. It is important to realize this when working with refugee children and adolescents.

Emotional Terminology

In the English language, a distinction is often made between fear as a reaction to a current threat that is perceived as more or less imminent, leading to an alarm reaction, and anxiety as a future-oriented emotion characterized by an elevated level of apprehension and lack of control [70]. However, this distinction is not easy to capture in languages with a different emotional lexicon. For example, during our own research with war-affected children in Burundi, we faced considerable challenges in the translation of research questionnaires on anxiety disorders into Kirundi, the national language that has a complicated vocabulary for emotional concepts. Terms such as "panic," "anxiety," and "fear" could not be easily differentiated in Kirundi [66]. After a careful translation and validation of the instruments [69], we had to make again many minor changes in the wording of the instruments in another study [12] in a different part of the country, likely due to variations in dialect and with change of language over time.

Cultural Idioms of Distress

Definitions of mental disorders are strongly connected to the ways people view the world and how they conceptualize personhood [36]. This leads to important variations in how people express that they are unhappy and distressed, for example, by using "cultural idioms of distress": common modes of expressing distress within a culture or community. Such cultural idioms link bodily distress and patterned dissociative behavior with social and psychological factors, and as such are important markers of depression and anxiety [34]. We illustrate this with a few examples of large refugee groups currently in the world: Rohingya (1.1 million), Syrians (6.7 million), and Afghans (2.7 million).

Rohingya refugees in Bangladesh and Malaysia most commonly use the term *waushanti* (or ashanti/oshanti) to indicate they are feeling emotionally not well. The term literally means "lack of peace" and is often translated as "sad" or "restless" but can refer to a variety of emotional states such as feeling stressed, grieving, and other forms of emotional pain [64]. When digging deeper in the language, there are Rohingya words that denote some aspects of depression such as *monmora* or *cinta lager* (feeling sad), *mon horaf lager* or *dil hous kous lager* (feeling low mood), and *chhoit lager* (not feeling well, losing interest in things, and restless mind). Most commonly, however, the experience of depression is expressed with terms such as *gaa cisciyaar* or *gaa bish lager* (pain in the body) and *gaa zoler* or *gaa furer* (burning sensation in the body) or *unniyashi lager* (feeling of suffocation) [64]. Similarly, Syrian Arabic has a range of idioms to indicate general distress ("heaviness in the heart, cramps in the guts" and other complaints); one idiom is *habit qalbi*, "failing or crumbling of the heart," which is linked to the physical sensations related to sudden fear. The syndrome *halat ikti'ab* resembles depression with concepts such as brooding, darkening of mood, aches, and a gloomy outlook and may be accompanied by a variety of medically unexplained somatic symptoms and fatigue, as well as signs of social isolation and avoiding to engage on conversations. Expressions often used by Syrian refugees to express helplessness are *mafi natija*, "there is no use," and *hasis hali mashlol*, "I feel like I'm paralyzed [28]. Among Afghans in Kabul, various idioms were identified such as *jigar khun* "bloody liver," occurring when a person has experienced painful event or chronic stress; *asabi* "being nervous"; and *fishar*, the feeling of emotional pressure and/or agitation, or conversely, of very low energy and motivation [42, 50]; while among Pashto speakers in Nangarhar, common idioms were *was-wasi* (constant worry, thinking a lot, social isolation, and repetitive actions), *wahmi,* (unreasonable fear, easily being frightened, and frightening dreams), and *peyran,* being possessed by spirits with pseudo seizures and a variety of somatic complaints [68].

Although these idioms of distress have not been as widely explored among refugee children, practitioners should be mindful that children are socialized in these idioms for expressing distress. It is not realistic for mental health practitioners to familiarize themselves in-depth with all languages and idioms of distress of refugees, but it is important to realize the quandaries of translation of emotional terms, the application of diagnoses, and the use of diagnostic and research instruments across cultures. It can help to ask interpreters to translate as literally as possible, and to consult overviews on cultural aspects of mental health of specific refugee groups such as the ones we mentioned for Syrian refugees [28] and Rohingya refugees [64], or the overview for Somali refugees [11].

Expression of Emotions and Cultural Norms

There are important normative differences between cultural contexts about how a child or young person should behave and should express their feelings. For example, in some cultures, children are discouraged to express negative emotional states such as anger or sadness in public, while on others the expression of negative emotions is more accepted. There are also often gendered patterns of what is perceived as normal. What in one culture may be seen as excessively shy can be perceived as perfectly normal in other cultures. Similarly, what in one cultural context can be seen as verbally aggressive and demanding behavior can be seen in another culture as within the normal border/population or individual norm. This is relevant for work with refugee children and emphasizes the need to put symptoms and behavior in context during assessment.

Assessment for Emotional Disorders in Refugee Children

Assessment of children for depression and anxiety disorders follows the general assessment principles described elsewhere in this volume (Chaps. 5 and 6, [61]). For children under 12 years, an assessment of the child should routinely be accompanied by parental assessment. Since many young children do not verbalize their emotional states, clinicians can inquire about sleep disturbances since this is almost always present in kids with anxiety [56]. Sleep disturbances are both manifestations of depression and anxiety, as well as perpetuating factors that maintain or worsen emotional health [13]. Since sleep disruptions may be a core feature of childhood anxiety disorders, children and caretakers may find it easier to discuss a child's sleep disruptions than to directly verbalize mood states.

In settings where screening tools are routinely being used as part of the assessment process, they can be applied for refugee children, but with certain caveats, such as ensuring that the child has sufficient understanding of the language in which the screener is offered and that the child realizes the purpose of the questionnaire. Refugee children may be unfamiliar with the use of such tools and could perceive it as an academic test or something they should perform well on. Culturally and linguistically adapted versions of screening tools should be used if available [4].

As with other mental health conditions, it is important to use various sources of information when assessing a child with a potential emotional disorder. Sources could include (1) observations by the caregivers or others such as teachers, social workers, etc., (2) complaints as expressed by the child, and (3) clinical observations made during the interview. An assessment should not narrowly focus on the symptoms that are brought forward (such as emotional symptoms and social functioning) but also touch upon potential comorbid issues such as substance use problems, self-harm, and suicidality and on issues around coping with difficulties.

Management of Emotional Disorders in Refugee Children and Adolescents

General Management Principles

Feeling irritable, helpless at times, fearful, and worried about one's future are all common experiences for refugee children and do not necessarily constitute a psychiatric disorder. However, interventions should be considered for those who have more severe symptoms that affect their ability to function socially and academically, leaving them to suffer in silence. On the one hand, rates of emotional disorders in children globally are rising, possibly caused by more attention to child problems or a trend to label behavioral variations as psychiatric diagnoses. On the other hand, the vast majority of children with mental health disorders do not receive any treatment while they could benefit from it [25]. Refugee children tend to have a much lower mental health care utilization and are therefore even more severely undertreated. This is a concern, as mood disorders remain a leading cause of adolescent suicide. A staged approach to mental health problems would take a life course and preventative approach to identifying symptoms that have potential to worsen [52]. A multilayered public health or "stepped care" approach to mental health care is necessary for refugee children; for those with mild depressive and anxiety symptoms, strengthened family and community support may be enough to assist the child. Moderate symptoms may require targeted psychological interventions, and severe symptoms that affect child functioning may require psychotropic medications [29, 67].

Mental health workers involved in the treatment of children or adolescents with emotional disorders should take time to build supportive and collaborative relationships with the child and the family or carers. Treatment should start with an explanation of the mental health care provider about the diagnosis. Such psychoeducation should target both the child and the caregivers and use appropriate language. Refugee children and families may have very different understanding of concepts such as "depression," "anxiety disorder," and "mental illness." Therefore, a clear explanation of the signs and symptoms of a depression/anxiety disorder is important – using careful language and where appropriate, referring to cultural idioms of distress, expected course of the illness, and the impact on different areas of social functioning, such as at school, at home, or with peers. It is essential to take sufficient time and to check whether child and caregiver understand and accept the diagnosis. If appropriate, such information can be given in group format, through group psychoeducation sessions or peer support groups.

It is important to provide general information about the benefits of regular exercise on emotional disorders, encourage the child to follow a structured and supervised exercise program where possible, and provide information about sleep hygiene [48]. A variety of interventions exist that are aimed at the promotion of emotional and social well-being of the child. These interventions are often multimodal, integrating a psychomotor component with play, games, and a broad range of artistic expressions. TeamUp is an example, helping refugee children to deal with anger and stress and interact respectfully with peers. It is active in the Netherlands, Uganda, Colombia, and the occupied Palestinian territory (oPt) (cf www.warchildholland.org). Another more recent and population wide initiative aims at interventions that strengthen resiliency and prevent the development of mental illness among refugee youth. Several of these interventions are based on principles of positive psychology and are less explicitly dealing with emotional disorders. These initiatives often use task sharing and task shifting to primary care professionals or lay people in the community.

Psychotherapeutic Interventions

The preferred treatment for emotional disorders are structured evidence-based psychotherapies such as cognitive behavioral therapy (CBT) and interpersonal therapy (IPT) [7, 53]. A major challenge is to adapt these methods to make them appropriate for age and cultural background [6, 47]. The theory underpinning cognitive behavioral therapies poses that cognitive distortions and behavioral or emotional avoidance are causing or sustaining the problem. CBT treatment focuses on changing cognitions, aiming to substitute negatively laden cognitions with neutral, realistic thoughts and on helping children overcome avoidance by confronting feared situations or thoughts and behavioral activation. Newer waves of CBT often incorporate elements of acceptance and commitment therapy and mindfulness techniques [62]. There is some evidence that involving parents in CBT sessions is effective [30]. CBT can also be used in school-based group interventions. Studies into the effects of such interventions are inconclusive [51, 65]. More specific studies are required to better understand what works and in which context. In settings with limited human resources, there have been successful research trials in which nonspecialized workers are trained and intensively supervised to provide CBT [45, 46], but there is a great need for more research in the provision of CBT-based interventions with refugees in low- and middle-income countries and how this can be integrated in routine systems of care. The World Health Organization (WHO) has developed the Early Adolescent Skills for Emotions (EASE) psychological intervention for young adolescents with internalizing problems. EASE is group-based (seven sessions for adolescents and three sessions for their caregivers) and can also be delivered by nonspecialist providers. It is currently tested in a trial in Lebanon and one in Jordan [9, 32, 58].

Family Interventions and Parenting Skills

In times of armed conflict, families are the most important source of resilience to come to terms with distress, adverse events, and secondary adversities [17]. The family may serve as a protective context for processing the consequences of adverse events and providing a safe place [44, 60]. Forced displacement can undermine attachment and family relations, while cohesive families ensure that children have access to both emotional support, individuality, and privacy [39]. Over the last years, parenting and school-based interventions for conflict-affected populations have become increasingly popular. Parenting-based interventions for refugee children aim to support parents to provide a social environment with structure, security, and emotional warmth and to provide a safe space that enables a child to come to terms with what has happened in the past. Longitudinal studies show that effective parenting practices provide a protective environment for their children. When parents are able to monitor their children, set limits, encourage development of skills and problem-solving, and in general transfer a positive outlook on life, their children are more likely to show resilience after violence and forced displacement [27]. Several promising studies among refugees and other war-affected populations show how parenting interventions can lead to reduction of harsh punishment practices, improved family dynamics and better child well-being [14, 33, 54, 59], but more evidence is needed to understand to what extent these effects are sustained over time and do in fact lead to improvements in mental health outcomes of the children and can be used successfully in routine care settings.

It is good practice to involve the family in the treatment of younger children. For adolescents this is more complicated. Research with involvement of families in the treatment of depressed persons shows promising results in terms of improved functioning of the depressed person and well-being of family members, but there is limited evidence on how to do this with adolescents [16, 31]. As far as we know, there is no rigorous research on the effects of parental involvement in the management of emotional disorders in refugee children or adolescents [2].

Medication for Emotional Disorders

For those refugee youth with serious depressive or anxious symptoms that are affecting their social and academic functioning, psychiatric medications may be warranted, though the use of antidepressant medication such as selective serotine reuptake inhibitors has been controversial. In 2004, the American Food and Drug Administration issued a "black box warning" on the safety and efficacy of antidepressants for children and adolescents. The World Health Organization advises not to use antidepressant medication in children under 12 years and cautions risk of increased suicidality [72]. The recent NICE guidelines use a minimum age of 8 years for the use of fluoxetine which is currently the only antidepressant registered for use in children between 8 and 12 years [48]. The choice to use medication for emotional disorders in children should only be taken after careful considerations of risks and benefits, discussion with the child and caregivers, and only in more severe cases and preferably in combination with psychotherapy and or family interventions [18, 40].

School-Based Interventions

There is surprisingly limited evidence on the effectiveness of school-based interventions for refugee or other war-affected children [63]. There is some evidence for the use of creative expressive techniques [57] or simplified CBT [26], but more research is needed in order to evaluate effectiveness. Another way of involving schools in mental health treatment of refugee children and adolescents is by training teachers or social workers to identify and refer children who likely have emotional disorders [20, 22].

Conclusion

Emotional disorders in refugee children are serious and are undertreated problems that warrant more attention. Child mental health professionals have much to offer these children, as long as they make serious attempts to understand the perspectives of refugee children and their families, and when they can combine individual approaches with family- and community-oriented methods.

References

1. American Psychiatric Association. Diagnostic and statistical manual of mental disorders. 5th ed. Washington, DC: Author; 2013.
2. Ballard J, Wieling E, Forgatch M. Feasibility of implementation of a parenting intervention with Karen refugees resettled from Burma. J Marital Fam Ther. 2018;44:220–34.
3. Baxter AJ, Scott KM, Vos T, Whiteford HA. Global prevalence of anxiety disorders: a systematic review and meta-regression. Psychol Med. 2013;43(5):897–910.

4. Bean T, Derluyn I, Eurelings-Bontekoe E, Broekaert E, Spinhoven P. Validation of the multiple language versions of the Hopkins symptom Checklist-37 for refugee adolescents. Adolescence. 2007;42(165):51–71. Retrieved from http://www.ncbi.nlm.nih.gov/pubmed/17536475.

5. Beesdo-Baum K, Knappe S. Developmental epidemiology of anxiety disorders. Child Adolesc Psychiatr Clin N Am. 2012;21(3):457–78.

6. Bernal G, Jiménez-Chafey MI, Domenech Rodríguez MM. Cultural adaptation of treatments: a resource for considering culture in evidence-based practice. Prof Psychol Res Pract. 2009;40(4):361–8.

7. Brent D, Maalouf F. Depressive disorders in childhood and adolescence. In: Thapar A, Pine DS, Leckman JF, Scott S, Snowling MJ, Taylor E, editors. Rutter's child and adolescent Psychiatyry. Chichester: Wiley; 2015. p. 874–92.

8. Bronstein I, Montgomery P. Psychological distress in refugee children: a systematic review. Clin Child Fam Psychol Rev. 2011;14(1):44–56. https://doi.org/10.1007/s10567-010-0081-0.

9. Brown FL, Steen F, Taha K, Aoun M, Bryant RA, Jordans MJ, Ghatasheh M. Early adolescent skills for emotions (EASE) intervention for the treatment of psychological distress in adolescents: study protocol for randomised controlled trials in Lebanon. Trials. 2019;20:545.

10. Caron C, Rutter M. Comorbidity in child psychopathology: concepts, issues and research strategies. J Child Psychol Psychiatry. 1991;32(7):1063–80.

11. Cavallera V, Reggi M, Abdi S, Jinnah Z, Kivelenge J, Warsame AM, et al. *Culture, context and mental health of Somali refugees: a primer for staff working in mental health and psychosocial support programmes*. Geneva: United Nations High Commissioner for Refugees; 2016.

12. Charak R, de Jong J, Berckmoes LH, Ndayisaba H, Reis R. Assessing the factor structure of the childhood trauma questionnaire, and multiple types of abuse and neglect among adolescents in conflict affected Burundi. Child Abuse Negl. 2017;72:383–92.

13. Charuvastra A, Cloitre M. Safe enough to sleep: sleep disruptions associated with trauma, posttraumatic stress, and anxiety in children and adolescents. Child Adolesc Psychiatr Clin N Am. 2009;18(4):877–91.

14. Chaudhury S, Brown FL, Kirk CM, Mukunzi S, Nyirandagijimana B, Mukandanga J, et al. Exploring the potential of a family based prevention intervention to reduce alcohol use and violence within HIV-affected families in Rwanda. AIDS Care. 2016;28:118–29.

15. Cheung AH, Zuckerbrot RA, Jensen PS, Ghalib K, Laraque D, Stein RE, et al. Guidelines for adolescent depression in primary care (GLAD-PC): II. Treatment and ongoing management. Pediatrics. 2007;120(5):e1313–26.

16. Dardas LA, van de Water B, Simmons LA. Parental involvement in adolescent depression interventions: a systematic review of randomized clinical trials. Int J Ment Health Nurs. 2018;27:557 70.

17. de Jong J. Family interventions and armed conflict. In: Halford K, van de Vijver F, editors. Culture and families: research and practice: Elsevier; 2020.

18. Dubicka B, Wilkinson PO. Latest thinking on antidepressants in children and young people. Arch Dis Child. 2018;103:720–1.

19. Eapen V, Graham P, Srinath S. Where there is no child psychiatrist: a mental healthcare manual. London: Royal College of Psychiatrists; 2012.

20. Ellis HB, Miller AB, Abdi S, Barrett C, Blood EA, Betancourt TS. Multi-tier mental health program for refugee youth. J Consult Clin Psychol. 2013;81:129–40.

21. Eruyar S, Maltby J, Vostanis P. Mental health problems of Syrian refugee children: the role of parental factors. Eur Child Adolesc Psychiatry. 2018;27:401–9.

22. Fazel M, Doll H, Stein A. A school-based mental health intervention for refugee children: an exploratory study. Clin Child Psychol Psychiatry. 2009;14:297–309.

23. Fazel M, Reed RV, Panter-Brick C, Stein A. Mental health of displaced and refugee children resettled in high-income countries: risk and protective factors. Lancet. 2012;379(9812):266–82. https://doi.org/10.1016/S0140-6736(11)60051-2.

24. Fazel M, Stein A. The mental health of refugee children. Arch Dis Child. 2002;87:366–70.

25. Ford T, Hamilton H, Meltzer H, Goodman R. Child mental health is everybody's business: the prevalence of contact with public sector services by type of disorder among British school children in a three-year period. Child Adolesc Mental Health. 2007;12(1):13–20.
26. Fox PG, Rossetti J, Burns KR, Popovich J. Southeast Asian refugee children: a school-based mental health intervention. International Journal of Psychiatric Nursing Research. 2005;11(1):1227–36.
27. Gewirtz A, Forgatch M, Wieling E. Parenting practices as potential mechanisms for child adjustment following mass trauma. J Marital Fam Ther. 2008;34:177–92.
28. Hassan G, Kirmayer L, Mekki-Berrada A, Quosh C, el Chamma, R, Deville-Stoetzel JB, et al. Culture, context and the mental health and psychosocial wellbeing of Syrians: a review for mental health and psychosocial support staff working with Syrians affected by armed conflict. 2015. Retrieved from Geneva: http://www.unhcr.org/55f6b90f9.pdf.
29. Inter-Agency Standing Committee. IASC guidelines on mental health and psychosocial support in emergency settings. IASC: Geneva; 2007.
30. Ishikawa SI, Okajima I, Matsuoka H, Sakano Y. Cognitive behavioural therapy for anxiety disorders in children and adolescents: a meta-analysis. Child Adolesc Mental Health. 2007;12(4):164–72.
31. Jones RB, Thapar A, Stone Z, Thapar A, Jones I, Smith D, Simpson S. Psychoeducational interventions in adolescent depression: a systematic review. Patient Educ Couns. 2018;101:804–16.
32. Jordans MJ, Tol WA. Mental health in humanitarian settings: shifting focus to care systems. Int Health. 2013;5(1):9–10. https://doi.org/10.1093/inthealth/ihs005.
33. Jordans MJ, Tol WA, Ndayisaba A, Komproe IH. A controlled evaluation of a brief parenting psychoeducation intervention in Burundi. Soc Psychiatry Psychiatr Epidemiol. 2013;48(11):1851–9. https://doi.org/10.1007/s00127-012-0630-6.
34. Kirmayer LJ. Cultural variations in the clinical presentation of depression and anxiety: implications for diagnosis and treatment. J Clin Psychiatry. 2001;62:22–30.
35. Kleinman A. Culture and depression. N Engl J Med. 2004;351(10):951–3. Retrieved from PM:15342799.
36. Kleinman A, Good B, editors. Culture and depression: studies in the anthropology and cross-cultural psychiatry of affect and disorder. Berkeley: University of California Press; 1985.
37. Lam TP, Goldberg DP, Dowell AC, Fortes S, Mbatia JK, Minhas FA, Klinkman MS. Proposed new diagnoses of anxious depression and bodily stress syndrome in ICD-11-PHC: an international focus group study. Fam Pract. 2012;30(1):76–87.
38. Lewis-Fernández R, Hinton DE, Laria AJ, Patterson EH, Hofmann SG, Craske MG, et al. Culture and the anxiety disorders: recommendations for DSM-V. Focus. 2011;9(3):351–68.
39. Lindblom J, Vänskä M, Flykt M, Tolvanen A, Tiitinen A, Tulppala M, Punamäki RL. From early family systems to internalizing symptoms: the role of emotion regulation and peer relations. J Fam Psychol. 2017;31(3):316.
40. Locher C, Koechlin H, Zion SR, Werner C, Pine DS, Kirsch I, et al. Efficacy and safety of selective serotonin reuptake inhibitors, serotonin-norepinephrine reuptake inhibitors, and placebo for common psychiatric disorders among children and adolescents: a systematic review and meta-analysis. JAMA Psychiat. 2017;74(10):1011–20.
41. Meyer SR, Steinhaus M, Bangirana C, Onyango-Mangen P, Stark L. The influence of caregiver depression on adolescent mental health outcomes: findings from refugee settlements in Uganda. BMC Psychiatry. 2017;17:405.
42. Miller KE, Omidian P, Rasmussen A, Yaqubi A, Daudzai H. Daily stressors, war experiences, and mental health in Afghanistan. Transcult Psychiatry. 2008;45(4):611–38. https://doi.org/10.1177/1363461508100785.
43. Montgomery E. Long-term effects of organized violence on young middle eastern refugees' mental health. Soc Sci Med. 2008;67:1596–603.
44. Mooren T, Bala J, Van der Meulen J. A family-centered approach to working with refugee children and adolescents. In: Song S, Ventevogel P, editors. Child, adolescent and family refugee mental health. Cham: Springer; 2020. pp. this volume.

45. Murray LK, Hall BJ, Dorsey S, Ugueto AM, Puffer ES, Sim A, et al. An evaluation of a common elements treatment approach for youth in Somali refugee camps. Global Mental Health. 2018;5:e16. https://doi.org/10.1017/gmh.2018.

46. Murray LK, Skavenski S, Kane JC, Mayeya J, Dorsey S, Cohen JA, et al. Effectiveness of trauma-focused cognitive behavioral therapy among trauma-affected children in Lusaka, Zambia: a randomized clinical trial. JAMA Pediatr. 2015;169(8):761–9. https://doi.org/10.1001/jamapediatrics.2015.0580.

47. Naeem F, Phiri P, Munshi T, Rathod S, Ayub M, Gobbi M, Kingdon D. Using cognitive behaviour therapy with south Asian Muslims: findings from the culturally sensitive CBT project. Int Rev Psychiatry. 2016;27:233–46.

48. National Institute for Health and Care Excellence. Depression in children and young people: identification and management. 2019. Retrieved from https://www.nice.org.uk/guidance/ng134.

49. Nielsen MB, Carlsson J, Rimvall MK, Petersen JH, Norredam M. Risk of childhood psychiatric disorders in children of refugee parents with post-traumatic stress disorder: a nationwide, register-based, cohort study. Lancet Public Health. 2019;4(7):e353–9.

50. Omidian P, Miller K. Addressing the psychosocial needs of women in Afghanistan. Critical Half. 2006;4:17–22.

51. Ooi CS, Rooney RM, Roberts C, Kane RT, Wright B, Chatzisarantis N. The efficacy of a group cognitive behavioral therapy for war-affected young migrants living in Australia: a cluster randomized controlled trial. Front Psychol. 2016;7:1641.

52. Patel V, Saxena S, Lund C, Thornicroft G, Baingana F, Bolton P, et al. The lancet commission on global mental health and sustainable development. Lancet. 2018;392:1553–98.

53. Pine DS, Klein RG. Anxiety disorders. In: Thapar A, Pine DS, Leckman JF, Scott S, Snowling MJ, Taylor E, editors. Rutter's child and adolescent psychiatry. 6th ed. Oxford: John Wiley & Sons; 2015. p. 822–40.

54. Puffer ES, Green EP, Chase RM, Sim AL, Zayzay J, Friis E, et al. Parents make the difference: a randomized-controlled trial of a parenting intervention in Liberia. Global Mental Health. 2015;2:e15.

55. Reed RV, Fazel M, Jones L, Panter-Brick C, Stein A. Mental health of displaced and refugee children resettled in low-income and middle-income countries: risk and protective factors. Lancet. 2012;379(9812):250–65. https://doi.org/10.1016/S0140-6736(11)60050-0.

56. Rey JM, Bella-Awusah TT, Jing L. Depression in children and adolescents. In: Rey JM, editor. IACAPAP e-textbook of child and adolescent mental health. Geneva: International Association for Child and Adolescent Psychiatry and Allied Professions; 2015.

57. Rousseau C, Drapeau A, Lacroix L, Bagilishya D, Heusch N. Evaluation of a classroom program of creative expression workshops for refugee and immigrant children. J Child Psychol Psychiatry. 2005;46:180–5.

58. Sijbrandij M, Acarturk C, Aktas M, Bryant RA, Burchert S, Carswell K, et al. Strengthening mental health care systems for adult and adolescent Syrian refugees in Europe and the Middle East: integrating scalable psychological interventions in 8 countries. Eur J Psychotraumatol. 2017;8(Sup2):1388102.

59. Sim A, Annan J, Puffer E, Salhi C, Betancourt T. Building happy families: impact evaluation of a parenting and family skills intervention for migrant and displaced Burmese families in Thailand. New York: International Rescue Committee; 2014.

60. Slobodin O, de Jong JT. Family interventions in traumatized immigrants and refugees: a systematic review. Transcult Psychiatry. 2015;52(6):723–42.

61. Song S, Ventevogel P. Principles of the mental health assessment of refugee children and adolescents. In: Song S, Ventevogel P, editors. Child, adolescent and family refugee mental health. Cham: Springer; 2020. pp. this volume.

62. Stallard P. Think good, feel good: a cognitive behavioural therapy workbook for children and young people. London: Wiley; 2019.

63. Sullivan AL, Simonson GR. A systematic review of school-based social-emotional interventions for refugee and war-traumatized youth. Rev Educ Res. 2016;86(2):503–30.

64. Tay AK, Islam R, Riley A, Welton-Mitchell C, Duchesne B, Waters V, Varner A, Silove D, Ventevogel P. Culture, context and mental health of Rohingya refugees: a review for staff in mental health and psychosocial support programmes for Rohingya refugees. Geneva: UNHCR; 2018.

65. Tol WA, Komproe IH, Jordans MJ, Ndayisaba A, Ntamutumba P, Sipsma H, et al. School-based mental health intervention for children in war-affected Burundi: a cluster randomized trial. BMC Med. 2014;12:56. https://doi.org/10.1186/1741-7015-12-56.

66. Ventevogel P. Borderlands of mental health: explorations in medical anthropology, psychiatric epidemiology and health systems research in Afghanistan and Burundi. (PhD). 2016. Universiteit van Amsterdam, Amsterdam.

67. Ventevogel P, Duchesne B, Hughes P, Whitney C. Mental health and psychosocial support (MHPSS). In: Abubakar I, Zumla A, editors. Clinical handbook of refugee health. London: Taylor & Francis; 2020.

68. Ventevogel P, Faiz H. Mental disorder or emotional distress? How psychiatric surveys in Afghanistan ignore the role of gender, culture and context. Intervention. 2018;16(3):207–14.

69. Ventevogel P, Komproe IH, Jordans MJ, Feo P, De Jong JTVM. Validation of the Kirundi versions of brief self-rating scales for common mental disorders among children in Burundi. BMC Psychiatry. 2014;14:36.

70. Wicks-Nelson R, Israel AC. Abnormal child and adolescent psychology. London: Routledge; 2015.

71. World Health Organisation. mhGAP intervention guide (mhGAP-IG) version 2.0 for mental, neurological and substance use disorders for non-specialist health settings. Geneva: WHO; 2016.

72. World Health Organization. Intervention guide for mental, neurological and substance use disorders in non-specialized health settings. Geneva: Author; 2010.

73. World Health Organization. International classification of diseases for mortality and morbidity statistics (11th Revision). 2018. Retrieved from https://icd.who.int/browse11/l-m/en.

74. World Health Organization, & United Nations High Commissioner for Refugees. mhGAP humanitarian intervention guide (mhGAP-HIG): clinical management of mental, neurological and substance use conditions in humanitarian emergencies. Geneva: WHO; 2015.

Substance Use Among Refugee and Conflict-Affected Children and Adolescents

M. Claire Greene and Jeremy C. Kane

Introduction

Interventions to prevent and treat substance use problems have recently emerged as a priority for adolescent health, particularly among vulnerable adolescents [41]. Despite this recognition, there remains a lack of knowledge regarding the burden of substance use problems among refugee and conflict-affected children and adolescents in low-, middle-, and high-income settings. In part this is because most existing data are limited to adults, and assessment tools for children and adolescents are specific to high-income contexts [51]. Data on children and adolescents who have been resettled in high-income settings reveal that alcohol and other drug use are rare relative to other psychopathology [7, 8]. However, in some refugee camps, the prevalence of alcohol and other drug use is comparable to children and adolescents in urban areas and higher than those in rural host communities [18]. Some have expressed concerns that alcohol and other drug use in some refugee camps is becoming normalized and increasing in prevalence, particularly during emerging adulthood, thus strengthening the need for prevention efforts during adolescence [18, 37].

Refugee and conflict-affected adolescents tend to display higher-risk patterns of substance use relative to adolescents who use alcohol and other drugs from host communities [25]. When asked about reasons for using alcohol and other drugs, refugee and conflict-affected adolescents in low- and high-income settings reported

M. C. Greene (✉)
Department of Psychiatry, Columbia University/New York State Psychiatric Institute, New York, NY, USA

Johns Hopkins Bloomberg School of Public Health, Baltimore, MD, USA
e-mail: Claire.Greene@nyspi.columbia.edu

J. C. Kane
Johns Hopkins Bloomberg School of Public Health, Baltimore, MD, USA

Department of Epidemiology, Columbia University, New York, NY, USA

© Springer Nature Switzerland AG 2020
S. J. Song, P. Ventevogel (eds.), *Child, Adolescent and Family Refugee Mental Health*, https://doi.org/10.1007/978-3-030-45278-0_11

that alcohol, specifically, is used to cope with trauma, boredom, frustration, as well as for social reasons [25, 33, 37]. The types of substances that are commonly used vary by population and world region [54]. For example, khat use is a common stimulate chewed in East Africa and the Middle East, while Yaba is a pill comprised of methamphetamine and caffeine that is more prevalent in South and Southeast Asia [13, 57] (see Table 11.1 for substance types and examples). Consequences attributable to substance use among refugee adolescents include an array of psychosocial consequences [25], but of particular concern to this population is impaired school performance and, in some cases, expulsion [48]. In qualitative research, school engagement and teacher involvement was protective against substance use among conflict-affected adolescents in Liberia, while risk factors include not attending school, poor relationships with peers and family, and poor socioeconomic conditions [46, 48], which is similar to what has been reported for refugee and immigrant adolescents resettled in high-income countries and youth more generally [28, 49].

Interventions

Providing treatment and prevention services for substance use disorder to refugee and conflict-affected children and adolescents necessitates unique considerations related to both their developmental and socio-cultural context. Recommendations from high-income settings suggest that adolescents that are using substances may benefit from interventions even if they do not meet criteria for a substance use disorder, because any use is considered cause for concern at this developmental period [3]. In general, earlier age of onset of substance use and disorder is a reliable indicator of severity for individuals with substance use problems. Thus, prevention and early intervention is critical in this age group. Contextual factors that challenge the implementation of substance use interventions for refugee children and adolescents include general mistrust in institutions that provide substance use services [37, 47], stigma and resistance to seeking care [38, 47], fragmentation of services for individuals with co-occurring health challenges [47], and, particularly for refugees who have been resettled in new contexts, health system-level barriers in the provision of care (e.g., language barriers, treatment programs unable to accommodate refugees who do not speak the local language or those with complex histories, and lack of provider training in culturally competent and trauma-informed care) [38, 47]. Despite these challenges, it is critical for providers working with refugees who have been resettled in high-income countries and those in low- and middle-income settings to be knowledgeable in intervention strategies that may be used to promote health as well as prevent and treat substance use problems in these populations.

Prevention Strategies

Prevention strategies aim to modify factors that increase risk for substance use and related problems. There are multiple types of prevention strategies, each of which

Table 11.1 Types of substances

Substance	Type	Common administration	Acute effects	Examples
Alcohol	Sedative	Swallowed	Coordination problems, disinhibition, drowsiness, euphoria, impaired memory and judgment	Beer, wine, liquor, home brew
Cannabis	Sedative, hallucinogen	Smoked, swallowed	Appetite, balance and coordination problems, distorted sensory perception, euphoria, slow reaction time	Marijuana, pot, hash, weed
Inhalants	Sedative, hallucinogen	Inhaled through nose or mouth	Disinhibition, headache, impaired memory, motor coordination problems, stimulation	Gases, glue, nitrites, paint thinner, whippets
Opioids	Sedative	Injected, smoked, snorted, swallowed	Confusion, coordination problems, dizziness, drowsiness, euphoria, sedation, slowed breathing	Codeine, heroin, methadone, morphine, opioids, opium, tramadol
Sedatives	Sedative	Swallowed	Confusion, coordination problems, euphoria, impaired judgment, slurred speech, relaxation	Benzodiazepines, Barbiturates
Stimulants	Stimulant	Injected, smoked, snorted, swallowed	Anxiety, hyperactivity, irritability, mental alertness, paranoia, reduced appetite, restlessness, tremors	Amphetamine, crack, cocaine, khat, methamphetamine, Yaba

targets different populations at risk of substance use disorder. Below we describe prevention interventions using the classifications recommended by the United Nations Office on Drugs and Crime: universal, selective, and indicated prevention [21, 55, 56].

Universal Prevention

Universal interventions are those that are given to the whole population regardless of individual risk [21]. School-, family-, peer-, and community-based universal prevention interventions for substance use have been developed and evaluated in immigrant adolescents and those facing adversity in low- and middle-income countries, although not refugee populations. School-based prevention strategies typically focus on teaching emotion regulation and socialization among primary school-aged children, followed by more explicit prevention of substance use for secondary school-aged adolescents [50]. The content of school-based prevention interventions vary substantially but are often made up of a combination of the following components: (1) social resistance skills training focused on increasing awareness of the social influences that support substance use and developing skills to resist these influences [10]; (2) normative education, which corrects myths and incorrect perceptions regarding substance use among peers [23]; and (3) competence enhancement which focuses on problem-solving, decision-making, general cognitive skills, self-control, self-esteem, coping skills, etc. [10, 23]. Evaluations of these interventions have produced mixed findings in high-income settings but tend to be more supportive of the skills-based over education-based interventions [14, 17]. An example of a universal prevention program for conflict-affected adolescents in Croatia to delay the initiation of drinking and reduce alcohol use among 6th–8th grade students is provided in Table 11.2 [1, 59]. A qualitative study in the Democratic Republic of Congo identified critical components for prevention efforts in conflict-affected adolescents. These included the involvement of community members to model appropriate behaviors, serve as mentors, empower families, involve schools and churches, provide work opportunities, organize youth groups, and provide other social and educational opportunities [32].

Family-based interventions are another universal prevention strategy that addresses issues in parenting, communication, and reducing substance use among family members and typically engages both the child and parent(s) [23]. Most immigrant studies that describe family-based prevention efforts delivered in high-income settings focus on family and parenting skills to prevent adolescent substance use. Findings from these studies underscore the importance of adaptation of these interventions to align with the cultural norms in the populations to whom they are delivered [2, 15, 34, 36]. Family-based interventions implemented in LMICs are summarized in Table 11.2 [11, 35, 39].

Peer-based interventions are less commonly implemented in high-income settings. We identified one example of a peer-based universal prevention program implemented in Uganda that targeted vulnerable children and adolescents living in slum communities. Youth were trained to educate and develop campaigns to teach

Table 11.2 Summary of research on prevention interventions

Author, Year	Population type (country)	Description of intervention	Findings
Universal prevention			
Abatemarco, 2004 [1]; West, 2008 [59]	Conflict-affected 6th–8th grade students (Croatia)	*Project Northland:* behavioral and educational curricula, peer activities, parental/community involvement	Reduction in increased intentions to use alcohol among adolescents, particularly females, and qualitative results revealed that program was particularly effective among early adolescents
Allen, 2013 [2]	Immigrant Latino parents of adolescents aged 10–14 years (USA)	8 group parenting sessions covering adolescent development, parenting across cultures, communication and relationships, conflict resolution, etc.	The intervention was feasible and acceptable to immigrant Latino parents. Preliminary results suggest significant improvements in parent reports of adolescent internalizing behaviors, marginal improvements in externalizing behaviors, but no change in substance use behaviors
Andrade, 2018 [4]	Latino immigrant youth (USA)	*Adelante:* social marketing campaign portraying adolescent narratives describing resilience despite adversity through print advertisements, social media, videos, blogs, and other platforms	No evaluation of campaign impact, but objective was to reduce substance use, sexual risk, and violence
Cluver, 2018 [11]	Families reporting conflict with their adolescent child (South Africa)	*Parenting for Lifelong Health: Sinovuyo Teen:* 14-session parent and adolescent program delivered by community members on topics relevant to family skill-building (e.g., problem management, communication, violence prevention)	The intervention improved parent-child interactions and reduced adolescent substance use. There was no effect of the intervention on mental health, behavioral outcomes, or community violence exposure
Kasirye, 2015 [29]	Adolescents living in slum communities (Uganda)	Peer-led prevention program involving monitoring substance use in their community and communicating information about substance use prevention to their peers	No evaluation of the effect of the intervention; however, involving adolescents and peers in prevention can improve implementation and acceptability

(continued)

Table 11.2 (continued)

Author, Year	Population type (country)	Description of intervention	Findings
Litrownick, 2000 [34]; Elder, 2002 [15]	Immigrant Hispanic adolescents and their caregiver (USA)	*Sembrando Salud:* 8-week school-based group intervention program (5 sessions adolescents only, 3 sessions adolescents + caregivers) covering behavioral health, problem-solving, developing parental support, improved communication, and booster phone calls	The intervention was associated with improved parent-child communication. However, there were no significant difference in smoking or drinking immediately post-intervention or at the 1- or 2-year follow-up assessment
Maalouf, 2014 [35]; McDonald, 2013 [39]	Children and families of 9 low- and middle-income countries	*Strengthening families (SF10–14):* 14 weekly family skills training sessions involving family meals, parent, and teen skills training *Families and Schools Together (FAST):* 8 weekly multifamily groups led by trained professionals focused on structured family activities	SF10–14 was associated with improved parental anger management, problem-solving among children, and family dynamics. FAST was associated with improved family dynamics, child behavior, peer relationships, parental involvement, and reduced family conflict, but results differed across countries
Marsiglia, 2016 [36]	7th grade students and parents in schools with a high proportion of foreign-born Latinos (USA)	*Keepin it REAL:* 10-week program delivered by teachers during school day that teachers drug-resistance training *Familias Preparando la Nueva Generacion:* 8 workshops for parents designed to empower parents and improve family functioning/communication	The combined school-based and parent intervention resulted in lower alcohol and tobacco use 18 months after baseline relative to adolescents/parent dyads who only received the school-based or the parenting intervention. This reduction was explained (i.e., mediated) by increased antidrug norms
Indicated prevention			
Pengpid, 2013 [45]	University students with hazardous alcohol use (South Africa)	*Screening and brief intervention:* 20-minute brief intervention with personalized feedback. Intervention based on the information-motivation-behavioral skills model	Students receiving the screening and brief intervention displayed a significantly greater reduction in hazardous alcohol use compared to students who received an educational leaflet

Abbreviations: *LMIC* low- and middle-income country, *USA* United States of America peers and other community members about substance use in order to prevent substance-related problems in their community [29]. These interventions have yet to be evaluated in refugee populations.

Social marketing strategies, a form of community-based universal prevention, have been developed for immigrant populations in high-income settings. These strategies are intended to reach difficult to reach populations, such as immigrant adolescents, with public health messaging. For example, one campaign portrayed adolescent narratives describing resilience despite adversity through print advertisements, social media, videos, blogs, and other platforms [4]. Many of these universal prevention strategies have not been rigorously, if at all, evaluated and substance use has yet to be included as a secondary outcome in many existing evaluations. Universal prevention strategies still serve a valuable role in refugee and conflict-affected children and adolescents health because they may strengthen characteristics protective against a variety of threats to health in these populations and modify the presence of known risk factors for substance use and related problems.

Selective Prevention

Selective interventions are those that are given to individuals at elevated risk of substance use disorder due to the presence of measurable risk factors [21]. For example, selective prevention interventions may target children and adolescents who have parents with a substance use disorder or youth exhibiting aggressive or externalizing behavioral problems [50]. In general, selective prevention interventions may comprise more directed parenting and family skills training or coping and behavioral (e.g., impulsiveness, anger) skills training for children and adolescents [50]. Selective prevention interventions are disproportionately unrepresented in research and practice focused on substance use in refugee, conflict-affected, and vulnerable populations [22]. Future efforts to better direct prevention strategies toward individuals at elevated risk for substance use disorder are needed to fill this gap in knowledge.

Indicated Prevention

Indicated interventions are those that prevent disorder among very high-risk individuals or those displaying early signs of disorder. For substance use, the objective of indicated prevention interventions is typically to prevent the transition from "use" to "disorder" [50]. For children and adolescents, indicated prevention strategies typically include mentoring and brief interventions (Fig. 11.1) [42, 62]. Motivational Enhancement Therapy (MET), the most common form of brief interventions, is a provider-delivered intervention that is intended to resolve ambivalence about abstinence, moderation, or engagement with treatment. It begins with an initial assessment followed by personalized feedback, discussion of treatment or substance-related goals, empathic listening, and elicitation of self-motivational statements that lead to a plan for changing substance use and related behaviors [5]. Brief interventions have been tested and evaluated in adult refugee populations [9, 16, 60], but not in children or adolescents. One school-based brief intervention trial in South Africa was identified; however, the intervention targeted university

ASSESSMENT

Is the child's alcohol or other substance use associated with physical, psychological, or other harm?
- Explore the use of alcohol or drugs including level of risk
- Explore friend's alcohol/drug use patterns
- Ask about amount and patterns of use, triggers to alcohol or drug use, and harm to self and others.

MANAGEMENT

1. Manage harmful effects of alcohol or drug use
2. Provide brief personalized feedback
3. Assess and facilitate motivation of child to stop or reduce alcohol or drug use
4. Discuss ways to reduce or stop harmful use
5. Offer psychosocial support
6. Regular follow-up

Fig. 11.1 Brief intervention for hazardous use of alcohol and other drugs

students in emerging adulthood. Although older than the scope of this chapter, this intervention may serve as a model for integrating indicated prevention into school-based settings for refugee and conflict-affected children and adolescents (see Table 11.2) [45].

Treatment Strategies

Treatment strategies for substance use problems are distinct from prevention strategies in that they are intended for children or adolescents who have met symptom criteria for a substance use problem. However, these interventions are sometimes also used as indicated prevention strategies (i.e., among those with preclinical or subthreshold disorder). In resource-limited settings such as refugee camps or LMIC generally, these interventions should likely be reserved for children and adolescents with higher-level problems and/or those who have not responded to lower-intensity interventions (e.g., brief interventions).

Cognitive Behavioral Therapy

According to Waldron and Kaminer [58], "cognitive behavioral models conceptualize substance use and related problems as learned behaviors that are initiated and maintained in the context of environmental factors" [58]. Although there can be variability in content across cognitive behavioral therapy (CBT) treatments for child and adolescent substance use, in general they include teaching clients to avoid stimulating cues and self-monitoring, coping skills training, and skills to change maladaptive thoughts and feelings that may lead to substance using behavior. Sessions can be delivered either individually or in-group format. Counselors often ask clients to complete homework assignments and conduct behavioral rehearsals with them (e.g., to build substance use refusal skills) [58]. For children with symptoms of post-traumatic stress, which is likely to be common in humanitarian settings, CBT may also be trauma-focused and include components of relaxation, trauma narratives, and gradual exposure [12, 27]. Finally, CBT may also be combined with previously described MET (see Box 11.1). CBT-based interventions in LMIC have tended to focus on adults [44] or non-substance use outcomes [40]. However, these studies have demonstrated the feasibility of training lay providers to deliver CBT-based interventions with effectiveness and fidelity to the treatment model. This is crucial for the applicability of CBT for adolescent substance use in conflict and refugee settings.

Trauma-focused cognitive behavioral therapy (TF-CBT) is an intervention that has been implemented and evaluated among vulnerable children in Zambia and has been shown to reduce substance use 1 year after TF-CBT compared to vulnerable adolescents who received psychosocial counseling. The reduction was particularly large among youth with post-traumatic stress symptoms [26]. The results of the Zambia trial and reviews conducted in the USA suggest that CBT has potential to be an effective treatment strategy for children and adolescents who are refugees and in humanitarian settings [58]. The primary focus of future studies in this area should be on feasibility and implementation of CBT-based interventions.

Box 11.1 Case Example

A 16-year-old Congolese boy lived in Uganda as a refugee with his family. At school, he became friends with peers who engaged in heavy substance use and over the course of a year, started to use marijuana and alcohol almost daily. After police found him intoxicated and unconscious on the road, his parents took him to a mental health counselor. He began individual weekly sessions on cognitive behavioral therapy that started with psychoeducation about the risks of substance abuse. Motivational interviewing was used to identify his stage of change, identify triggers to his using substances, and brainstormed relapse prevention strategies. The next phase was skills coaching, where they discussed stress management and how to deal with interpersonal stress. The third phase was centered on understanding and addressing traumatic experiences, grief, and loss. They also included his mother in psychoeducation, relapsed prevention, and developed a safety plan. Over about 6 months, the teen was better able to understand the motivations behind his use, addressed triggers, and identified alternative strategies to use. He developed a new set of friends and became more engaged in school work.

Contingency Management

Contingency management (CM) is based on operant conditioning theory, which suggests that the use of substances is continued due to both the physiological effects of the substance and the nonphysiological (i.e., social) reinforcements that accompany use [53]. The theory behind CM is that substance use may be reduced through positive reinforcements with immediate and tangible incentives. Incentives (e.g., food, non-food items) may be used when certain treatment goals are achieved, such as medication adherence, attendance at counseling appointments, and negative urine screens. Negative reinforcement (e.g., involvement of criminal justice, grounding) or negative punishment (e.g., reduction in rewards that may be provided for achieving goals) may also be used; however, positive reinforcement is preferred [53]. CM is typically combined with psychosocial (e.g., CBT) or medication treatments. For example, an adolescent may receive a reward for attending a scheduled CBT session. CM principles can also be applied by parents of the adolescents in addition to counselors [53]. CM is still in early stages of evaluation for use with adolescents in high-income countries and has not been used among adolescents in LMIC or humanitarian settings.

Family-Based Interventions

Family-based interventions (i.e., the inclusion of caregivers in treatment) to address adolescent substance use are common approaches implemented in high-income countries [6, 24]. Interventions that specifically feature family involvement include Brief Strategic Family Therapy, Family Behavior Therapy, Functional Family Therapy, Multidimensional Family Therapy, and Multisystemic Therapy. These approaches include the child's caregivers/parents and potentially other family members and friends/peers. Details of these approaches are beyond the scope of this chapter but are available in a review by Hogue and Liddle [24]. In general, objectives of these approaches include improving communication, managing conflict, addressing co-occurring mental, behavioral and learning disorders, managing problems with work or school attendance, and strengthening supportive peer networks. A review by Hogue and Liddle found that these approaches collectively were effective in reducing adolescent substance use and that engagement and retention in the interventions was high, which is an important finding given that retention will certainly be a challenge among families in humanitarian and refugee settings. Although well-established and widely recommended in the USA and high-income countries, the use of family-based treatment approaches has not been rigorously tested in LMIC or among refugees.

Adolescent Community Reinforcement Approach

An important consideration in treatment approaches for adolescent substance use is whether the intervention is equipped to address co-occurring mental health and psychosocial problems, which commonly are comorbid with substance use. The adolescent community reinforcement approach (A-CRA) was developed to address both substance use and other psychiatric problems among adolescents by combining elements of CBT and family therapy [20]. The intervention may also include caregivers and is comprised of the following components: problem-solving, goal setting, communication skills, anger management, medication monitoring, identifying thoughts, feelings and behaviors that trigger substance use, relapse prevention, encouraging pro-social activities, teaching caregiver skills, and improving the adolescent-caregiver relationship. The approach is meant to be delivered flexibly with the counselor choosing aforementioned components based on the adolescent's needs. A-CRA needs effectiveness testing in high-income, lower-income, and humanitarian settings. The original A-CRA manual is available online [19].

12-Step Facilitation

12-step programs for substance use, such as Alcoholics Anonymous or Narcotics Anonymous, are widely used interventions both in high- and lower-income countries. Advantages of these programs are that they are very low cost, flexible, and provide adolescents with a strong support network. On the other hand, because the programs are peer-led, there is no clinical oversight and the effectiveness of the programs has not been rigorously studied among children and adolescents [30, 31]. Given their popularity (including in LMIC) and the access to a peer/social support community, these programs warrant further investigation.

Pharmacotherapy

Pharmacological treatments for substance use disorders among adolescents have been used much less often than behavioral and family-based approaches described above; however, investigations in this area are increasing [61]. According to the National Institute on Drug Abuse in the USA, there are currently no FDA-approved medications for the treatment of substance use disorder among adolescents. Among adults, commonly prescribed medications include buprenorphine, methadone, and naltrexone for opioid use and acamprosate, disulfiram, and naltrexone for alcohol use; and there are no medications approved for marijuana, cocaine, or methamphetamine use disorder [43]. Evidence of effectiveness and safety of these medications among adolescents is very preliminary and there are concerns that side effects may differ among adolescents compared to adults [43, 61]. Given the limited availability of evidence and the feasibility issues of delivering pharmacological treatment in refugee and humanitarian contexts, it is likely that this approach can only be used in rare cases—among adolescents with very severe substance use disorders and in situations where a trained provider is available to monitor treatment progress, side effects, and any safety concerns. Dosage recommendations for managing alcohol withdrawal and are available in the mhGAP Humanitarian Intervention Guide [62].

Conclusions

This chapter summarized interventions for substance use problems among children and adolescents, including prevention and treatment approaches. The review presented here suggests that there are evidence-based interventions within each of these approaches that can effectively address substance use among adolescents. However, there is essentially no extant literature on the effectiveness, feasibility, or acceptability of interventions among refugee populations, in humanitarian contexts, or among younger children [14, 22]. It is important also to distinguish intervention studies delivered to refugee children and adolescents as compared to non-refugee populations, given that refugees are likely to have elevated exposure to potentially traumatic events, may have different ongoing insecurity related to their legal status, and different sources of ongoing adversity (e.g., fractured support systems, discrimination, lack of livelihoods) [8]. The Mental Health Standard in the 2018 Sphere Handbook includes substance use as one of its nine key actions and specifically calls for efforts to minimize harm related to alcohol and drug use, as well as training providers in detection and brief intervention, harm reduction, and management of withdrawal and intoxication [52]. Urgent efforts are needed to adapt, test, and implement effective interventions, including those recommended in the Sphere Handbook and other guidelines, to reduce the burden of substance use problems among refugee children and adolescents globally.

References

1. Abatemarco DJ, West B, Zec V, Russo A, Sosiak P, Mardesic V. Project Northland in Croatia: a community-based adolescent alcohol prevention intervention. J Drug Educ. 2004;34(2):167–78.
2. Allen ML, Hurtado GA, Yon KJ, Okuyemi KS, Davey CS, Marczak MS, et al. Feasibility of a parenting program to prevent substance use among Latino youth: a community-based participatory research study. Am J Health Promot. 2013;27(4):240–4. https://doi.org/10.4278/ajhp.110204-ARB-52.
3. American Society for Addiction Medicine. ASAM patient placement criteria for the treatment of substance related disorders. 2nd ed. Chevy Chase: American Society of Addiction Medicine; 2001.
4. Andrade EL, Evans WD, Barrett ND, Cleary SD, Edberg MC, Alvayero RD, et al. Development of the place-based Adelante social marketing campaign for prevention of substance use, sexual risk and violence among Latino immigrant youth. Health Educ Res. 2018;33(2):125–44. https://doi.org/10.1093/her/cyx076.
5. Barnett E, Sussman S, Smith C, Rohrbach LA, Spruijt-Metz D. Motivational Interviewing for adolescent substance use: a review of the literature. Addict Behav. 2012;37(12):1325–34. https://doi.org/10.1016/j.addbeh.2012.07.001.
6. Becker SJ, Curry JF. Outpatient interventions for adolescent substance abuse: a quality of evidence review. J Consult Clin Psychol. 2008;76(4):531–43. https://doi.org/10.1037/0022-006X.76.4.531.
7. Betancourt TS, Newnham EA, Layne CM, Kim S, Steinberg AM, Ellis H, Birman D. Trauma history and psychopathology in war-affected refugee children referred for trauma-related mental health services in the United States. J Trauma Stress. 2012;25(6):682–90. https://doi.org/10.1002/jts.21749.

8. Betancourt TS, Newnham EA, Birman D, Lee R, Ellis BH, Layne CM. Comparing trauma exposure, mental health needs, and service utilization across clinical samples of refugee, immigrant, and U.S.-origin children. J Trauma Stress. 2017;30(3):209–18. https://doi.org/10.1002/jts.22186.

9. Bolton P, Lee C, Haroz E, Murray L, Dorsey S, Robinson C, et al. A transdiagnostic community-based mental health treatment for comorbid disorders: development and outcomes of a randomized controlled trial among Burmese refugees in Thailand [Randomized Controlled Trial; Research Support, U.S. Gov't, Non-P.H.S.]. PloS Med. 2014;11(11):e1001757. https://doi.org/10.1371/journal.pmed.1001757. (Accession No. Cn-01112532).

10. Botvin GJ. Preventing drug abuse in schools: social and competence enhancement approaches targeting individual-level etiologic factors. Addict Behav. 2000;25(6):887–97. Retrieved from https://www.ncbi.nlm.nih.gov/pubmed/11125777.

11. Cluver LD, Meinck F, Steinert JI, Shenderovich Y, Doubt J, Herrero Romero R, et al. Parenting for Lifelong Health: a pragmatic cluster randomised controlled trial of a non-commercialised parenting programme for adolescents and their families in South Africa. BMJ Glob Health. 2018;3(1):e000539. https://doi.org/10.1136/bmjgh-2017-000539.

12. Cohen JA, Mannarino AP, Deblinger E. Treating trauma and traumatic grief in children and adolescents. New York: Guilford Press; 2006.

13. Das KN. Stateless Rohingya refugees sucked into booming Bangladesh drug trade. Reuters. 2017. Retrieved from https://in.reuters.com/article/myanmar-rohingya-bangladesh-drugs-idINKBN1662M8.

14. Das JK, Salam RA, Arshad A, Finkelstein Y, Bhutta ZA. Interventions for adolescent substance abuse: an overview of systematic reviews. J Adolesc Health. 2016;59(4S):S61–75. https://doi.org/10.1016/j.jadohealth.2016.06.021.

15. Elder JP, Litrownik AJ, Slymen DJ, Campbell NR, Parra-Medina D, Choe S, et al. Tobacco and alcohol use-prevention program for Hispanic migrant adolescents. Am J Prev Med. 2002;23(4):269–75. Retrieved from https://www.ncbi.nlm.nih.gov/pubmed/12406481.

16. Ezard N, Debakre A, Catillon R. Screening and brief intervention for high-risk alcohol use in Mae La refugee camp, Thailand: a pilot project on the feasibility of training and implementation. Intervention. 2010;8(3):223.

17. Flynn AB, Falco M, Hocini S. Independent evaluation of middle school-based drug prevention curricula: a systematic review. JAMA Pediatr. 2015;169(11):1046–52. https://doi.org/10.1001/jamapediatrics.2015.1736.

18. Glick P, Al-Khammash U, Shaheen M, Brown R, Goutam P, Karam R, et al. Health risk behaviours of Palestinian youth: findings from a representative survey. East Mediterr Health J. 2018;24(2):127–36. Retrieved from https://www.ncbi.nlm.nih.gov/pubmed/29748941.

19. Godley SH, Meyers RJ, Smith JE, Karvinen T, Titus JC, Godley MD, et al. The adolescent community reinforcement approach for cannabis users, Cannabis Youth Treatment (CYT) Series, vol. 4. Rockville: Center for Substance Abuse Treatment, Substance Abuse and Mental Health Services Administration; 2001.

20. Godley SH, Smith JE, Passetti LL, Subramaniam G. The Adolescent Community Reinforcement Approach (A-CRA) as a model paradigm for the management of adolescents with substance use disorders and co-occurring psychiatric disorders. Subst Abus. 2014;35(4):352–63. https://doi.org/10.1080/08897077.2014.936993.

21. Gordon RS Jr. An operational classification of disease prevention. Public Health Rep. 1983;98(2):107–9. Retrieved from http://www.ncbi.nlm.nih.gov/pubmed/6856733.

22. Greene MC, Ventevogel P, Kane JC. Substance use services for refugees. Bull World Health Organ. 2019;97:246–246A.

23. Griffin KW, Botvin GJ. Evidence-based interventions for preventing substance use disorders in adolescents. Child Adolesc Psychiatr Clin N Am. 2010;19(3):505–26. https://doi.org/10.1016/j.chc.2010.03.005.

24. Hogue A, Liddle HA, Becker D. Multidimensional family prevention for at-risk adolescents. In: Kaslow FW, Patterson T, Kaslow FW, Patterson T, editors. Comprehensive handbook of psychotherapy: cognitive-behavioral approaches, vol. 2. Hoboken: Wiley; 2002. p. 141–66.

25. Horyniak D, Higgs P, Cogger S, Dietze P, Bofu T. Heavy alcohol consumption among marginalised African refugee young people in Melbourne, Australia: motivations for drinking, experiences of alcohol-related problems and strategies for managing drinking. Ethn Health. 2016;21(3):284–99. https://doi.org/10.1080/13557858.2015.1061105.
26. Kane JC, Murray LK. Implementation of evidence-based mental health treatments in Zambia. Paper presented at the Zambia Ministry of Health Research Dissemination Meeting, Lusaka, Zambia, 2018.
27. Kane JC, Murray LK, Cohen J, Dorsey S, Skavenski van Wyk S, Galloway Henderson J, et al. Moderators of treatment response to trauma-focused cognitive behavioral therapy among youth in Zambia. J Child Psychol Psychiatry. 2016;57(10):1194–202. https://doi.org/10.1111/jcpp.12623.
28. Kane JC, Johnson RM, Iwamoto DK, Jernigan DH, Harachi TW, Bass JK. Pathways linking intergenerational cultural dissonance and alcohol use among Asian American youth: the role of family conflict, parental involvement, and peer behavior. J Ethn Subst Abus. 2018:1–21. https://doi.org/10.1080/15332640.2018.1428709.
29. Kasirye R. Efficacy of a peer interactive youth-led drug prevention programme: a UYDEL-UNODC project. International Journal of Prevention and Treatment of Substance Use Disorders. 2015:69–78.
30. Kelly JF, Urbanoski K. Youth recovery contexts: the incremental effects of 12-step attendance and involvement on adolescent outpatient outcomes. Alcohol Clin Exp Res. 2012;36(7):1219–29. https://doi.org/10.1111/j.1530-0277.2011.01727.x.
31. Kelly JF, Dow SJ, Yeterian JD, Myers M. How safe are adolescents at Alcoholics Anonymous and Narcotics Anonymous meetings? A prospective investigation with outpatient youth. J Subst Abus Treat. 2011;40(4):419–25. https://doi.org/10.1016/j.jsat.2011.01.004.
32. Kohli A, Remy MM, Binkurhorhwa AK, Mitima CM, Mirindi AB, Mwinja NB, et al. Preventing risky behaviours among young adolescents in eastern Democratic Republic of Congo: a qualitative study. Glob Public Health. 2017:1–13. https://doi.org/10.1080/17441692.2017.1317009.
33. Levey EJ, Oppenheim CE, Lange BC, Plasky NS, Harris BL, Lekpeh GG, et al. A qualitative analysis of factors impacting resilience among youth in post-conflict Liberia. Child Adolesc Psychiatry Ment Health. 2016;10:26. https://doi.org/10.1186/s13034-016-0114-7.
34. Litrownik AJ, Elder JP, Campbell NR, Ayala GX, Slymen DJ, Parra-Medina D, et al. Evaluation of a tobacco and alcohol use prevention program for hispanic migrant adolescents: promoting the protective factor of parent-child communication. Prev Med. 2000;31:124–33.
35. Maalouf W, Campello G. The influence of family skills programmes on violence indicators: experience from a multi-site project of the United Nations Office on Drugs and Crime in low and middle income countries. Aggress Violent Behav. 2014;19(6):616–24. https://doi.org/10.1016/j.avb.2014.09.012.
36. Marsiglia FF, Ayers SL, Baldwin-White A, Booth J. Changing Latino adolescents' substance use norms and behaviors: the effects of synchronized youth and parent drug use prevention interventions. Prev Sci. 2016;17(1):1–12. https://doi.org/10.1007/s11121-015-0574-7.
37. Massad SG, Shaheen M, Karam R, Brown R, Glick P, Linnemay S, Khammash U. Substance use among Palestinian youth in the West Bank, Palestine: a qualitative investigation. BMC Public Health. 2016;16:800.
38. McCleary JS, Shannon PJ, Cook TL. Connecting refugees to substance use treatment: a qualitative study. Soc Work Public Health. 2016;31(1):1–8. https://doi.org/10.1080/19371918.2015.1087906.
39. McDonald L, Doostgharin T. UNODC global family skills initiative: outcome evaluation in Central Asia of Families and Schools Together (FAST) multi-family groups. Soc Work Soc Sci Rev. 2013;16(2):51–75.
40. Murray LK, Skavenski S, Kane JC, Mayeya J, Dorsey S, Cohen JA, et al. Effectiveness of trauma-focused cognitive behavioral therapy among trauma-affected children in Lusaka, Zambia: a randomized clinical trial. JAMA Pediatr. 2015;169(8):761–9. https://doi.org/10.1001/jamapediatrics.2015.0580.

41. Nagata JM, Hathi S, Ferguson BJ, Hindin MJ, Yoshida S, Ross DA. Research priorities for adolescent health in low- and middle-income countries: a mixed-methods synthesis of two separate exercises. J Glob Health. 2018;8(1):010501. https://doi.org/10.7189/jogh.08.010501.
42. National Institute on Alcohol Abuse and Alcoholism. Alcohol screening and brief intervention for youth: a practitioner's guide. Bethesda: NIAAA; 2012.
43. National Institute on Drug Abuse. Principles of adolescent substance use disorder treatment: a research-based guide. Rockville: National Institute of Health; 2014.
44. Papas RK, Sidle JE, Gakinya BN, Baliddawa JB, Martino S, Mwaniki MM, et al. Treatment outcomes of a stage 1 cognitive-behavioral trial to reduce alcohol use among human immunodeficiency virus-infected out-patients in western Kenya. Addiction. 2011;106(12):2156–66. https://doi.org/10.1111/j.1360-0443.2011.03518.x.
45. Pengpid S, Peltzer K, Van der Heever H, Skaal L. Screening and brief interventions for hazardous and harmful alcohol use among university students in South Africa: results from a randomized controlled trial. Int J Environ Res Public Health. 2013;10(5):2043–57. https://doi.org/10.3390/ijerph10052043.
46. Petruzzi LJ, Pullen SJ, Lange BCL, Parnarouskis L, Dominguez S, Harris B, et al. Contributing risk factors for substance use among youth in postconflict Liberia. Qual Health Res. 2018;28(12):1827–38. https://doi.org/10.1177/1049732318761863.
47. Posselt M, McDonald K, Procter N, de Crespigny C, Galletly C. Improving the provision of services to young people from refugee backgrounds with comorbid mental health and substance use problems: addressing the barriers. BMC Public Health. 2017;17(1):280. https://doi.org/10.1186/s12889-017-4186-y.
48. Pullen SJ, Petruzzi L, Lange BC, Parnarouskis L, Dominguez S, Harris B, et al. A qualitative analysis of substance use among Liberian youth: understanding behaviors, consequences, and protective factors involving school youth and the school milieu. Int J Ment Health Psychiatry. 2016;2(1). https://doi.org/10.4172/2471-4372.1000116.
49. Rastegar D, Fingerhood M. The American Society of Addiction Medicine handbook of addiction medicine. New York: Oxford; 2016.
50. Robertson EB, David SL, Rao SA. Preventing drug use among children and adolescents. 2nd ed. Bethesda: National Institute on Drug Abuse; 1997.
51. Salas-Wright CP, Vaughn MG. A "refugee paradox" for substance use disorders? Drug Alcohol Depend. 2014;142:345–9. https://doi.org/10.1016/j.drugalcdep.2014.06.008.
52. Sphere Association. The sphere handbook: humanitarian charter and minimum standards in humanitarian response. 4th ed. Geneva: Sphere Association; 2018.
53. Stanger C, Budney AJ. Contingency management approaches for adolescent substance use disorders. Child Adolesc Psychiatr Clin N Am. 2010;19(3):547–62. https://doi.org/10.1016/j.chc.2010.03.007.
54. United Nations High Commissioner for Refugees, & World Health Organization. Rapid assessment of alcohol and other substance use in conflict-affected and displaced populations: a field guide. Geneva: World Health Organization; 2008.
55. United Nations Office on Drugs and Crime. International standards for the treatment of drug use disorders. UNODC. 2016. Retrieved from http://www.unodc.org/documents/International_Standards_2016_for_CND.pdf.
56. United Nations Office on Drugs and Crime. International standards on drug use prevention, Second updated edition. UNODC. 2018. Retrieved from https://www.unodc.org/documents/prevention/standards_180412.pdf.
57. UNODC. World drug report 2013. United Nations; 2013.
58. Waldron HB, Kaminer Y. On the learning curve: the emerging evidence supporting cognitive-behavioral therapies for adolescent substance abuse. Addiction. 2004;99 Suppl 2:93–105. https://doi.org/10.1111/j.1360-0443.2004.00857.x.
59. West B, Abatemarco D, Ohman-Strickland PA, Zec V, Russo A, Milic R. Project Northland in Croatia: results and lessons learned. J Drug Educ. 2008;38(1):55–70. https://doi.org/10.2190/DE.38.1.e.

60. Widmann M, Apondi B, Musau A, Warsame AH, Isse M, Mutiso V, et al. Comorbid psychopathology and everyday functioning in a brief intervention study to reduce khat use among Somalis living in Kenya: description of baseline multimorbidity, its effects of intervention and its moderation effects on substance use. Soc Psychiatry Psychiatr Epidemiol. 2017;52(11):1425–34. https://doi.org/10.1007/s00127-017-1368-y.

61. Winters KC, Tanner-Smith EE, Bresani E, Meyers K. Current advances in the treatment of adolescent drug use. Adolesc Health Med Ther. 2014;5:199–210. https://doi.org/10.2147/AHMT.S48053.

62. World Health Organization, & United Nations High Commissioner for Refugees. mhGAP Humanitarian Intervention Guide (mhGAP-HIG): clinical management of mental, neurological and substance use conditions in humanitarian emergencies. Geneva: WHO; 2015.

Children and Adolescents with Developmental Disabilities in Humanitarian Settings

12

Vanessa Cavallera, Ramzi Nasir, and Kerim Munir

Background

Introduction and Definitions

Child development is the learning process that every child goes through to enable him/her to master important skills (developmental milestones) for life. These include thinking and cognition, language and communication, and motor skills. Developmental disability (DD) is an umbrella term for an impairment or delay of skills in the above domains usually due to lifelong conditions that are acquired in childhood. A person is considered carrying a disability when they have difficulties functioning or participating in normal daily activities (which can be due to the severity of their condition, lack of appropriate supports, inappropriate social attitudes, or government policies) [1].

This chapter is aimed primarily at humanitarian workers in all sectors (including health, mental health, social services, protection, or education) who come into direct contact with children and families, or who are sought when concerns about development are raised.

Significance of the Problem and Unique Vulnerabilities

Reliable measurements of the number of children with DD are lacking but are estimated to range between 10% and 20% of children globally, with higher

V. Cavallera (✉)
Independent Consultant, Milan, Italy

R. Nasir
Consultant in Developmental Behavioral Pediatrics, London, UK

K. Munir
Boston Children's Hospital, Harvard Medical School, Boston, MA, USA

© Springer Nature Switzerland AG 2020
S. J. Song, P. Ventevogel (eds.), *Child, Adolescent and Family Refugee Mental Health*, https://doi.org/10.1007/978-3-030-45278-0_12

percentages for specific types of DD [2–6]. Among refugee populations, recent records from the Syria crisis estimated that one in five refugees is affected by physical, sensory, or intellectual impairment and that 13.4% of them have intellectual impairment [7, 8]. Despite the presence of a protective legal framework (Box 12.1), children with DD are often a low priority in humanitarian settings and therefore extremely vulnerable to death and injury with long-term implications for the health and well-being.

Box 12.1 Legal Framework: Disability in the Context of Human Rights
Children with disabilities are often discriminated against, and they undergo human rights violations. However, like for any child with a more obvious physical disability, there is a legal framework in place to protect them:

- Convention on the Rights of the Child (CRC) [9]
- Convention on the Rights of Persons with Disabilities (CRPD): promotes, protects, and ensures the human rights for all people with disabilities, with a specific attention to children (Article 7, 23, and 24) [10]
- UN General Assembly Resolution A/65/452 [11]
- WHO Executive Board Report by the Secretariat (EB133/4) Comprehensive and coordinated efforts for the management of autism spectrum disorders [12]
- World Health Assembly (WHA) Resolution WHA67/2014/REC/1 on autism spectrum disorders (WHA67.8) Comprehensive and coordinated efforts for the management of autism spectrum disorders (ASD) [13]
- Charter on the Inclusion of Persons with Disabilities in Humanitarian Action Launched at the World Humanitarian Summit in Istanbul, Turkey (23 and 24 May 2016)

It is important to also remember that there are common cultural misconceptions[1] associated with DD that put these children as well as their families at increased risk of human rights violation and reduced access to services [14–17].

When to Suspect a Child Has a Developmental Disability

Children with DD do not present with a label, and it might take several encounters with a child or family to realize there might be something different about the child (e.g., slower learning than other children of the same age and difficulties in

---

[1] For example, in some cultures, a DD is considered a curse or result of black magic or a punishment for caregivers' actions.

carrying out everyday activities considered normal for the age).[2] Caregivers are usually the first to notice differences in their child's development, and any concerns they express should be taken seriously. In certain situations, caregivers might also play down the child's difficulties for a variety of reasons, and not share their concerns until a certain amount of trust has been built with the worker. Oftentimes, children are brought to professionals because of concerns about behaviors or recurrent health problems without specific mention of the developmental delays.

Common Types of Developmental Disability

Children with Difficulty in Understanding and Thinking Skills (Cognitive Development)

Children with cognitive difficulties may (i) act and play like younger children; (ii) have a reduced understanding and ability to follow requests/instructions than other children; (iii) show reduced independence skills (e.g., eating, dressing, toileting, and taking care of hygiene. For older children: keeping themselves safe, managing their time); and (iv) present learning difficulties in school.[3] However, the above difficulties may have other causes and should not be automatically attributed to reduced cognitive difficulties (see assessment section below).

Children with Communication Difficulties

Children acquire communication skills in a predictable order. These skills include the ability to speak, use nonverbal communication strategies (e.g., eye contact, hand gestures), and the ability to engage socially with others. These skills are acquired early in life through a generally predictable sequence, although there might be cultural variations (Box 12.2). Children are suspected of having communication difficulties when delays are noted in the milestones listed in Box 12.2. Note: The sequences in milestones acquisition outlined in Box 12.2 are from the United States

---

[2] See:

(i) CDC *Developmental milestones* at https://www.cdc.gov/ncbddd/actearly/pdf/checklists/Checklists-with-Tips_Reader_508.pdf

(ii) mhGAP Humanitarian Intervention Guide *Box ID 1: Developmental milestones: warning signs to watch for* (p.44) at http://apps.who.int/iris/bitstream/handle/10665/162960/9789241548922_eng.pdf;jsessionid=71BD9206C489806502219F30861C39E7?sequence=1

(iii) *Where There is No Psychiatrist* at https://www.cambridge.org/core/books/where-there-is-no-psychiatrist/47578A845CAFC7E23A181749A4190B54

[3] Academic difficulties ought not be confused with intellectual disability, even though these may represent warning signs (see section below).

and are based on US population standards. At the time of writing, there are no agreed upon international standards that can be applied globally although there are efforts underway to create them. Additionally, there are variations in timing and quality of the skills that children demonstrate at specific ages which may also vary depending on specific personal characteristics, context and environment, as well as co-occuring conditions. Therefore, we recommend that these milestones are only used to acquaint the reader with trajectories of development, but we caution that they should not be used as a tool to assess children or interview caregivers (see Sect. 13.4.1 below).

Box 12.2 Communication Developmental Milestones [18, 19]

	Social communication	Language
Up to 6 months	Show an interest in looking at faces Responds to other people's emotions Responds to own name Likes to play with others, especially parents	Cooing babbling Copies sounds Vocalizes differently to indicate happiness and unhappiness
By 12 months	Uses simple gestures, like shaking head "no" or waving "bye-bye" Plays games such as "peek-a-boo" and "pat-a-cake" Responds to simple spoken requests	Says "mama" and "dada" and exclamations like "uh-oh!" Says first words
By 18 months	Plays simple pretend, such as feeding a doll Points to show others something interesting Likes to hand things to others as play	Says several single words
By 2 years	Follows simple instructions Gets excited when with other children Points to things or pictures when they are named	Says sentences with two to four words Knows names of familiar people and body parts Repeats words overheard in conversation
By 3 years	Shows affection for friends without prompting Copies adults and friends Plays make-believe with dolls, animals, and people Joins in play with other children	Can name most familiar things Carries on a conversation using two to three sentences
By 4 years	Tells stories Would rather play with other children than by themselves Cooperates with other children and shares Takes turns in games without assistance from an adult	Knows some basic rules of grammar, such as correctly using "he" and "she"

Children with Autism Spectrum Disorder (ASD)   Children with ASD display a wide range of speech and social communication difficulties as the main feature. They additional show a range of odd, repetitive behaviors and interests (Box 12.3).

Box 12.3 Red Flags for Autism Spectrum Disorders [18]

Impairment in social interaction	Lack of/delay in milestones in Box 12.2
Impairment in communication	Lack of/delay in milestones in Box 12.2 Unusual repetitive speech Reduced eye contact and use of gesture
Repetitive behaviors and restricted interests	Repetitive movements with objects (e.g., spinning or lining up objects) Repetitive movements or posturing of body (e.g., hand flapping) Unusual sensory exploration Excessive interest in particular toys or activities
Emotional regulation	Distress over removing objects or change in routine Difficulty calming when distressed Abrupt shifts in emotional states Unresponsive to interactions
Sensory difficulties	Specific aversion or over attraction to certain smells, tastes, sounds, textures, or visual objects

---

Children with Other Developmental Difficulties

Children with Difficulties in Movement   These are commonly associated with communication and learning difficulties and include difficulties with eating/swallowing, use of hands, and walking. The assessment and management of motor difficulties is a broad topic and beyond the scope of this chapter. Children should be referred to health and therapy specialists for further assessment.

Children with Behavioral or Emotional Difficulties   Children with difficulties communicating or understanding may often feel frustrated, anxious, or depressed. These emotions often present as behavioral challenges, for example, not listening, crying for no reason, fear of separation from caregivers, and aggression to self or others.

Children with Delays in Multiple Domains   Some children may present with various combinations of the above categories.

Assessment

In humanitarian settings, assessment decisions must be practical and focus on the most pressing needs of the child and family. Focus on what you can do for the child and family within your abilities, and what requires referral, keeping in mind what additional needs might arise. A clinical diagnosis is not usually necessary or feasible in this setting and should only be made by a *trained* clinician.

Caregiver Interview

Often caregivers notice that the child is having some difficulties, but they may not be able to detect the specific problem or where to get help. This is particularly true for milder cases of children with DD. Caregivers should be asked about their concerns and any acute or pre-existing situation as well as current needs [20]. Paying attention to addressing the caregiver's worries and concerns during the assessment is important to also build a partnership with the caregiver and alleviate their anxiety. Therefore, sufficient time should be allocated to conduct the assessment and discuss its outcome. It is important to keep in mind that DDs are a sensitive topic in many settings, and the humanitarian workers should be aware of common community beliefs around these issues and how to sensitively talk about them without labelling or stigmatizing any child.

We recommend an open-ended conversational style to enquire about caregiver concerns. For example, it is better to ask: "Do you have concerns or worries about how your child communicates?", rather than "How many words does your child know?" This type of questioning allows the caregiver to share their concerns openly and provides better understanding of the child's difficulties in the context of their own culture and environment. These questions can also be asked in comparison with other children of the same age in the same country. Asking about specific milestones in a checklist manner can provide misleading information (either falsely reassuring or causing unwarranted alarm). This approach is particularly important for those who do not have training in assessing children's development. In cases where the humanitarian worker is not familiar with the local language or culture, it is essential to use local, culturally competent interpreters to avoid misunderstandings and cultural biases. Based on the responses, general advice can be given to the family (see below) or make professional referrals.

Direct observation of the child (e.g., his/her interactions with adults or other children and with the humanitarian worker) can also be helpful but should be interpreted with caution as children may behave differently in different environments

Example of questions to caregivers of children can be found in Box 12.4.

Box 12.4 Example of Questions to Caregivers of Children [21]

Do you have concerns about your child's behavior, communication, interactions, self-care skills, etc.?
Is your child behaving like others of the same age?
How much help is the child currently receiving to do daily activities (depending on the age of the child, e.g., dressing, toileting, feeding, helping with chores, schoolwork)?
How does your child communicate with you?
Is the child able to ask for what he/she wants?

Younger children	Older children/adolescents*
Does the child smile at you? Does the child react to his/her name? How does the child talk to you?	Is the child able to help in and carry out everyday household activities [give examples appropriate to the context]?
What kinds of things can your child do alone (sitting, walking, eating, dressing, or toileting)?	Is the child going to school? How is she/he doing in school? Is she/he able to finish the schoolwork?
How does your child play? Is your child able to play well with other children of the same age?	Does the child often have difficulties in school because she/he cannot understand or follow instructions?
	Is there one particular subject in which she/he is weaker?
	*These questions can and should also be asked directly to the child/adolescent if his age and developmental stage allow

Direct Child Assessment

If possible and appropriate to your role, the child should also be assessed directly by following communication tips in Box 12.5.

Box 12.5 Practical Tips for Approaching and Communicating with Children with Developmental Disabilities [20, 22, 23]
Environment

- Ensure a private/separate space for the child and his/her family (protected from unexpected stimuli).
- Use signs and communication materials that are understandable to all.

Communication with the child

- Identify a caregiver or a community member who can facilitate communication with the child.
- Be patient.
- Do not make assumptions and confirm that you understand what the child has expressed.
- Give clear instructions in a calm voice with a positive attitude (calm and soft-spoken demeanor).
- Give clear details about changes in schedules and places.
- Communicate in an accessible way (e.g., by using drawings or objects, using simple words).

Basic Health Assessment Hearing and vision impairment may often contribute to learning and communication difficulties and can be assessed following simple steps (Box 12.6)

Box 12.6 Assessing the Child for Visual and/or Hearing Impairment [21, 24]

For vision assessment, see if the child fails to:	For hearing assessment, see if the child fails to:
Look at your eyes	Turn head to see someone behind them
Follow a moving object with the head and eyes	when they speak
Grab an object	Show reaction to loud noise
Recognize familiar people	Make a lot of different sounds (Tata, dada, baba), if an infant
If the child is not able to do the above refer the child to a specialist (if available)	

If *trained health-care professionals* are available, a comprehensive developmental history should be collected, and children should be assessed for co-occurring health conditions that might be treatable (e.g., malnutrition, epilepsy, anemia, thyroid disease, chronic infections) or that might recur in the family (e.g., genetic condition or recurrent environmental exposures during pregnancy). As DD are chronic conditions, lifelong health monitoring is important to assess changes in functioning and secondary health problems [25]. It's important to also note that children with difficulties communicating or understanding may present with:

- Malnutrition, obesity, dental, and digestive difficulties (constipation or diarrhea): due to poor feeding, a restricted diet, or eating non-food objects
- Accidental or non-accidental injury due to maltreatment or low safety awareness
- Late diagnosis of treatable conditions due to difficulty reporting symptoms or neglect by caregivers

Assessment of Trauma Reactions

Children with DD are more vulnerable to mental health difficulties, including symptoms of anxiety and depression. Additionally, in humanitarian settings, it is important to be aware of specific ways such children react to trauma (Box 12.7).

Box 12.7 Understanding Trauma Responses in Children with Developmental Disabilities	
Disproportionate impact of loss, grief, and traumatic exposure of children with DD	Children with DD are more likely than other children to experience post-traumatic reactions Children with DD may perceive events such as multiple relocations, loss of school, loss of teacher, and loss of a pet as equivalent to death: they are therefore more vulnerable to "traumatic grief" [26] Children with DD face challenges in talking about their loss especially in the context of cognitive limitations in finding meaning from their loss [26, 27] Separation and loss of primary caregivers is also associated with destabilizing impact of secondary changes in the child's living conditions and how the child is nurtured → It is important to provide consistent attachment figures to provide comfort and alleviate distress

Misconceptions	Children with DD
	  Are not capable of emotional insight and less likely to suffer from trauma
	  Are more likely to forget trauma
	  Who do not use speech cannot be in treatment in psychotherapy or trauma-focused cognitive behavioral therapies (TF-CBT)

Environmental Assessment

The contextual and environmental situation of the child and his/her family should also be assessed, with particular attention to exploring: (i) ongoing exposure to violence, maltreatment, and risks to the child/adolescent (see Box 12.8); (ii) opportunities for the child/adolescent to play or participate in family, community, and social life; and (iii) caregivers' needs [21]. Lastly, in the assessment phase, it is crucial to look beyond the child and his/her family, by also mapping all support, resources, and services available to the child and the family [22].

Assessing the Impact of the Humanitarian Context It is also essential to remember that conflict, disaster, and displacement have an impact on pre-existing DD. These consequences (Box 12.9) should be considered during the assessment and management set up to mitigate them.

Box 12.8 Exposure to Violence or Maltreatment
Individuals with DD are at high risk for maltreatment or abuse that can occur in various forms:

Physical: for example, using physical violence
Sexual: for example, sexual activity with a child
Emotional: for example, making a child feel worthless or unloved
Neglect: for example, failing to keep a child healthy, clean, or sending them to available educational settings

Signs of maltreatment or abuse can be obvious or subtle: for example, physical injuries, sexually transmitted disease, pregnancy, or behavioral changes (e.g., withdrawal, aggression, sexualized behaviors, self-harm)

Box 12.9 Additional considerations in Humanitarian Contexts [20, 22, 23, 28, 29]
- Fewer established relationships and therefore disproportionate unfavorable response to any loss or injury of key figures
- Increased level of dependency on others
- Difficulties removing themselves from harm and anticipate danger and warning signs
- Difficulties in recognizing and expressing additional injuries or conditions developed during/after the humanitarian situation
- High vulnerability to unusual and unexpected stimuli occurring in emergency situations
- Difficulties in coping with the humanitarian emergency and adapting to new living environments
- More pronounced and more protracted symptoms of grief and bereavement (discussed in other parts of this book) compared to other children in these situations
- Greater neurobiological vulnerability to psychological stress and development of heightened anxiety states
- Lack of protective networks due to break down of families and social system with resulting greater risks of violence, exploitation, abuse, and even death
- Harsher family conditions due to increased difficulties in accessing humanitarian aid and support/supplies (full-time supervision of child needed, stigma and consequent hiding of the child, specific supplies needed for extreme preferences)

- Exclusion from mainstream humanitarian interventions
- Significant decline in adaptive behavior, communication, and socialization skills during the weeks following the humanitarian crisis and aggravation of underlying disability and symptoms (hyperactivity and impulsiveness, inattentiveness, fussiness, and peculiar behaviors) with consequences on both the child (e.g., failure to obtain necessary information and increased dependence) as well as others (e.g., violent outbursts) due to the unstable surroundings and lack of medications
- Regression to previous developmental stages (as with children with no disabilities or children with pre-existing DD)

Management and Practical Tips

Sometimes in camp or resettlement settings, children may actually be able to access better services than they were able to in their places of origin [30]. Therefore, the transition from an emergency phase to a more stable situation (Box 12.10) can provide opportunities for children with DD and ensuing mental health services in general. The identification of children with DD is critical for service provision but also for the development of policies and strategic planning [3]. Moreover, humanitarian workers need to be aware of the local perceptions of DD and sensitive to their own biases to ensure these children and their families are protected and supported in the right way.

Box 12.10 General Management of Developmental Disability by Emergency Phase in a Humanitarian Crisis

Emergency phase

Use accessible warning systems and safety procedures
Make the child feel safe by facilitating stability of the adults around them and of the fundamental elements of daily life (e.g., environmental safety, food, clothing, and shelter)
Support adaptation of children with DD to the new situation and changing environments
Provide, as feasible, partitioned-off spaces or private rooms in temporary housing
Link children and caregivers with services and activities
Avoid exposure to broadcasts of the emergency situation to the extent possible
Identify a focal point for disability that will support the mainstreaming of the inclusion of persons with disabilities throughout the humanitarian response and address specific needs (e.g., ensure accessible camps and services) [22, 23, 31]

Post-emergency phase

Activate community resources and community-based protection for children with DD [23]
Ensure children with DD have access to "child friendly" safe areas where they can feel comfortable, move around, and play freely [21]

Child- and Caregiver-Focused Interventions

The provision of early interventions and supports should focus on both the family and the child. The caregivers are the key partners for delivering interventions and providing support to children with DD. After the assessment and the identification of the child's needs, learning about available resources and services is the first step to understand what you can do to support these families and where you might refer them if needed. The following are practical tips that can help in providing support to children with DD and their families [21, 24, 25]:

- Avoid giving the child a specific label or diagnosis. At the stage of intervention, it is important for the non-specialist humanitarian worker to recognize that DD is a possibility, share that information with the family, and provide basic support.
- Address the psychosocial impact of the child's disorders on the caregiver.
- Praise the caregiver and the children for their efforts and strengths.
- Link caregivers with supporting services and networks (parent groups, peer support, etc.), respite care (center-based, home-based, community-based, or any combination), and/or support primary caregivers in burdening chores to allow them to care for the child [23].
- Explain that children with DD should not be blamed for having a disability.
- Offer ideas about how caregivers can help their children learn (Box 12.11).
- Link the child and the family with recreation services (to include children in regular programs, and/or targeted activities as depending on context).
- Recognize urgent situations and seek appropriate consultation (e.g., a child who is being maltreated or deteriorating over time).

If services and capacity is available:

- Link caregivers with places/services where they can go for advice.
- Link caregivers with provision of counselling.
- Linking caregivers with provision of therapy and education to maximize the child's function and skills.
- Link caregivers with parent skills trainings or other brief psychological treatments. An important resource currently piloted in a variety of settings (including humanitarian settings) is the WHO's Caregiver Skills Training program [32].
- Teach caregivers stress management.[4]

---

[4] One simple exercise is to breathe into a count of 4, hold it in for 8, and breathe out 8. Repeat this cycle 3 times.

Box 12.11 Advice to Caregivers to Support Their Children [20–22, 24, 33]

Well-being and parenting	• Spend time with the child in enjoyable activities • Play and communicate with the child • Show understanding and respect • Have realistic expectations and be supportive • Protect the child from any form of maltreatment and abuse • Anticipate further major life changes and provide support
How to manage the child	• Get to know the child well (what makes them happy, what stresses them, what are their strengths and weaknesses) • Give loving attention, including engaging and playing with the child every day • Facilitate return to predictable daily routines (regular sleeping, play, etc.) in spite of the disruption that occurred • Learn how the child communicates and responds (using words, gestures, non-verbal expression, and behaviors) • Be aware of general hygiene • Assign simple tasks to do to the child that match their ability level, one at a time, and break complex activities down into simple steps (reward the child at every step) • Ensure the child attends school/community activities setting as much as possible

Addressing challenging behaviors	• Be consistent about what the child is allowed and not allowed to do
	• Give clear, simple, and short instructions
	• Praise or reward the child when you observe good behavior, and distract him/her from things they should not do
	• Give no reward when behavior is problematic, or punish mildly (e.g., withholding rewards and fun activities)
	• Put off discussions with the child until you are calm
	• Avoid using criticism, yelling, and name-calling
	• Use time-out: when the child misbehaves, tell him/her to go away (e.g., to another room) and come back after a prescribed amount of time
	  – It should not be explained as a punishment but as a negative consequence of the child's disruptive behavior
	  – The place chosen should not be fun or interesting (e.g., a bedroom full of toys), and the time period should, as a simple rule, not be more than the age of the child in minutes (so a 7-year-old should have a 7-min period)
	  – It is important to talk to the child after the "time-out" period and discuss why she/he needed to have "time-out," which behavior led to him/her having "time-out" and ways in which they could avoid this in the future

Teaching self-care and communication techniques	• Support children and adolescents in developing a book, a board, or cards with pictures or drawings related to daily activities, feelings, and items (like utensils, favorite games, or whether they are feeling hot or cold), so they can use it to communicate their needs or desires • Use objects that represent different activities to support the child's understanding and ability to anticipate what will come next and help build routine

Interventions to Support Child in the Community

Reach out to children with DD and their families directly to ensure inclusion Children with DD are often hidden within communities and may need extra support to access services and activities due to security or to attitudinal and environmental barriers [34]. However, the United Nations Convention on the Rights of Persons with Disabilities (CRPD) requires States Parties to ensure that persons with disabilities are protected in situations of risk or humanitarian crisis [10]. Their inclusion in routine humanitarian programming is critical and should not be something "special" or separate. Special attention should be placed in the education settings and other activities in the community (such as child friendly spaces that are widely used in humanitarian settings to provide a temporary, safe environment in which children can experience a supportive and developmentally appropriate setting in situations of extreme adversity) [35–37]. In practice, however, despite calls for such activities to be made inclusive for all children, these interventions are rarely accessible for children with developmental disabilities. Children with disability of all ages benefit and have the right to attend educational settings: do enquire about educational and early childhood education settings and assure child is able to attend those.

Use participatory approaches Children with DD and their families should be involved in program design and evaluation to understand their needs and interests and to develop strategies to overcome barriers to participation. These approaches may include ranking exercises, photo elicitation and story-telling, as well as qualitative methods (e.g., focus group discussions and one-on-one interviews) [34]. These consultations also contribute to the children's empowerment by recognizing the critical value of their inputs and their role as active contributors to their community.

Build on strengths and minimize vulnerabilities Children with DD have strengths and vulnerabilities like any other child which may be overlooked when focusing on the disability-related traits only. Children with DD rarely think of themselves as disabled and aspire to fulfil their own dreams and to participate in normal family and community life [3]. Enabling them to be part of decision-making processes and leading activities increases their confidence and promotes development of life and leadership skills [34].

Advocate for the needs of children with DD and sensitize communities on such issues It is important for humanitarian workers to promote understanding among the surrounding communities to allow for acceptance of the individual and his/her family [20]. Advocacy approaches include meeting with relevant stakeholders, lobbying, meeting with communities, training persons with disabilities in representation, producing awareness raising materials, using media such as radio, public gatherings, letter writing campaigns, bottom-up community-driven approaches, collaboration with influential organizations, and gaining support from experts and international institutions [30]. Specific awareness campaigns should also be promoted among public and private institutions, in order to identify and train stakeholders [23].

Promote a healthy and nurturing environment for all children Children should be surrounded by a stable environment that ensures children's good health and nutrition, protects them from threats, and gives young children opportunities for early learning, through interactions that are emotionally supportive and responsive[5] [18].

Explore existing systems of care and policies The multidisciplinary needs of children with DD require coordination and collaboration between different professionals, organizations, and sectors (e.g., health, social care, education, and mental health). On a systems level, different sectors and organizations need to develop policies and procedures that facilitate external collaboration. On an individual level, professionals working with children with DD and their families need to develop an understanding of the vast network of organizations and professionals available in the local context. It is important to discuss what is typically done to support children and what services and policies exist. As the needs of children with DD are often neglected, humanitarian workers often will need to advocate for these individuals for both adherence to policies and access to services. This should be considered an essential part of planning (e.g., in this regard, it may be important to consider having a separate individual in charge of advocacy).

Collect data on children and adolescent with developmental disabilities (and all disabilities in general) In order for advocacy efforts to be successful, data on persons with disabilities should be collected and introduced in routine data collection processes, and the surveillance system should be strengthened in this direction [8, 22]. Monitoring and reporting procedures on violations against children should also include specific data on children with DD who are more at risk of violence, abuse, and trafficking [30]. Lack of accurate data on their number and locations adversely affects the strategic planning and placement of those children in both general and specialized prevention, intervention, and general support [8].

---

[5] See:

(i) Nurturing Care Framework at http://www.who.int/maternal_child_adolescent/child/nurturing-care-framework/en/
(ii) Care for Child Development Package at https://www.unicef.org/earlychildhood/index_68195.html

Facilitate resettlement of children and families with DD It is important for humanitarian workers to be aware of regulations for fast-tracking asylum procedures for refugee children with DD and their families with DD. Humanitarian workers should also make sure, in case asylum is granted, that all medical and other relevant information follow the child to destination to help the child access services during resettlement.

Follow-Up and Referral

Humanitarian workers should refer children to specialists for further assessment and advice on management plan if [20, 21]:

- There is no improvement
- Symptoms gradually deteriorate
- Physical health is affected
- There is predicted danger to the child

Acknowledgments We'd like to acknowledge for review of chapter Dr. Karen Olness (Case Western Reserve University), Dr. Daniel Martinez Garcia (Medecins Sans Frontieres), Dr. Ana Maria Tijerino (Medecins Sans Frontieres), Dr. Ilgi Ertem (Ankara University), as well as the review and encouragement of Dr. Judy Palfrey (Boston Children's Hospital, Harvard University)

References

1. World Health Organization (WHO). International classification of functioning, disability and health: children and youth version. Geneva: WHO; 2007.
2. World Health Organization. Autism spectrum disorders. Fact Sheet [Internet]. WHO; 2017 [cited 2017 Dec 18]. Available from: http://www.who.int/mediacentre/factsheets/autism-spectrum-disorders/en/.
3. World Health Organization (WHO). Early childhood development and disability: a discussion paper. Geneva: WHO; 2012.
4. Maulik PK, Mascarenhas MN, Mathers CD, Dua T, Saxena S. Prevalence of intellectual disability: a meta-analysis of population-based studies. Res Dev Disabil. 2011;32(2):419–36.
5. Munir KM. The co-occurrence of mental disorders in children and adolescents with intellectual disability/intellectual developmental disorder. Curr Opin Psychiatry. 2016;29(2):95–102.
6. Matson JL, Kozlowski AM. The increasing prevalence of autism spectrum disorders. Res Autism Spectr Disord. 2011;5(1):418–25.
7. HelpAge International. Hidden victims of the Syrian crisis: disabled, injured and older refugees. 2014.
8. Jabri S. The children with autism spectrum disorders in Syrian crisis: challenges and recommendations. Int J Emerg Ment Health Hum Resil. 2015;17(4):676–7.
9. United Nations. Convention on the rights of the child [Internet]. 1989 [cited 2018 Nov 22]. Available from: https://www.ohchr.org/en/professionalinterest/pages/crc.aspx.
10. United Nations. Convention on the rights of persons with disabilities (CRPD) [Internet]. New York; 2006 [cited 2018 Nov 22]. Available from: https://www.un.org/development/desa/disabilities/convention-on-the-rights-of-persons-with-disabilities.html.

11. United Nations. Promotion and protection of the rights of children: report of the third committee. In: Sixty-fifth General Assembly of the United Nations (A/65/452) New York [Internet]. 2010 [cited 2018 Nov 22]. Available from: http://www.un.org/en/ga/third/65/reports.shtml.

12. World Health Organization. Comprehensive and coordinated efforts for the management of autism spectrum disorders. In: Executive Board, 133rd session (EB133/4). Geneva; 2013 Apr.

13. World Health Organization. Comprehensive and coordinated efforts for the management of autism spectrum disorders. In: Sixty-seventh World Health Assembly (WHA67/2014/REC/1). Geneva; 2014 May.

14. Al-Salehi SM, Al-Hifthy EH, Ghaziuddin M. Autism in Saudi Arabia: presentation, clinical correlates and comorbidity. Transcult Psychiatry. 2009;46(2):340–7.

15. Baker DL, Miller E, Dang MT, Yaangh C-S, Hansen RL. Developing culturally responsive approaches with southeast Asian American families experiencing developmental disabilities. Pediatrics. 2010;126(Suppl 3):S146–50.

16. Ravindran N, Myers BJ. Cultural influences on perceptions of health, illness, and disability: a review and focus on autism. J Child Fam Stud. 2012;21(2):311–9.

17. Soltani S, Takian A, Akbari Sari A, Majdzadeh R, Kamali M. Cultural barriers in access to healthcare services for people with disability in Iran: a qualitative study. Med J Islam Repub Iran. 2017;31:51.

18. Centers for Disease Control and Prevention (CDC). Milestones checklists [Internet]. CDC; 2018 [cited 2018 Nov 6]. Available from: https://www.cdc.gov/ncbddd/actearly/pdf/checklists/Checklists-with-Tips_Reader_508.pdf.

19. NHS Foundation Trust. Social Communication Developmental Milestones Final.pdf [Internet]. [cited 2018 Nov 6]. Available from: https://www.humber.nhs.uk/Downloads/Services/Childrens%20therapies/SLT/Milestones/Social%20Communication%20%20Developmental%20Milestones%20Final.pdf.

20. Nakamura K, editor. Key points for supporting children/persons with developmental disorders in disasters. A guide for everyone on how to respond to persons with developmental disorders. Vol. rehabilitation manual 32. Japan: National Rehabilitation Center for Persons with Disabilities. Collaborating Centre for Disability Prevention and Rehabilitation; 2016.

21. World Health Organization, Mental Health Gap Action Programme, World Health Organization. mhGAP Intervention Guide for mental, neurological and substance use disorders in non-Specialized health settings: mental health gap action programme (mhGAP). [Internet]. Version 2.0. WHO; 2016 [cited 2018 Mar 26]. Available from: http://www.ncbi.nlm.nih.gov/books/NBK390828/.

22. UNICEF. Including children with disabilities in humanitarian action: general guidance. UNICEF; New York, USA 2017.

23. Working Table MAECI – RIDS (Italian Network on Disability and Development). Humanitarian aid and disability Vademecum. Ministry of Foreign Affairs and International Cooperation, Directorate General for Development Cooperation (DGDC); 2015 Oct.

24. World Health Organization, United Nations High Commissioner for Refugees. MhGAP humanitarian intervention guide (mhGAP-HIG): clinical management of mental, neurological and substance use conditions in humanitarian emergencies. 2015.

25. Therapeutic Guidelines Limited. Management guidelines: developmental disability [Internet]. Version 3. Melbourne: Therapeutic Guidelines Limited; 2012 [cited 2018 Oct 10]. Available from: https://tgldcdp.tg.org.au/fulltext/quicklinks/management_guideline.pdf.

26. Brickell C, Munir K. Grief and its complications in individuals with intellectual disability. Harv Rev Psychiatry. 2008;16(1):1–12.

27. Gray JA, Abendroth M. Perspectives of US direct care workers on the grief process of persons with intellectual and developmental disabilities: implications for practice. J Appl Res Intellect Disabil JARID. 2016;29(5):468–80.

28. Olness K, Mandalakas A, Torjesen K. How to help the children in disasters. 4th ed. Health Frontiers: Kenyon; 2015.

29. Kerns CM, Newschaffer CJ, Berkowitz SJ. Traumatic childhood events and autism spectrum disorder. J Autism Dev Disord. 2015;45(11):3475–86.

30. Rohwerder BL. Intellectual/developmental disabilities and conflict – advocacy of the forgotten [Master of arts in post-war recovery studies]. [New York]: University of York. Post-War Reconstruction and Development Unit – Department of Politics; 2011.

31. Rohwerder B. Intellectual disabilities in humanitarian assistance policy and practice: the need to consider the diversity within disability. In: Mitchell D, Karr V, editors. Crises, conflict and disability ensuring equality. 1st ed. London: Routledge; 2014.

32. Tekola B, Girma F, Kinfe M, Abdurahman R, Tesfaye M, Yenus Z, et al. Adapting and pre-testing the World Health Organization's Caregiver Skills Training programme for autism and other developmental disorders in a very low-resource setting: findings from Ethiopia. Autism. 2019;16:1362361319848532.

33. Valenti M, Di Giovanni C, Mariano M, Pino MC, Sconci V, Mazza M. L'autismo nel post-terremoto: l'esperienza dell'Aquila come base per una linea guida operativa. Epidemiol Prev. 2016;40(2):49–52.

34. Women's Refugee Commission. Including adolescent girls with disabilities in humanitarian programs: principles and guidelines [Internet]. New York; 2015 Sep [cited 2018 Sep 13]. Available from: https://www.womensrefugeecommission.org/images/zdocs/Girls-w-Disabilities-Principles%2D%2D-Guidelines.pdf.

35. Alliance for Child Protection in Humanitarian Action, editor. Standard 10: mental health and psychosocial distress. In: Child protection minimum standards in humanitarian action. 3rd ed: Alliance for Child Protection in Humanitarian Action; 2019.

36. Inter-Agency Standing Committee. Inter- Agency Standing Committee guidelines on inclusion of persons with disabilities in humanitarian action. Geneva: IASC; 2019.

37. Munir K, Ergene T, Tunaligil V, Erol N. A window of opportunity for the transformation of national mental health policy in Turkey following two major earthquakes. Harv Rev Psychiatry. 2004;12(4):238–51.

Severe Mental Disorders and Neuropsychiatric Conditions in Refugee Children and Adolescents

13

Nancy H. Liu and Neerja Chowdhary

Context

The number of refugees has been increasing (United Nations [71]), and over half are under the age of 18 [70]. The refugee experience during youth can significantly impact the development of SMD and ESD, as well as subsequent access to support and resources. We provide an overview of the incidence, risk and resilience factors, and key considerations in the clinical assessment and management of SMDs and ESDs associated with the child and adolescent refugee experience.

Prevalence of SMDs and ESDs in Refugee Children and Adolescents

The Global Burden of Diseases, Injuries, and Risk Factors Study (GBD) produces assessments of prevalence, incidence, and years lived with disability (YLDs) for diseases and injuries for all countries from 1990 to the present [27]. The global prevalence of SMD and ESD in children and adolescents (i.e., defined as those less than 20 years old) from the 2016 GBD report is presented below in Table 13.1.

N. H. Liu (✉)
Department of Psychology, University of California, Berkeley, Berkeley, CA, USA
e-mail: nancy.liu@berkeley.edu

N. Chowdhary
Department of Mental Health and Substance Abuse, World Health Organization, Geneva, Switzerland
e-mail: chowdharyn@who.int

© Springer Nature Switzerland AG 2020
S. J. Song, P. Ventevogel (eds.), *Child, Adolescent and Family Refugee Mental Health*, https://doi.org/10.1007/978-3-030-45278-0_13

Table 13.1 Global prevalence and disability-adjusted life years (DALYs) of SMD in <20 years old

Condition	DALYs (per 100,000)	Prevalence (cases per 100,000)
Schizophrenia	8.4 (5.28–12.79)	12.5 (8.85–17.24)
Bipolar disorder	54.64 (32.69–85.47)	259.58 (195.85–332.71)
Epilepsy	198.53 (157.32–250.51)	343.43 (273.89–425.26)

Severe Mental Disorders

In emergency settings specifically, reviews suggest that among adults, approximately 2% of refugees meet criteria for a psychotic disorder (i.e., schizophrenia, schizoaffective disorders, delusional disorders, or other psychotic disorders) [14]. Another review for protracted refugee settings reports a lifetime prevalence of psychosis in adults around 3.3% [37]. A review for conflict settings that uses a broader category of severe disorders (i.e., schizophrenia and bipolar disorder, as well as severe anxiety, severe post-traumatic stress disorder [PTSD], and severe depression) estimates the point prevalence for adult refugees as 5.1% [9]. As noted in these reviews, significant heterogeneity exists across studies, likely due to sampling and methodological issues, and reliable data on children and adolescents are limited. We do know that children and adolescents who are refugees are about 2 to 4 times more likely to develop psychosis (both affective and non-affective) than those in the general population [3, 28, 47]. Additionally, immigrants have a 2 times risk for non-affective psychosis and about 3 times risk for affective psychosis compared to those without this migration history [62].

Epilepsy and Seizure Disorders

Epilepsy is one of the most common neurological diseases and affects people of all ages, races, social classes, and geographical locations. In 2016, epilepsy accounted for more than 13 million disability-adjusted life years (DALYs) and was responsible for 0.5% of the total disease burden. In children and young adults, epilepsy caused the most burden compared with any other neurological condition as estimated by the GBD study [15].

An analysis of health data from 90 refugee camps across 15 LMICs reported that among children under 5 years of age, epilepsy and seizure disorders (82.74% male/82.29% female) also accounted for the largest proportion of mental, neurological, and substance use disorder (MNS) visits [31]. Children with epilepsy often have coexisting physical or mental health conditions which can increase their health-care needs. Intellectual disability (full-scale intelligence quotient <70 and deficits in adaptive behavior) is the most common comorbidity in children with epilepsy (30–40%). Common mental health comorbidities in ESDs include attention deficit hyperactivity disorder (ADHD), autism spectrum disorder, and depressive and anxiety disorders. Other comorbidities include migraines, sleep problems, and language impairments [76].

Risk and Resilience Factors for SMDs and ESDs in Refugee Children and Adolescents

Being a refugee is not the only nor the most important risk criterion for developing an SMD; rather, a combination of premorbid factors (e.g., family history and/or prior adversity) and exposure to stressors during the refugee experience may lead to development of SMD. Although the etiology of SMD in refugee populations is multifactorial, refugee-specific experiences of adversity, limited material resources, social exclusion, and discrimination may play a critical role in developing SMD and ESDs and ongoing challenges associated with daily functioning. We describe risk factors for SMD followed by those for ESD and end with resilience factors for both SMDs and ESDs among child and adolescent refugees.

Adversity

Children and adolescent refugees face significant adversity which likely influences the development of SMD. The refugee experience often includes multiple adversities and losses that can occur pre-displacement (e.g., poverty in the country of origin), during displacement (e.g., conflict, dislocation, loss of loved ones), and/or resettlement during post-displacement (e.g., difficulty transitioning to a new culture). Although this is described as a linear process, we recognize that millions of refugee youth who are in refugee settlements in LMICs will never be resettled.

Although the majority of displaced children and adolescents demonstrate resilience, about 11% go on to develop PTSD—about ten times more likely than the age-matched general population [14]. Traumatic experiences can increase risk for psychosis in individuals who are refugees, especially within the early post-migratory years for the first generation [51]. In non-refugee populations, this also holds true: acute stress reaction or PTSD diagnoses are associated with a 2.3 to 3.8 times risk for schizophrenia spectrum or schizophrenia disorder and a 4.2 times risk for bipolar disorder, even after controlling for parental mental disorder [50]. There was a 15-fold increase in SMD in the first year after the traumatic stress disorder, and although decreasing over time, risk stayed significant for 5 years [50].

In non-refugee populations, childhood adversity is associated with the later onset of bipolar disorder [19] and substantially increases the risk for psychosis [72]. It is well-documented among non-refugee individuals with SMD, and about 50% of individuals with psychosis reported childhood sexual or physical abuse [55].

Traumatic experiences appear associated with a dose-dependent relationship, with more trauma exposure leading to more disability [66]. Immigrants with refugee status appear more likely to experience psychosis, in part due to violence, conflict, and compounded adversity [52, 67]. Symptoms may be part of the more general stress of uprooting and migration or related to cumulative trauma that may tip an individual toward sufficient risk for developing SMD [51]. For those with family history and genetic predisposition for SMD, stress can affect the neurobiological processes in those already at high risk for psychosis [1]. Thus, adverse experiences appear significantly related to the prevalence of SMD among refugee populations.

Refugee youth are also vulnerable to ongoing adversity *after developing* an SMD. They may be at higher risk for neglect, exploitation, and unreliable access to care [63]. Thus, although adversity is a risk factor for the development SMD, it continues to be a problem even after an SMD diagnosis and into adulthood [46], highlighting the vulnerability of these individuals both before and after an SMD diagnosis.

Social Disadvantage

Although research has explored migration, generational status, refugee status, and ethnic minority status as specific risk factors for developing psychosis [7, 8, 33], one explanation that combines these lines of research is the social defeat hypothesis, which proposes that social disadvantage may explain the effect of migration on psychosis, especially adversity and social exclusion [61]. Social disadvantage experiences common to the refugee experience which increases risk for SMD include social isolation, loss of social and family supports, discrimination and marginalization in the host country, unemployment, scarcity and economic disadvantage, unemployment or interrupted education, lack of stable housing, and poor physical health [10].

Substance Use

The link between cannabis and psychosis is well-documented, and a recent systematic review highlights that higher cannabis use is associated with an increased risk for psychosis [39]. It is possible that cannabis may interact with childhood adversity to lead to psychosis [29]. Cannabis is also linked to manic symptoms, its use associated with a threefold risk of the new onset of manic symptoms [21]. Although less established but not uncommon in refugee populations, khat—a stimulant commonly used in East African and Arab countries—appears relevant to risk for psychosis, especially among those with pre-existing vulnerability [49, 73].

Ecological Models

Multisystem ecological models focus on a comprehensive understanding of the refugee experience, incorporating past adversity, ongoing daily stressors and social disadvantage (e.g., unsafe living environments, inability to meet basic needs, lack of employment/education, isolation from traditional social supports), and background disruptions of core psychosocial systems [63]. In addition to genetic and premorbid adverse factors, the risk factors associated with the refugee experience such as

Table 13.2 Reducing risk for epilepsy and seizure disorders in refugee youth

These potentially preventable causes of epilepsy make it important to focus on reducing epilepsy risk in the following ways:

Risk factor	Prevention
Perinatal risk factors	Adequate perinatal care can reduce new cases of epilepsy caused by birth injury
Central nervous system infections	Prevention and treatment of infectious diseases such as malaria and neurocysticercosis
Traumatic brain injury	Preventing head injury is the most effective way to prevent post-traumatic epilepsy
Fevers	The use of drugs and other methods to lower the body temperature of a feverish child can reduce the chance of febrile seizures

trauma, cannabis use, disadvantaged social status, and environmental factors [54] facing refugee youth may heighten the overall risk of developing SMDs among this population.

Risk Factors for ESDs

Major modifiable risk factors for epilepsy include perinatal risk factors, central nervous system (CNS) infections, and traumatic brain injury (TBI), which, together along with stroke, account for an estimated 25% of epilepsy cases [76]. See Table 13.2 for a list of modifiable risk factors along with practical tips to reduce ESDs in refugee youth.

Perinatal Risk Factors

These include gestational age at delivery, birth weight, maternal health conditions such as nutritional status, pre-eclampsia, the presence and skill of birth attendants, method of delivery, perinatal infection (e.g., human immunodeficiency virus [HIV]), and other adverse events and conditions.

Central Nervous System Infections

These comprise three main categories: bacterial meningitis, viral encephalitis, and neurocysticercosis. Bacterial meningitis and viral encephalitis combined account for approximately 2–3% of epilepsies in HIC and about 5% of epilepsies in LMIC. In some LMIC where the *Taenia solium* (pork tapeworm) is endemic, roughly one-third of epilepsies are attributed to neurocysticercosis. Malaria is one of the most common parasitic diseases worldwide. Its neurological form, known as cerebral malaria, is a potential cause of ESDs in malaria-endemic regions of the world.

Traumatic Brain Injury

TBI is the cause of epilepsy in 4% of cases in LMIC and 5% of cases in HIC. Road traffic injuries, falls, and violence are the most common causes of TBI. The risk of ESDs is higher in people with severe versus mild TBI (increased almost 20-fold).

Resilience Factors for SMDs and ESDs

Several host country factors relate to lower rates of mental disorders. These include being employed, having appropriate and stable living arrangements, and feeling accepted in the host country [6]. As the age of onset for SMDs tends to be around late secondary school or early employment years, children and adolescents with SMD often discontinue their education or never integrate into employment, disrupting social integration. Therefore, continued engagement in the educational and employment processes may be protective. In the early stages of SMD, early engagement with work, social supports, and connection treatment that addressed several domains (e.g., social supports, medication, coping supports, social integration) is associated with good outcomes for those with SMD [32]. In addition, community engagement, employment and education stability, supportive family communication, and religion are also associated with better outcomes and protective against relapse [17, 60].

Challenges and Proposed Solutions to Care Associated with SMDs and ESDs in Refugee Children and Adolescents

There are several challenges associated with care for refugee youth with SMDs and ESDs. These include scarcity, access to basic resources, and barriers to accessing care, even when services are available due to stigma associated with being both a refugee and having an SMD [63]. Therefore, it is helpful for humanitarian workers to become familiar with common reasons for misdiagnoses, cultural frameworks and explanatory models, and the value and limitations of recognizing emerging symptoms and first episodes in refugee youth. WHO, through the mental health Gap Action Programme (mhGAP), has produced guidelines.

for the management of mental, neurological, and substance use conditions. These can be used by non-specialists to provide SMD and ESD care (e.g., nurses or community health workers (CHW) in resource poor areas) [75].

Assessment and Diagnosis

SMDs are commonly misdiagnosed. This might be especially the case among refugee youth, given that the age of onset for SMDs is around late adolescence to early adulthood. Misdiagnoses can include non-recognition (i.e., not diagnosing SMD when it is present), misidentification (e.g., grief as psychosis), and overdiagnosis (i.e., giving a diagnosis when SMD is not present). Recognition of SMDs in refugee children and adolescents can be challenging, as symptoms such as social withdrawal, lack of interest, or anxiety may be early indicators of SMD but also overlap closely with normal developmental reactions to stressful situations.

It is recommended that humanitarian workers use validated and culturally sensitive tools, especially those developed for these settings [74] and those with clear diagnostic criteria and a cultural formulation which incorporates explanatory models of SMD and ESDs [34] to guide diagnosis and reduce biases. Beyond cultural factors, situational factors to consider include psychotic-like symptoms related to trauma exposure that are highly prevalent in low-income, post-conflict settings [64]. Given the accumulation of stressors common to the refugee experience, it is important to recognize comorbidities like extreme stress, grief, anxiety, and depression that are commonly present with SMD and ESD.

Cultural Sensitivity and Explanatory Models

Understanding explanatory models (i.e., attributions of symptoms) can help with overcoming mistrust, stigma associated with SMDs and ESDs, and lack of knowledge of services. For refugee youth in particular, sensitivity to explanatory models is important for improving help-seeking behaviors [58], including increasing adherence and compliance and ability to benefit from treatment [5, 38, 41]. For SMDs, common attributions include (1) supernatural reasons such as demon possession, evil spirits, jinn [35], and witchcraft; (2) psychosocial factors, such as interpersonal stressors, general stressors, and excessive thinking [78]; and (3) biological factors, such as those described by many Western societies. For ESDs, common stigmatizing misconceptions include views that individuals with ESDs are contagious, crazy and possessed by demons, bewitched, or punished by gods [76]. Matching treatments to explanatory models allow them to be culturally meaningful [11] and increase acceptance, engagement, and satisfaction with treatment [41].

If available, interviews should occur in the native language of the patient and include someone familiar with the culture (i.e., a cultural broker) to clarify the cultural context of the problems. And, if using interpreters, sensitivity to confidentiality issues should be prioritized at the outset of interviews. Beyond this, culturally sensitive approaches to assessment [2] include:

- Incorporate the patient and caregivers' explanatory models for symptoms
- Elaborate these explanations for symptoms
- Confirm the diagnosis of SMD and ESD
    - If present, then subsequent connection to treatment
    - If not present, re-interpreting symptoms as due to social vulnerability factors and prominent cultural idioms

Prodrome Symptoms of SMD in Refugee Youth

The age of onset for SMDs is around late adolescence to early adulthood. In one study among refugee youth, the age of onset for psychosis was 21 years [28]. Prodrome symptoms refer to symptoms prior to the onset of SMD. Although prodrome symptoms do not necessarily go on to become SMD and are still under investigation [22], humanitarian workers should be familiar with common prodrome symptoms, especially among those refugee youth with a family history of SMD. Psychosis prodrome symptoms can include deterioration in functioning, unusual thought content, high levels of suspicion or paranoia, social impairment, and substance abuse [1]. Bipolar disorder prodrome symptoms include anxiety and depression, unstable mood (including irritability), and subthreshold or low-level manic symptoms (i.e., shifts in mood and energy). Sleep disturbance appears common among children and adolescents with SMD, which may contribute to emotion regulation and resultant mood [25].

Stigma and Recovery

After diagnosis, patients, family members, and humanitarian workers alike may have views that SMDs are untreatable or associated with a chronic trajectory. For these individuals, it is important to highlight evidence of recovery [4]. For example, more people recover from SMDs than was once previously thought [23, 24], and about 15% of individuals have a single episode of schizophrenia with complete remission [57]. In Europe, 10–20% are employed [40]. Instilling hope and motivation appears associated with better functioning outcomes in young people with SMD [18].

Individuals with SMDs and ESDs are at increased risk of neglect, exploitation, and abuse. Given the limited mental health resources available to refugees and delayed access to care in situations of mass displacement, the WHO's mhGAP community toolkit can be helpful for normalizing SMD and ESD symptoms and mobilizing community and social resources [77]. Developing partnerships with traditional health practitioners may help to reach more people with SMD and ESD and is a strategy to improve access to effective treatment and alter misconceptions and stigmatizing practices.

Access to Medications

Lack of access to medications and fractured medicine supplies is frequent challenges in humanitarian settings. Children with ESDs in particular require regular treatment for many years, sometimes for a lifetime. An abrupt withdrawal of antiseizure medicines can have life-threatening consequences, including status epilepticus. Therefore, it is essential to ensure that access to these medicines is sustained over time to permit uninterrupted treatment.

Providing Care for SMDs and ESD in Refugee Youth: What Can Be Done

We provide some guidance and considerations below to identifying and providing care for refugee youth with SMDs and ESDs, which are aligned with the actions described in the Inter-Agency Standing Committee (IASC) Guidelines [30]. Interventions designed for refugee children should aim to prevent psychological distress and impairment and to promote optimal emotional, social, and cognitive development. We also recognize these are not possible in all settings. The following are recommended principles to keep in mind, and as noted by Silove et al. [63], creative solutions to actual implementation are sorely needed. Below is a brief overview and summary of these principles.

Address Basic Needs and Safety First

- Prioritizing the impact of the post-migration environment is critical. Providing safety, increased access to services, and opportunities to work or study can improve resilience and the general trajectory of children and adolescents [63].
- Coordination of services, both basic and health needs, is especially important for marginalized groups. Providing resources and information to help navigate the system and about entitlements and services can help with connection and may be facilitated through the use of technology.

Implement Culturally Sensitive Outreach

- Outreach programs can prioritize trust and cultural sensitivity to increase access to care. Barriers to care often include language, belief systems, cultural expectations, distrust of the system, and unfamiliarity with the way mental health works [20, 59], and lack of connection to care can lead to increased risk of marginalization.

Integrate Mental Health with Community, Physical Health, and Other Resources

- The provision of mental health and psychosocial support services at the community level needs to be part of broad integrated platforms—population, community, health, social, and educational services—that provide basic services and security, promote community and family support through participatory approaches, and strengthen coping resources. These improve the daily functioning and well-being of individuals with SMD and ESD and protect the most vulnerable from further adversity while also empowering individuals to take charge of their lives and view themselves as valuable members of society. For refugee youth in particular, providing these basic needs, ensuring safety, and being integrated into mainstream society improve outcomes [13].

- Programs can help refugees overcome barriers to physical and mental health care. Multidisciplinary and multilevel approaches that integrate physical and mental health needs are important for this population, given that individuals with SMD live 15–20 years less than the general population [68], and this may be worse in LMICs (e.g., Ref. [16]). Integrating mental health treatment with physical health treatment allows for all services to be provided and may assist with helping to reduce the excess mortality among this population [36].

Facilitate Accurate Diagnoses by Non-specialists

- Assessment guidelines like those in WHO's mhGAP intervention guide for mental, neurological, and substance use disorders for use in non-specialized health settings (mhGAP-IG), version 2.0 [75], can be helpful for the correct identification of SMDs and ESDs.
- For SMD, integrating cultural sensitivity, explanatory models, cultural brokers, caregivers, family history, cumulative adversity, and common prodrome symptoms can reduce misdiagnoses.
- Psychosis may have significant overlap with dissociative disorders, and adversity and psychosis are tightly intertwined; however in general, patients with schizophrenia spectrum disorders on average have more negative symptoms (e.g., withdrawal, lack of interest, isolation) and cognitive deficits, whereas those with dissociative disorders have more dissociative and positive symptoms (e.g., hallucinations, paranoia) and exhibit intact cognitive functions [56]. Both appear implicated in adversity however, and these are reminders of the inherently fuzzy boundaries between diagnoses.
- Bipolar disorder is marked by manic or hypomanic episodes and is often accompanied by depressed moods. Mania refers to an experience that lasts for at least 1 week and is characterized by extremely good, excited, or irritable moods, as well as increased self-confidence, decreased need for sleep, talking faster or more loudly, racing thoughts, distractibility or inability to think clearly, increased goal-directed behavior, feelings of tension and restlessness that can cause excessive physical activity, and excessive involvement in pleasurable activities that may not be safe or responsible (e.g., spending money, risky sexual activity, making decisions quickly without thinking through consequences).
- For ESDs, differentiating seizures from fainting spells or pseudoseizures can reduce misdiagnoses. Fainting spells often are associated with flushing, sweating, pallor, and occasionally a feeling of vision darkening prior to the episode. Pseudoseizures are typically associated with a stress trigger. Episodes are often prolonged and can involve jerking of the body with eyes closed and, unlike an epileptic seizure, rapid return to baseline after the episode.

Provide Effective Mental Health Treatments

- In addition to access to and organization of services, the delivery of effective mental health interventions is important for refugee youth with SMD and ESD [20, 53, 59]. Effective treatments include psychosocial and pharmacological methods as described in the mhGAP-IG, mhGAP humanitarian intervention guide (mhGAP HIG), and mhGAP community toolkit [75, 77].
- Training and supervision programs can help with developing a good understanding of the background and experience of refugee groups and equipping them to provide the best possible advice and treatment in a culturally appropriate manner, given different values systems [45].
- Cognitive behavioral treatments (CBT) can be helpful for SMD [65], especially those in the early stages of the disorder [44]. CBT is also effective for comorbidities like depression and anxiety. Self-help versions of CBT treatment such as problem management plus (PM+) may be helpful among refugee youth [69]. In instances when caregivers may be unavailable, obtain informed consent, and provide treatment to the youth, adapting language to appropriate levels of understanding.

Incorporate Family Support, Employment/Education Support, and General Health Promotion

To the degree possible, try to provide the following support for refugee youth with SMDs:

- Family and caregiver supports are an important component of refugee youth mental health [75]. Good clinical practices include assessing needs of caregivers while also allowing opportunities for the youth to express concerns privately. Family-based promotion programs based on CBT principles and family psychoeducation are effective for SMD [42, 48]. Such programs emphasize healthy family environments and communication skills that are protective and reduce relapse, especially when criticism and hostility are reduced and clear, supportive, validating, and calm environments and communication skills are available.
- Focusing treatment on predictors of social outcomes can be impactful, as clinical outcomes do not always correlate with social outcomes [23]. Factors in SMD that are most predictive of improved outcomes, e.g., negative symptoms (inexpressive faces, monotone speech, lack of motivation) and cognitive symptoms, appear to have the most impact on employment/education, reintegration with society, and social functioning over time [43]. Explore available resources within the family, school, and community.
- Given the high risk of vulnerability for those with SMD and ESD, youth-focused suicide prevention programs [26], substance use programs [12], and protections from victimization and marginalization can be protective of these groups.

- Health promotion for individuals with SMD should focus on:
  - Healthy diet (e.g., increased fruits and vegetables) and scheduling regular exercise through games and physical activity (ideally with supportive others)
  - Sleep that aims for 8 to 9 hours of sleep per night with regular bed and wake times across the week
  - Social integration that includes engagement with school, employment, and regular daily rhythms and schedules that include stress reducing activities
  - Reducing use of substances like tobacco, cannabis, khat, and alcohol which may include social support, replacement activities, and psychoeducation around relapse

References

1. Addington J, Heinssen R. Prediction and prevention of psychosis in youth at clinical high risk. Annu Rev Clin Psychol. 2012;8:269–89.
2. Adeponle AB, Groleau D, Kirmayer LJ. Clinician reasoning in the use of cultural formulation to resolve uncertainty in the diagnosis of psychosis. Cult Med Psychiatry. 2015;39(1):16–42.
3. Anderson KK, Cheng J, Susser E, McKenzie KJ, Kuryak P. Incidence of psychotic disorders among first-generation immigrants and refugees in Ontario. Can Med Assoc J. 2015;187:E279–86.
4. Bellack AS. Scientific and consumer models of recovery in schizophrenia: concordance, contrasts, and implications. Schizophr Bull. 2006;32:432–42.
5. Bhui K, Bhugra D. Explanatory models for mental distress: implications for clinical practice and research. Br J Psychiatry. 2002;181:6–7.
6. Bogic M, Njoku A, Priebe S. Long-term mental health of war-refugees: a systematic literature review. BMC Int Health Hum Rights. 2015;15:29.
7. Bourquet F, van der Ven E, Malla A. A meta-analysis of the risk for psychotic disorders among first- and second-generation immigrants. Psychol Med. 2011;41:897–910.
8. Cantor-Graae E, Selten JP. Schizophrenia and migration: a meta-analysis and review. Am J Psychiatr. 2005;162:12–24.
9. Charlson F, van Ommeren M, Flaxman A, Cornett J, Whiteford H, Saxena S. New WHO prevalence estimates of mental disorders in conflict settings: a systematic review and meta-analysis. Lancet. 2019;394:192–4.
10. Dapunt J, Kluge U, Heinz A. Risk of psychosis in refugees: a literature review. Transl Psychiatry. 2017;7:e1149.
11. Dickson K, Bangpan M. What are the barriers to, and facilitators of, implementing and receiving MHPSS programmes delivered to populations affected by humanitarian emergencies? A qualitative evidence synthesis. Global Mental Health. 2018;5:e21.
12. Elbogen EB, Johnson SC. The intricate link between violence and mental disorder. JAMA Psychiat. 2009;66:152–61.
13. Fazel M, Patel V, Thomas S, Tol W. Mental health interventions in schools in low-income and middle-income countries. Lancet Psychiatry. 2014;1:388–98.
14. Fazel M, Wheeler J, Danesh J. Prevalence of serious mental disorder in 7000 refugees resettled in western countries: a systematic review. Lancet. 2005;365:1309–14.
15. Feigin VL, et al. Global, regional, and national burden of neurological disorders, 1990-2016: a systematic analysis for the Global Burden of Disease Study 2016. Lancet Neurol. 2019;18:459–80.
16. Fekadu A, Medhin G, et al. Excess mortality in severe mental illness: 10-year pouplation-based cohort study in rural Ethiopia. Br J Psychiatry. 2015;206:114.

17. Fleischhacker WF, Arango C, Arteel P, et al. Schizophrenia—time to commit to policy change. Schizophr Bull. 2014;40:S165–94.
18. Fulford D, Piskulic D, Addington J, Kane JM, Schooler NR, Mueser KT. Prospective relationships between motivation and functioning in recovery after a first episode of schizophrenia. Schizophr Bull. 2018;44:369–77.
19. Garno JL, Goldberg JF, Ramirez PM, Ritzler BA. Impact of childhood abuse on the clinical course of bipolar disorder. Br J Psychiatry. 2005;186:121–5.
20. Giacco D, Matanov A, Priebe S. Providing mental healthcare to immigrants: current challenges and new strategies. Curr Opin Psychiatry. 2014;27:282–28.
21. Gibbs M, Winsper C, Marwaha S, Gilbert E, Broome M, Singh SP. Cannabis use and mania symptoms: a systematic review and meta-analysis. J Affect Disord. 2015;171:39–47.
22. Hafeman DM, Merranko J, Axelson D, Goldstein BI, et al. Toward the definition of bipolar spectrum disorders in at-risk youths. Am J Psychiatr. 2016;173:695–704.
23. Harding CM, Brooks GW, Ashikaga T, Strauss JS, Breier A. The Vermont longitudinal studies of persons with severe mental illness, II: long-term outcome of subjects who retrospectively met DSM-III criteria for schizophrenia. Am J Psychiatr. 1987;144:727–35.
24. Harrow M, Grossman LS, Jobe TH, Herbener ES. Do patients with schizophrenia ever show periods of recovery? A 15-year multi-follow-up study. Schizophr Bull. 2005;31:723–34.
25. Harvey AG, Mullin BC, Hinshaw SP. Sleep and circadian rhythms in children and adolescents with bipolar disorder. Dev Psychopathol. 2006;18:1147–68.
26. Hauser M, Galling B, Correll CU. Suicidal ideation and suicide attempts in children and adolescents with bipolar disorder: a systematic review of prevalence and incidence rates, risk factors, and targeted interventions. Bipolar Disorder. 2013;15:507–23.
27. Hay SI, Abajobir AA, Abate KH, et al. Global, regional, and national disability-adjusted life-years (DALYs) for 333 diseases and injuries and healthy life expectancy (HALE) for 195 countries and territories, 1990–2016: a systematic analysis for the Global Burden of Disease Study 2016. Lancet. 2017;390:1260–344.
28. Hollander AC, Dal H, Lewis G, Magnusson C, Kirkbride JB, Dalman C. Refugee migration and risk of schizophrenia and other non-affective psychoses: cohort study of 1.3 million people in Sweden. Br Med J. 2016;352:i1030.
29. Houston JE, Murphy J, Adamson G, Stringer M, Shevlin M. Childhood sexual abuse, early cannabis use, and psychosis: testing an interaction model based on the National Comorbidity Survey. Schizophr Bull. 2008;34:580–5.
30. Inter-Agency Standing Committee. IASC guidelines on mental health and psychosocial support in emergency settings, 2007. 2007. Available at: https://interagencystandingcommittee. org/mental-health-and-psychosocial-support-emergency-settings-0/documents-public/iasc-guidelines-mental. Last accessed 15 Oct 2019.
31. Kane JC, Ventevogel P, Spiegel P, Bass JK, van Ommeren M, Tol WA. Mental, neurological, and substance use problems among refugees in primary health care: analysis of the health information system in 90 refugee camps. BMC Med. 2014;12:228.
32. Kane JM, Robinson DG, Schooler NR, et al. Comprehensive versus usual community care for first-episode psychosis: 2-year outcomes from the NIMH RAISE early treatment program. Am J Psychiatr. 2016;173:4.
33. Kirkbride JB, Barker D, Cowden F, et al. Psychoses, ethnicity and socioeconomic status. Br J Psychiatry. 2008;193:18–24.
34. Kirmayer LJ, Thombs BD, et al. Use of an expanded version of the DSM-IV outline for cultural formulation on a cultural consultation service. Psychiatr Serv. 2008;59:683–6.
35. Lim A, Hoek HW, Blom JD. The attribution of psychotic symptoms to jinn in Islamic patients. Transcult Psychiatry. 2015;52(1):18–32.
36. Liu NH, Daumit GL, Dua T, Aquila R, Charlson F, Cuijpers P, et al. Excess mortality in persons with severe mental disorders: a multilevel intervention framework and priorities for clinical practice, policy and research agendas. World Psychiatry. 2017;16:30–40.
37. Llosa AE, Ghantous Z, Souza R, et al. Mental disorders, disability and treatment gap in a protracted refugee setting. Br J Psychiatry. 2014;204:208–13.

38. Makanjuola V, Esan Y, Oladeji B, Kola L, et al. Explanatory model of psychosis: impact on perception of self-stigma by patients in three sub-Saharan African cities. Soc Psychiatry Psychiatr Epidemiol. 2017;51:1645–54.
39. Marconi A, Di Forti M, Lewis CM, Murray RM, Vassos E. Meta-analysis of the association between the level of cannabis use and risk of psychosis. Schizophr Bull. 2016;42:1262–9.
40. Marwaha S, Johnson S. Schizophrenia and employment – a review. Social Psychiatry and Psychiatric Epidemiology. 2004;39:33–49.
41. McCabe R, Priebe S. Explanatory models of illness in schizophrenia. Br J Psychiatry. 2004;185:25–30.
42. Miklowitz DJ, Scott J. Psychosocial treatments for bipolar disorder: cost-effectiveness, mediating mechanisms, and future directions. Bipolar Disorder. 2009;11:110–22.
43. Milev P, Ho BC, Arundt S, Andreasen NC. Predictive values of neurocognition and negative symptoms on functional outcome in schizophrenia: a longitudinal first-episode study with 7-year follow-up. Am J Psychiatr. 2005;162:495–506.
44. Morrison AP, French P, Stewart SLK, Birchwood M, Fowler D, Gumley AI, et al. Early detection and intervention evaluation for people at risk for psychosis (EDIE-2): a multisite randomized controlled trial of cognitive therapy for at risk mental states. Br Med J. 2012;344:e2233.
45. Mosko MO, Gil-Martinez F, Schulz H. Cross-cultural opening in German outpatient mental healthcare service: an exploratory study of structural and procedural aspects. Clin Psychol Psychother. 2012;20:434–46.
46. Mueser KT, et al. Interpersonal trauma and posttraumatic stress disorder in patients with severe mental illness: demographic, clinical, and health correlates. Schizophr Bull. 2004;30:35–57.
47. Norredam M, Garcia-Lopez A, Keiding N, Krasnik A. Risk of mental disorders in refugees and native Danes: a register-based retrospective cohort study. Soc Psychiatry Psychiatr Epidemiol. 2009;44:1023–9.
48. O'Brien MP, Miklowitz DJ, Candan KA, et al. A randomized trial of family focused therapy with populations at clinical high risk for psychosis: effects on interactional behavior. J Consult Clin Psychol. 2014;82:90–101.
49. Odenwald M. Chronic khat use and psychotic disorders: a review of the literature and future prospects. Sucht. 2007;53(1):9–22.
50. Okkels N, Trabjerg B, Arendt M, Pedersen CB. Traumatic stress disorders and risk of subsequent schizophrenia spectrum disorder or bipolar disorder: a nationwide cohort study. Schizophr Bull. 2017;43:180–6.
51. Parrett NS, Mason OJ. Refugees and psychosis: a review of the literature. Psychosis. 2010;2(2):111–21.
52. Porter M, Haslam N. Predisplacement and postdisplacement factors associated with mental health of refugees and internally displaced persons: a meta-analysis. J Am Med Assoc. 2005;294:602–12.
53. Priebe S, Sandhu S, Dias S, et al. Good practice in health care for migrants: views and experiences of care professionals in 16 European countries. BMC Public Health. 2011;11:187.
54. Radua J, Ramella-Cravaro V, Ioannidis JPA, et al. What causes psychosis? An umbrella review of risk and protective factors. World Psychiatry. 2018;17:49–66.
55. Read J, van Os J, Morrison A, Ross C. Childhood trauma, psychosis and schizophrenia: a literature review with theoretical and clinical implications. Acta Psychiatr Scand. 2005;112:319–45.
56. Renard SB, Huntjens RJC, Lysaker PH, Moskowitz A, Aleman A, Pijnenboarg GHM. Unique and overlapping symptoms in schizophrenia spectrum and dissociative disorders in relation to models of psychopathology: a systematic review. Schizophr Bull. 2017;43:108–21.
57. Rosen K, Garety P. Predicting recovery from schizophrenia: a retrospective comparison of characteristics at onset with people with single and multiple episodes. Schizophr Bull. 2005;31:735–50.
58. Rousseau C, Key F, Measham T. The work of culture in the treatment of psychosis in migrant adolescents. Child Clinical Psychology & Psychiatry. 2005;10:305–17.

59. Sandhu S, Bjerre NV, Dauvrin M, et al. Experiences with treating immigrants: a qualitative study in mental health services across 16 European countries. Soc Psychiatry Psychiatr Epidemiol. 2013;48:105–16.
60. Sariah AE, Outwater AH, Malima KIY. Risk and protective factors for relapse among individuals with schizophrenia: a qualitative study in Dar es Salaam, Tanzania. BMC Psychiatry. 2014;14:240.
61. Selten JP, Booij J, Buwalda B, Meyer-Lindenberg A. Biological mechanisms whereby social exclusion may contribute to the etiology of psychosis: anarrative review. Schizophrenia Bulletin. 2017;43:287–92.
62. Selten JP, van der Ven E, Termorshuizen F. Migration and psychosis: a meta-analysis of incidence studies. Psychol Med. 2019:1–11.
63. Silove D, Ventevogel P, Rees S. The contemporary refugee crisis: an overview of mental health challenges. World Psychiatry. 2017;16(2):130–9.
64. Soosay I, Silove D, Bateman-Steel C, Steel Z, Bebbington P, Jones PB, et al. Trauma exposure, PTSD and psychotic-like symptoms in post-conflict Timor Leste: an epidemiological survey. BMC Psychiatry. 2012;12(1):229.
65. Stafford MR, Jackson H, et al. Early interventions to prevent psychosis: systematic review and meta-analysis. Br Med J. 2013;346:f762.
66. Steel Z, Silove D, Phan T, Bauman A. Long-term effect of psychological trauma on the mental health of Vietnamese refugees resettled in Australia: a population-based study. Lancet. 2002;360:1056–62.
67. Steel Z, Chey T, Silove D, Marnane C, Bryant RA, van Ommeren M. Association of torture and other potentially traumatic events with mental health outcomes among populations exposed to mass conflict and displacement: a systematic review and meta-analysis. J Am Med Assoc. 2009;302:537–49.
68. Thornicroft G. Physical health disparities and mental illness: the scandal of premature mortality. Br J Psychiatry. 2011;199:441–2.
69. Tol WA, Augustinavicius J, Carswell K, et al. Translation, adaptation, and pilot of a guided self-help intervention to reduce psychological distress in South Sudanese refugees in Uganda. Global Mental Health. 2018;5:e25.
70. United Nations High Commission for Refugees (UNHCR). Figures at a glance. 2019. Retrieved from: https://www.unhcr.org/pages/49c3646c11.html.
71. United Nations Office for the Coordination of Humanitarian Affairs. 2019 global humanitarian overview. Geneva: OCHA; 2019.
72. Varese F, Smeets F, Drukker M, et al. Childhood adversities increase the risk of psychosis: a meta-analysis of patient-control, prospective- and cross-sectional cohort studies. Schizophr Bull. 2012;38:661–71.
73. Widmann M, Warsame AH, Mkulica J, von Beust J, et al. Khat use, PTSD and psychotic symptoms among Somali refugees in Nairobi—a pilot study. Front Public Health. 2014;2:1–10.
74. World Health Organization and United Nations High Commissioner for Refugees. mhGAP Humanitarian Intervention Guide (mhGAP-HIG): clinical management of mental, neurological and substance use conditions in humanitarian emergencies. Geneva: WHO; 2015.
75. World Health Organization. mhGAP intervention guide for mental, neurological and substance use disorders in non-specialized health settings: mental health Gap Action Programme (mhGAP)—version 2.0. Geneva: WHO; 2016.
76. World Health Organization. Epilepsy: a public health imperative. Geneva: WHO; 2019. Available at https://www.who.int/mental_health/neurology/epilepsy/report_2019/en/.
77. World Health Organization. mhGAP community toolkit: field test version. Geneva: WHO; 2019.
78. Yang LH, Phillips MR, Lo G, Chou Y, Zhang X, Hopper K. "Excessive thinking" as explanatory model of schizophrenia: impacts on stigma and "moral" status in China. Schizophr Bull. 2010;36:836–45.

Part IV

Transforming Theory into Intervention Programs

What My Grandmother Would Have Taught Me: Enhancing Resilient Behavior in Unaccompanied Young Males in Denmark – A Pilot Project

14

Anne-Sophie Dybdal

Background

In 2015, approximately 5000 refugees and migrants, mainly from Syria and Afghanistan, came to Denmark in 1 week, crossing the border from Germany. This drew massive media and political interest and was the event that, in modern times, became a turning point in the Danish public awareness of the geopolitical context for refugees and migrants in Europe. Public pressure grew on politicians and authorities to strengthen the management of asylum cases, some calling for stricter legislation, others for better quality of services.

The following year, 2016, Danish media focused massively on young male asylum seekers in conflict with Danish law as well as some unfortunate incidents involving conflicts with local populations, and there was a growing public concern about the quality and adequacy of the support provided within the asylum system. This growing focus sparked an interest from Danish government to fund interventions with young unaccompanied asylum seekers, especially for what was seen as troubled, hard-to-reach males.

Based on lessons learnt from international programs, and the Danish refugee response in 2015, Save the Children partnered with the Himmerland Asylum Center and the Danish Immigration Service to design a project which aimed at supporting the well-being of, and address behavior concerns in a group of youth, living in the asylum center while waiting for their asylum application to be processed. It was designed in the fall of 2016 and implemented from January to April 2017. The project was designed as a variation of the Save The Children "Youth Resilience Programme" [14].

A.-S. Dybdal (✉)
Save The Children Denmark, Frederiksberg, Denmark
e-mail: ASD@redbarnet.dk

© Springer Nature Switzerland AG 2020
S. J. Song, P. Ventevogel (eds.), *Child, Adolescent and Family Refugee Mental Health*, https://doi.org/10.1007/978-3-030-45278-0_14

Objective

The overall objective of the pilot project was to address well-being and behavior concerns for the targeted youth. The main focus would be on selected areas of emotional control, decision-making, basic life skills, and skills for navigating the complex stressors of the asylum process, disturbing experiences during the flight and adaptation to Danish society.

The reason for the focus on males was threefold: (1) only 10, 0.29% of the unaccompanied minors in Denmark were female, (2) all reported incidents of clashes with local populations and reports of behavior problems included males, and (3) the partner asylum center only had male residents.

The Youth

All names in this chapter are pseudonyms. The persons quoted have been given a pseudonym that indicates the place of origin. All quotes were noted during the sessions by the program assistant in Danish (it was translated from the mother tongue of the person by professional translator). These are available in the Danish project report. No recordings were made, due to issues of fear in the participants.

About 60 youths were living in the center at the time of the project, and participation in the project was voluntary. Forty of them wished to participate and were subsequently divided into two groups of 20 persons. All participants claimed to be between 14 and 18 years. The team did not question this because age determination is a crucial part of the asylum process, and we could be seen as interfering with the claim for asylum made by the individuals. Many of them dreamt of subsequent family reunification after obtaining asylum. "When I get asylum hopefully my mother and my sisters will come to live with me" (Jawad, 16 years).

85% originated from Afghanistan, others from Somalia, Eritrea, Syria, Iraq, and North Africa. A few had experienced a short journey; others had been on the move for several years. The group of Afghan youth had all passed through Iran, and most of these had been working to pay their way. Some said that they had worked as construction workers, others as farm day laborers; others did not wish to disclose how they had survived. "Bad things happened but now I am safe, God willing" (Saddar, 15 years).

Most had gone to school in their country of origin, at least for a few years. The youth from the Horn of Africa in particular seemed well educated. There were a few in the group who had difficulties reading in their own language and had not gone to school for more than a few years. Three of the participants seemed to have quite serious cognitive impairments and motor skills delays. This was not routinely addressed in the center during the asylum phase but would be part of an integration plan and special needs education plan upon granted asylum.

The team did not have the details of the individual asylum claims and deliberately chose not to screen for post-traumatic stress disorder (PTSD), as this could involve probing into their personal stories and risk interfering with the asylum process. One participant from Somalia had been to prison in Somalia, and when confidence was built with the team and with the group, he disclosed that he had been tortured, rolling up his sleeve and showing the scars from cigarette burns. His testimony resonated with several of the youth.

"I do not trust men, but maybe I trust you...a little bit" (Abdi, 15 years, to male team member).

The project aimed to be inclusive with regard to sexuality, disability, and ethnicity. There were no youth with physical disabilities in the center at the time of the project. None of the young men directly identified themselves as LGBT (Lesbian, Gay, Bi sexual and Transsexual). The team later learned that LGBT youth are commonly offered extra protection and placed in other types of alternative care.

The Center

The asylum center staff was comprised of men and women with diverse backgrounds, but very few with a background in social work, education, or youth programs. All residents had an assigned contact person among the staff, but due to shifts and lack of time, there was not time for lengthy conversations, consistent bedtime routines, or help with tasks such as cooking.

The center was placed in a former boarding school in a remote rural area on the west coast of Denmark, in the middle of farmland and nature. The sea was within walking distance and a forest just outside the door. The inhabitants of the center were allowed freedom of movement, but because of the remote location, the youth depended on center staff for transportation. Trips and events were planned, and some had signed up for sports activities in the nearby community. The youth slept in shared rooms, in bunk beds. There was no supervised bedtime routine, and lights often were turned on all night because of night terrors. Youth complained about noise at night from peers who ran the corridors, unable to sleep.

Twice a week there was an organized shopping trip to town where the youth were expected to use a food allowance to buy food, clothes, and hygiene items.

Some found ways of travelling by bus to the nearby town to go out, also at night to visit discotheques and meet Danish youth. It was in these situations that there have been conflicts with young Danes – especially over girls and behavior that was seen by Danes as provocative and threatening. There is no legal obligation for youth to be chaperoned outside asylum centers. All minors have the right to a mentor/legal guardian, and in our project, those who were lucky enough to have one from the local area that was active and available were sometimes taken for trips and family events. These youth knew more about Danish culture than others and allegedly felt less bored and lonely.

Assessment

Tools

Prior to the project design, an assessment was conducted, using a mixed-method approach that included questionnaires, focus groups, key informant interviews with youth, center staff, and supervisory authority.

The assessment aimed to understand the wellbeing, resources, risks, and resilience of the youth. We also aimed to understand the underlying complexity behind the social dynamics as well as the behaviours and expressions of emotions of the youth.

Questions for the questionnaire were selected from an early version of the pre- and post-assessment tool (PPAT) [13], based on the Child and Youth Resilience Measure (CYRM) [16], and used to monitor and evaluate structured resilience-building interventions in humanitarian responses.

Findings

The assessment process was quite challenging, but although the formal results were difficult to conclude from, our observation of the youth's reaction to the assessment process itself, helped us understand more about their functioning and understanding. There were three main challenges:

1. Many of the youth had never been in a situation where adults had asked them for their opinions or perceptions. "This is strange, I do not remember any older people (meaning adults) asking for my opinion unless they wanted to scold me" (Ruben, 14 years). Practicing verbalizing ideas and experiences became, in itself, a focus in the resilience-building activities.
2. Many had little experience with introspection and reflection. Being asked to reflect on one's own subjective experience requires a meta-cognitive level of abstraction, thinking about thinking so to speak. For the team this was crucial information, and we considered it one of the most important insights for designing the activities. This cognitive skill is the foundation for cracking cultural codes and identifying positive coping mechanisms and critical thinking. Therefore, we selected this skill as a main theme in the workshops.
3. Being asked to reflect on the relative strength of an opinion or experiences was very difficult for most of the group. Some demonstrated an all-or-nothing response, which came across clearly in their communication and behavior patterns. "Susanne is a dumb one, she told me I must go to school. I will never talk to her again" (Hassan, 16 years).

   As the assessment process progressed, it became clear to us that our target group had complex patterns of functioning. They generally came across as street-wise and able to cope with serious adversity but also seemed quite immature in terms of emotional management and interpersonal relationships.

All stakeholders were quite consistent in how they reported the well-being of, risks and protective factors for, the youth. The insecurity of the asylum process was mentioned by all stakeholders as the top source of stress and behavior problems. The uncertainty in the asylum process poses in itself a risk for deteriorating mental health [3]. All stakeholders agreed that boredom and restlessness were also a reason for irritability, and that limited contact with the local population added to the isolation. Staff noted that many residents in the center came across as passive and were late for appointments. "It is as though they have given up" (Søren, 39 years, male staff). The youth themselves reported that it was a lack of sleep that made them late, and they also complained about difficulties in concentration and memory.

Staff, management, and youth all reported that there were regular conflicts, especially among the youth. Staff attributed conflict between youth to culture: "Their culture is very aggressive" (Lone, 27 years, female staff). Conflicts between the youth were commonly explained by youth themselves as a "fair reaction to annoying behavior of others."

Friendships and solidarity between the youth were seen by all stakeholders as a huge resource and protective factor. All participants agreed that friendships provided protection (from bullying) advice, emotional support, and encouragement. Whenever a young person was granted asylum, there was a sense of solidarity and shared joy and relief with the person but also sadness, and the team witnessed goodbyes where the best friends left behind showed strong reaction to separation. "I have said so many goodbyes, it is like someone is holding my head under water" (Hassan, 14 years).

Risks and Protective Factors

Resilience should always be seen in a context – resilient to what? [15]. The project did not see resilience as a personality trait but a set of behaviors, social/emotional experiences, relationships to others, and ability to navigate the risks in their environment. We divided the risks and protective factors into three domains: the environment; the interactions between the youth, as well as between youth and staff; and finally risks that were related to individual functioning.

The Environment

The immediate risks in the environment were described by youth and staff as prejudice and tensions with some parts of the local population, limited opportunities for stimulation and activity, the asylum process in itself, and risks of exploitation. The project was inspired by research pointing to the complex nature of interrelated factors that influence the resilience process in youth, as pointed out for example by Mohammed and Miles (2017) [11]. We learnt that attempts had been made to groom youth by gang members and others from outside the center. Grooming refers to the process where a person in a position of power manipulates a vulnerable person to overstep their boundaries and engage in sexual exploitation, criminal activity, and hazardous labor or other exploitative activity.

A strong protective factor was the mentors/legal guardians who actually spent time with "their" minor. There were also examples of local youth who reached out for friendship. The easy access to nature around the center was also regarded as a resource by staff, management, and social workers, but not by the youth themselves. They actually found nature frightening. The assessment clearly showed that lack of understanding of Danish law and understanding of social norms was a major source of frustration for the youth. Understanding the norms and legal aspects of sexuality, social interaction, gender, work, and private property is imperative to be able to navigate and benefit from social resources. In the questionnaire only 5 out of 40 indicated that they knew where to get help outside the center, although more than 30 agreed or strongly agreed that they knew where to get help for their problems inside the center. Mental health services were available by referral from center doctor to specialized care.

Interactions Between Youth and with Staff in the Asylum Center

An asylum center is in many ways an emotionally and socially complex entity. The youth found great comfort and support in friendships, some of them very intense, some noting that their friend was the only person they trusted in the world. This also made them vulnerable to separation and loneliness. We noted that a youth in crisis needs friends as well as a person that can separate their own feelings from that of the other and provide mature, balanced support. All respondents mentioned the subject of masculinity and sexuality several times, both as a problem and as a resource. The team understood that the risks here were that the masculine role could turn into a stereotype, not allowing the young men to express feelings or seek emotional support outside of their close friendships. "What do you mean talk about it, do I look like a girl?" (Sharif, 16 years). Center management and the social workers speculated that stereotyped gender roles would also create clashes with Danish peers and be an obstacle to interaction and understanding with the local youth.

The team found that stereotypes and clichés were not conducive to positive interaction with staff, who felt provoked and also resorted to their own stereotypes in their interpretation of behavior. "These young men are all trying to be alpha males, domineering and aggressive. I try not to let them win the power struggles they often initiate" (Bo, 41, male staff member).

Sexuality was a key topic. The team observed a range of sexualized behaviors between the boys. It was seen during the assessment and later during the sessions and appeared to be triggered in the group by insecurity and tension. Several of the young men disclosed that adults had "done bad things to them, including touching embarrassing parts of the body" (Ghazan, 14 years). This had happened before, during, and after the flight, so it was not limited to a survival strategy during the travel. For some it highlighted a more profound history of abuse, exploitation, and a "sexual economy" where sexuality was part of the exchange of favors, a way of expressing intimacy, as well as a way to exercise power and dominance. The team was aware that the body image and boundaries of abused youth can be distorted, (Hjort and Harway, 1981) [9] and discussed boundaries and sexuality with staff.

Individual Functioning

As it was not the focus of this project to provide psychological treatment, no psychometric test was used. With a focus on personality traits that have relevance for resilience processes [8], we noted that the group of youth generally appeared as quite robust, with sense of humor, creativity, and quite eloquent problem-solving skills. They also generally were impulsive, with high levels of arousal, suspicious, and aggressive. The team was not able to determine if this could be attributed to the flight and separation from family only or if there was a more profound history of abuse or deprivation in early childhood. The team were aware that the previous quality of parenting, as pointed out by Amstrong et al. (2005), could be the source of some of the maladative behaviour we observed [1]. We tried to avoid labelling them as "traumatized" or victims but at the same time acknowledging that the massive adversity and the risks that they had experienced had affected their personal functioning and ways of interacting with the world around them. A few of the participants were seemingly quite well functioning. During the assessment, almost 85% of youth expressed that they had sad feelings and sleeplessness on a daily basis.

Adjusting the Objective and Intervention Design

A particular challenge when working with "hard-to-reach" youth is to establish trust, create relevance, and build a working relationship. The participants in the group had clearly stated that they did not need "yet another psychologist who wants to talk about the past or fix us." In the Danish asylum system, there is reluctance to apply a trauma-focused intervention while the asylum seeker is still under the immense pressure of the asylum process. The preference is to focus on basic stress and/or grief management and support to coping strategies allowing for possibilities of referrals to special care in cases of mental health concerns, and our approach was in line with this. We decided to build our intervention around the three components: internal resources, interpersonal skills, and basic skills and knowledge needed to master and navigate the context.

The team did its best to maintain a realistic and modest level of expectation to behavior change outcomes, focusing on "small resilient movements" within the domains of resilience that include basic services, sense of belonging, and self-management. This model of practical work to enhance resilient behavior offered by Hart (2017), was used as inspiration to manage expectations and explore how the different domains of resilience for our target group were interlinked. For example, the meals were linked to nutrition education, learning how to cook and also a sense of belonning to the group and managing a role and impulse control in the task [7].

For the group in this project, some of the behaviors and strategies that had helped them survive and make it to Denmark were now an obstacle for their healthy coping and wellbeing. Based on the findings in the assessment, the team decided to design the intervention to address the issues that created the greatest risks (aggressive and impulsive behavior) and strengthen the key resources and protective factors (such as friendship and creative problem solving). As the project progressed, we adjusted and adapted the content and style to ensure that the interventions were relevant and engaging for all the group [10].

Staff members joined the groups to build good working relationships with the youth and to enable them to repeat and follow up on activities outside of the structured sessions, for example, activities in nature and sleep hygiene sessions. Participating in the sessions also gave the staff an opportunity to see the resources and potential in the youth and thus create new narratives about the participants and their motives. Together with the youth, the team chose to apply a variety of methods; some lent from social work using creative methodologies.

1. Nature-based activities, as proposed by Berman et al. [2]
2. Rap music [4]
3. Structured play, noncompetitive facilitated games
4. Psychoeducation
5. Somatosensory regulation
6. Reflection and role plays
7. Group work in smaller and larger groups
8. Action theater (theater of the oppressed)
9. Group discussions
10. Uncle speeches – concrete guidance on specific topics like drugs, done by rap musician on the facilitation team – invented by the youth themselves
11. Lego (tdm) brick methods for modelling and cognitive stimulation (for attention, memory, and concentration)

Prior to the workshops with youth (refer to Table 14.1), staff were given a 4-day training on key topics, including child development in adversity; effects of being an

Table 14.1 Overview of workshops

Number and title	Methodology
Establishing the group	Outdoors. Cooking a meal over an open fire. Structured noncompetitive games
Sleep hygiene and stress management	Outdoors and indoors. Breathing and muscle relaxation exercises
Me and my strengths	Outdoors and indoors Rap music based
Me and my feelings	Indoors Group work, stories, games, and rap music
Boundaries and grooming	Indoors
Friendship – Me and my close relationships	Indoors Stories and examples (from youth), discussions, resource maps
Communication and conflict management	Indoors
Positive communication	Indoors and outdoors Exercises, structured games, and discussions
Gender and sexuality	Indoors discussions, action theater
Goodbye	Cooking a meal together, evaluation, looking back, and saying goodbye

asylum seeker/refugee on child wellbeing; resilience; psychological first aid for child practitioners [5]; use of nature and rap music as pedagogical tools; and fun, safe, inclusive interaction with vulnerable children [6].

The core team was composed of two men and two women, a rap musician, a nature guide, a clinical psychologist, and a project assistant.

Feedback from Youth

All agreed that they had enjoyed the varied use of methodologies and were especially happy with the sessions on grooming and sexuality. Several of them also mentioned the stress management and sleep hygiene sessions as their favorites. No one had been in a fight or other types of conflict with the local community since the sessions started. Not all youth who had participated in the baseline were in the last meeting. Some had left soon after the baseline because they had been relocated, granted asylum, or disappeared after their application was rejected. Teachers and staff in the center said that there were fewer conflicts, higher school attendance, and fewer incidents of verbal abuse of staff, including verbal abuse with a sexualized content, and staff reported that the behavior was less "provocative" than before the sessions.

Discussion

Why did the project work? Although we will not know if the changes in behavior and well-being will sustain over time, we are convinced that this model of intervention was relevant and applicable in other contexts for a number of reasons:

1. Participatory approach. Youth were directly involved in the selection of themes and methodology. This enhanced motivation to participate and ensured that the skills they practiced were directly relevant to their lives. This helped the establishment of a good working relationship with the team.
2. Inclusion of basic themes. The choice to start the sessions with basic orientation on sleep hygiene, etc. proved efficient. When our participants were able to take control over their sleep, they not only felt much better; they also acquired a sense of mastery and gained trust that the workshops could offer important benefits for them. "Ah, Uncle, it is your fault that I am sleeping late" (Amail, 16 years old, laughing to team member).
3. Combining different resilience resources. Youth responded very well to the opportunity to the alteration between introspection and practice of concrete social skills. Especially for our target group who were living with a very uncertain future, the management of daily challenges and preventing further deterioration was the first priority. Inspired by Sanders et al. (2015), the issue of culture and behaviour was built into al activities, we dicussed culture and reflected on understanding and how to adjust and navigate without loosing a sense of dignity and cultural identity [12].

4. Creative activities. The use of nature, play, and music provided variation and a nonthreatening atmosphere. It was also a way to practice impulse regulation, verbalization, and allowing for fun. This was particularly useful for the youth who had little education and were not at ease in a traditional learning environment. Learning through play and exploring music as a way to practice cognitive and social skills were much appreciated by youth (and staff who later used it for language classes). Rhythm, clapping, singing, and dancing did, in itself, have a comforting, regulating effect on the participants.

5. Building trust. The group was managed with strict and clear ground rules which were consistently applied. We believe that the most important benefits of the intervention may not have been the content in itself but the structure, predictability, and safety of the group. We deliberately composed the team to allow for identification with different facilitators and to provide role models of different types of Danish adults.

An asylum center is a small community in itself, and we applied the principles for community-based mental health and psychosocial support [17], working on youth, caregiver, and systems simultaneously, knowing that the asylum center must compensate for the missing family, community, language, and culture. A lesson learnt in this project is that more focus should have been given to the surrounding community, and we recommend that mental health and psychosocial support programs for unaccompanied asylum-seeking youth includes components of community mobilization, mentorships, and interventions to connect youth in centers with youth from the host community. We deliberately avoided a trauma focus but focused on building resilience, aiming for small resilient movements. It is our belief that this particular group was not ready or able to benefit from a more traditional psychological group intervention, but we would recommend that a program of this kind includes more orientation on mental health concerns and where to seek support. The Danish system has a mental health safety net, and youth have access to skilled professionals – only they may not want to use them because of the trust issues mentioned. In retrospective, we could have improved the links with the mental health providers.

Staff supervision is essential. Staff have a practical and a pastoral role, and in reality, they are reparenting the youth they work with.

Any psychosocial intervention with the target group we worked with would need to consider the capacity of the staff and the opportunities for supervision and guidance. We also stipulate that psychosocial support should be provided with a clear view that many of the previous and current concerns and stressors are protection related.

Offering nonspecialized, structured, and targeted psychosocial support for asylum-seeking youth is not new in Denmark, but working with youth with behavior challenges in a group is. We have proposed a model that leans to social work and builds trust gradually. We wanted to provide comfort, hope, and positive opportunities to keep youth protected and to facilitate their development and well-being, using pathways that were suited for their background and capabilities, the simplest being perhaps the most effective. "Most of what I learnt is really what my grandmother would have taught me," *Badam* (16 years old).

References

1. Armstrong M, Birnie-Lefcovitch S, Ungar M. Pathways between social support, family well being, quality of parenting, and child resilience: what we know. J Child Fam Stud. 2005;14:269–81.
2. Berman M, Kross E, Krpan KM, Askren MK, Burson A, Deldin PJ, Kaplan S, Sherdell L, Gotlib IH, Jonides J. Interacting with nature improves cognition and affect for individuals with depression. J Affect Disord. 2012;140(3):300–5.
3. Bjertrup P, Bouhenia M, Mayaud P, Perrin C, Farhat JB, Blanchet K. A life in waiting: Refugees' mental health and narratives of social suffering after European Union border closures in march 2016. Soc Sci Med. 2018;215:53–60.
4. DeCarlo A, Hockman E. RAP therapy: a group work intervention method for urban adolescents. Social Work with Groups. 2004;26:45–59.
5. Dybdal A-S, Melin M, Terlonge P. Psychological first aid training manual for child practitioners. Save The Children KLS, Grafisk Hus; 2013.
6. Dybdal A-S, Øllgaard R. Fun Safe Inclusive, a half-day training module on facilitation skills. Save The Children KLS, Grafisk Hus; 2016.
7. Hart A. Interactive resilience framework. Posted by Boingboing; 2017. Retrieved from https://www.boingboing.org.uk/use-resilience-framework-academic-resilience/.
8. Hart A, Thomas H, Blincow D. Resilient therapy-working with children and families: Routledge Taylor & Francis Group; 2007.
9. Hjorth C, Harway M. The body-image of physically abused and normal adolescents. J Clin Psychol. 1981;37:863–6.
10. Liebenberg L, Theron C. Innovative qualitative explorations of culture and resilience. In: Theron L, Liebenberg L, Ungar M, editors. Youth resilience and culture: Springer Press; 2015.
11. Mohamed S, Miles T. The mental health and psychological well-being of refugee children and young people: an exploration of risk, resilience and protective factors. Educ Psychol Pract. 2017;33(3):249–63.
12. Sanders J, Munford R. The interaction between culture, resilience, risks and outcomes: a New Zealand study. In: Theron L, Liebenberg L, Ungar M, editors. Youth resilience and culture: Springer Press; 2015.
13. Save The Children. PPAT, pre and post assessment tool. 2019. In press.
14. Tengnas K, Dybdal A-S. The youth resilience programme: psychosocial support in and out of schools. Save The Children, KLS, Grafisk Hus; 2015.
15. Ungar M. Introduction to the volume. In: Ungar M, editor. The social ecology of resilience. A handbook of theory and practice. New York: Springer-Verlag; 2012.
16. Ungar M, Liebenberg L. The child and youth resilience measure (CYRM). Resilience Research Center, Dalhousie University; 2009.
17. United Nations Children's Fund. Operational guidelines on community based mental health and psychosocial support in humanitarian settings: three-tiered support for children and families (field test version). New York: UNICEF; 2018.

A Family-Centered Approach to Working with Refugee Children and Adolescents

15

Trudy Mooren, Julia Bala, and Yoke Rabaia

Introduction

There are several reasons for adopting a family lens in working with refugee populations. First, for most refugee parents, a major reason for seeking safety at the cost of leaving familiar surroundings, families, and friends is to safeguard the well-being and future prospects of their children [14]. Parental guidance and support, effective caregiving, and family cohesion are important protective factors enhancing positive adjustment of the children during and following adverse experiences [17, 45]. Parents and children can be each other's main sources of social support. Second, together, parents and children have access to their family coping resources and belief systems that may be unfamiliar to new social surroundings. Third, refugees are frequently moved to new locations, in particular during the asylum-seeking period in Western countries. Collective reception centers may close, forcing inhabitants to live elsewhere. While refugee youth may receive treatment from professionals (teachers, doctors, therapists), they will live with family members. Investing in healthy family adjustment may be worthwhile considering these constant changes. Overall, considering the cascade of disruptions in refugee lives, the family may be one of the few stable factors. Strengthening in supportive skills within families is therefore an attractive and sustainable approach.

T. Mooren (✉)
ARQ Centrum'45, Diemen, The Netherlands
e-mail: t.mooren@centrum45.nl; G.T.M.Mooren@uu.nl

J. Bala
ARQ National Psychotrauma Centre, Diemen, The Netherlands

Y. Rabaia
Institute of Community and Public Health, Birzeit University, Birzeit, Palestine

© Springer Nature Switzerland AG 2020
S. J. Song, P. Ventevogel (eds.), *Child, Adolescent and Family Refugee Mental Health*, https://doi.org/10.1007/978-3-030-45278-0_15

Refugee Families' Experiences

Most refugee families arriving in host countries or regions have been subjected to war-related violence (bombardments, displacement, harassments) and personal losses. Family members' lives have been severely disrupted due to disintegration of social structures, such as unavailability of work, school, and health care. Being forced to flee causes a discontinuity of social ties, within and outside the family. In particular after a residency permit has been obtained, but during long-lasting asylum procedures as well, people establish and start families in the host country, which has legal consequences. Life continues while displaced, even though opportunities to build social networks are more restricted. There is general consensus among the majority of people that children should not be separated from parents and are entitled to receive protection, shelter, and education regardless of legal status [7]. Nevertheless, exceptions to these rules do occur.[1]

> **Case Example: A Mixed Nationality Refugee Couple Settled in the Netherlands**
> A mixed Azeri-Georgian refugee couple had settled in the Netherlands. Their two daughters were born in the Netherlands. After acquiring the necessary documents, the couple was officially married. Dutch authorities intended to decline their asylum request but had no options to send them to either Azerbaijan or Georgia as a family. Neither country would accept the partner other than on the base of a tourist visa (which allows for a stay of only limited duration). The threat of being separated caused great distress in this family. Finally, after 8 years, they were granted residency in the host country.

Models of Family Adaptation

Systems theory in general and Bronfenbrenner's ecological model are useful frameworks to understand how a family adapts to turmoil and crises. From a social systems perspective, families are considered systems, as they form natural networks of relationships that strive to maintain a steady state [38]. A system may be any "set" of interrelationships – this is not bound to a nuclear family, for example. Pathology or well-being is affected by family relationships. During and following traumatic events, reactions of family members may help or hinder the well-being and development of children who were exposed to these events. One person's intensive (posttraumatic) stress reactions can influence all family members and the family as a whole [20]. Families structure themselves to achieve continuity across contexts as well as across developmental changes [16, 50]. After fleeing their country and leaving the extended family behind, a flexible refugee family will be able to adjust to the

---

[1] See f.i., Kerig [26]. Also, in the Netherlands, an Armenian mother was sent back to her country of origin, while her two children remained in the Netherlands hiding.

new environment, change in relationships, and division of tasks and roles. The ecological model of Bronfenbrenner and Morris [6] postulates that an individual's functioning will be impacted by different circles or layers of social interference. A child is dependent first of all of its family members (nuclear or extended), secondly of the social surroundings such as school, street, church. A next circle of social impact will be the wider community and so forth. These circles of social influence will interact with each other. These theoretical notions will be illustrated below when we describe how conflict and migration impact families.

Case Example: A Family from Azerbaijan

A family from the Caucasus applied for asylum 5 years ago in the Netherlands. They live in a densely populated collective refugee center with people from many different nationalities. The husband, wife, and 12-year-old and 16-year-old sons live in two small rooms. The husband left his country since he refused to support his manager in a political activity. He was taken hostage, maltreated, and miraculously escaped to a neighboring country. His father-in-law advised him not to return after fearing his safety, and his wife and sons sought shelter in a small village. When the eldest son became sick and needed hospital care, the police discovered their presence. Four police officers broke into the house, abducted the two boys and severely abused the mother, who lost consciousness. One year later, she and both sons were reunited with their father in the host country.

Upon reunion, family dynamics had changed. Both sons, in particular the eldest, and their mother, silently expressed their anger toward the father, blaming him for their current hopeless situation. The youngest boy copied the coping behavior of his mother – at times apathetic, quiet, and anxious, without motivation to play or attend school. He and his mother had frequent nightmares. Parents were unable to console their children or each other. Nothing of their traumatic experiences had been shared among each other. The parents felt terribly ashamed about their experiences and were incapable of or did not think it would be possible to talk about it with each other ever.

Context

Families, like individuals, cannot be seen irrespective of their context. Models of family development, adaptation, and psychopathology are relevant across a range of cultural and ethnic groups [31]. What defines a nuclear or extended family is dependent upon cultural customs and values. In some cultures, families are construed by interrelationships of three generations where grandparents are actively involved in the caretaking of their grandchildren. The cultural and social contexts in which families are embedded inform the sense of purpose that guides the family, including family structure, parents' socialization goals, family practices and rituals, and the emotional tone of family relations [24]. For some refugee men, the risk of being unemployed and not being able to provide the family with sufficient means can have a negative impact on self-esteem. This can, but not necessarily always does, may lead to violence against women and children [43]. For refugee women, having been exposed to sexual violence can lead to shame, a strong urge to hide, and a sense of a sense of urgency to restore families' values or pride [43]. The meaning and significance of violence and forced migration need to be understood within the sociopolitical and cultural frameworks of both the region of origin and the host country. Because these meaning structures change constantly meaning structures change constantly as result of migration and acculturation processes [2]. Parental practices and beliefs often undergo changes in time during the cultural transition after migration [4, 22].

Consequences of Armed Conflict and Migration on Families

After severe circumstances such as those caused by violence, war, or migration, mental health difficulties can develop. Based on interviews with Syrian parents and children in Lebanon, Sim, Fazel, Bowes, and Gardner [40] mention three categories of burden as a consequence of war and displacement: economic hardship and adaptation, psychological difficulties, and lack of safety. In the parent-child relationships, these may be associated with reduced parental supervision and parent-child interaction, increased harsh parenting, and increased parental control, respectively. These themes are interrelated and make up the daily difficulties some families face as a result of their changed circumstances.

First, low socioeconomic status has been identified as a risk factor for decreased quality of family functioning. Having little income forces parents to take on extra work obligations (when allowed), and may decrease the opportunity to provide in their children's needs. Due to limited financial resources of the families, opportunities to offer children activities (such as sports or arts, school trips, or holiday activities) are restricted, and parents are dependent upon the local authorities to grant these. Being a single mother and suffering from severe migraine, an Armenian lady sent her 10-year-old son for medical examination to the hospital by himself. She was available to the doctor by phone.

Second, with regard to psychological difficulties, it has been clearly demonstrated that among refugees, individual family members are at a high risk of suffering from intrusive, avoidant, and arousal symptoms to such an extent that a posttraumatic stress disorder (PTSD) is present. Frequently, PTSD goes together with comorbid disturbances such as depressive mood, or anxiety symptoms, in adults as well as children [19, 28]. Some responses to trauma, such as nightmares, flashbacks, and substance abuse, will have an impact on the relationship with family members. Being agitated, easily aroused, having nightmares, difficulty concentrating, being restless, depressed, and not being able to perform duties can all directly impact daily interactions with family [3]. The relation between psychological difficulties in parents, for instance, parental PTSD-symptoms and psychological distress, and behavioral problems in children has been reported repeatedly (e.g., [15]), either directly or mediated by changed parenting style, e.g., more harsh parenting [5] and violence [44].

Thirdly, several changes of residence and perceived discrimination [17] can threaten or undermine adaptive family safety and functioning.

> **Case Example: Family from Azerbaijan (Continued)**
> The youngest son fainted while showering. He lost consciousness and fell on the floor. His mother heard him falling, ran to the shower, panicked, and ran outside and left the building. His brother was able to help by turning down the water and bringing the boy outside the shower. Afterward, his mother felt guilty about not being able to help her son. She reported feeling overwhelmed by a sense of powerlessness that was reminiscent of the traumatic incidents in her home country. At that time, she had not been able to prevent her sons from being kidnapped. The older boy was upset and angry at his mother, believing her to be unable to care for her sons.

Changed Relationships and Functions

Parenting behavior may be impacted both by posttraumatic and displacement stressors leading to diminished sensitivity, emotional availability, or increased violence [5, 11, 46]. Forcibly displaced parents, overwhelmed by worries and uncertainties, preoccupied with internal and external problems can perceive their parenting competencies as negative and may feel guilty [13]. For example, the mother of a 12-year-old boy from Eritrea regrets that she was not able to pay attention to her child. It was a painful experience for her realizing she had not reacted to her son when he told her about success in school, because she had been lost in her thoughts. In the case example of the family from Azerbijan, the father felt guilty of leaving his family behind and did his best to arrange everything for his wife and two sons. While he effectively took care of many things (for instance, he did the groceries and cooded dinner daily) for his family, he also continued to be blamed by them.

The division of roles and tasks can be changed due to disruptions and losses in the family. Children, who are generally faster in learning the new language in a host country, become important helpers when dealing with authorities. Children can be at risk of being "parentified" if they take on parental responsibilities which are inappropriate for their developmental level. However, many children also take pride in being able to help their families [27].

Communication

Communication patterns can help or hinder the adaptation process. Families vary in the extent to which they talk about past experiences [10]. In some families, family members who have been lost or left behind, and the events that occurred, are constant subject of communication with daily following of hometown news on the television. In other families, only silent reminders of all changes have a place in family life: the expression on mothers' face after she made a phone call to her sister, a letter from immigration services on the table, and a picture of a lost son on the cupboard. But no stories are told or shared. The timing and the manner of disclosure are relevant depending on severity of the parent's symptoms and their inclination to discuss the trauma [10].

Making Sense of Experiences

Adjustment is fostered when there is room to create a meaningful explanation of traumatic events and disruptive changes – when family members manage to "make sense of experience." Making meaning of adversity helps to normalize and contextualize distress and facilitate appraisal and views as meaningful, comprehensive, and changeable [50]. Parents vary in their attempts to explain their traumatic experiences or the reason of their flight out of their home to children. For example, some children were told they were going to visit family or relatives when they actually fled their town. Parents may consider it too dangerous to inform their children before leaving, attempting to protect them and themselves, and in order not to jeopardize their flight. Family secrets, divergent beliefs, and family rules prohibiting disclosure may inhibit shared family meaning [35]. Avoiding discussion about traumatic experiences, flight or loss can interfere with the process of co-construction of meaning within the family. Not knowing what and why something happened may lead children to fantasize that they are to blame and that they made a mistake or said something wrong or feel disappointed. For example, a girl who had escaped Teheran with her mother had been told they would go on a trip abroad. Only after a while she understood it would be an indefinite departure. Her mother had feared she would have told someone about their departure and didn't want her deceased husband's family to know.

Resilience

Resilience or the ability to "bounce back" refers to a dynamic interactive process, implying continuous interactions of within and between multiple systems around a family [45, 48]. The dynamic interaction of protective factors and processes at individual, family, and community level is aimed to foster positive adaptation [8, 39]. Many refugee families demonstrate their capacity to function adaptively in the face of adversity [9, 49] by (1) organizational patterns (flexibility, connectedness, mobilizing social and economic resources), (2) communication and problem-solving (distancing, separatedness, independency [37]), and (3) belief systems that influence how family members make meaning of adversity, preserve hope, and harness spirituality to serve as a source of strength and even to achieve posttraumatic growth and transcendence. Refugee mothers from Eritrea/Ethiopia in a multifamily group believe that their faith, the ability to value what they have, hope, and care for children and mutual support are strenghtening them to finding ways to go on even though they are still living under difficult circumstances and without certainty about stay permit.

The Potential of Family Groups

Chronic adversity without sufficient adult support leads to a constant activation of the stress response system of children, which increases the risk for psychological problems and stress-related diseases in later life [41]. Preventive mental health interventions that aim to stop, lessen, or delay possible negative individual mental health and behavioral sequelae through improving family and community protective resources in resettled refugee families are needed [53]. In ARQ Centrum'45, a mental health care institute in the Netherlands, mental health care, we have adapted multifamily therapy (MFT) [1] for use as a preventive program in different settings [33, 51]. The aims of this program vary according to the needs of participants but always entail:

- Strengthening the resources within families and coping capacities to deal with stressors
- Fostering a social network around families
- Enhancing positive parenting and parent-child relationships

A focus on families is considered a powerful approach for preventive mental health interventions [18], and family groups offer many possibilities for empowering and strengthening protective processes within and between families.

Multifamily Groups

The multifamily approach combines group and family interventions for four to eight families, sharing similar problems. In a natural, safe, playful context, families are encouraged to interact and help each other solve problems, learn new skills, and experiment with new behavior. Multifamily groups can be considered as both a method and a setting. Family groups can be carried out in various context and locations (clinics, schools, asylum centers, or other places) (see Box 15.1). A flexible setting allows working with family groups but also splitting up into sub-groups (e.g., children of similar age, mothers, fathers, parents) when needed. Creating a context for problems can open possibilities for tailoring the approach: defining which problems need to be addressed, who to be included, the number of sessions and deciding whether an open or a closed group would be more preferable [1]. In a preventive multifamily group called "Good parenting in difficult times," which Mooren and Bala [33] implemented in a center for asylum seekers faced with a long-lasting asylum procedure without a certain outcome, parents found it important to learn how to cope with stress and protect children from their own stress reactions.

While open in setting, family groups as a method have a rather strict, clearly defined structure: an introductory icebreaking activity, an energizing activity, and then a core exercise centered on a theme that is significant to the group, ending with a pleasant and interactive reflection (see Box 15.2). A reflection exercise is intended to make participants think, evaluate, and consider what they have experienced in the

---

Box 15.1 How to Plan a Group
- Who would be the participants of the group?
- What is a central problem/topic for the group?
- What are the goals? Which interventions to choose?
- How many sessions need to be planned?
- Which problems would be treated in the group with families and which problems need to be planned to separate parents and children?
- How many facilitators are needed?
- Will it be an open or closed group?
- Which room/space will be appropriate for the group sessions?
- Are there contra-indications for participation; if so – which are they?

Box 15.2 Icebreakers and Exercises

Examples of icebreakers	Examples of core activities
Musical chairs	Sources of stress and coping (metaphor: The bucket and the treasure box).
Stone, paper, scissors/rabbit, arrow, wall (or any other children's game that are known)	Playing a game (memory).
Pulling or jumping rope	Drawing what's (thoughts, ideas, wishes) in the head of your parent/child.
Creating a spider network (a rope is being thrown to each of the participants standing in a circle; while they throw the rope, they hold on to it, thereby creating a web) exchanging compliments and symbolizing their being connected in the group	Drawing an animal that a person identifies with (because of positive characteristics or talents) on paper, attach it to your body and walk around as if at a social gathering. Participants will explain the reason of their animal choice to others. They may subsequently group themselves according to similarities and differences of the sorts. When working with families or teams, a next question may relate to strengths and weaknesses that are represented in the teams (what additional characteristics would be needed to empower the family or team?).
	Social gathering or reception party with participants writing compliments for each other. They are asked to write it on post-it and stick them to other persons.
	Step in your child's/parents' shoes – outline shoes on piece of paper and step on the paper of your child/parent.

group. What do they want to remember, continue practicing or doing, what has been a take-home-message? Anyone who has familiarity in working with groups and/or families can be a group facilitator, so these can be social workers, teachers, or psychotherapists. Group facilitators take a specific position within these group sessions: they are responsible for session programming, but during the meetings, they keep a predominantly background position. They offer activities and maintenance of rules that apply to group work (safety, structure), facilitate interactions between families, and stimulate reflexive thinking [1]. While a facilitator is responsible for the context, parents are responsible for their children at all times [1].

In between exercises that function as icebreaker or facilitate reflection are core thematic activities. These address themes that are relevant for the group concerned, e.g., reducing home violence, dealing with uncertainty (having no legal permit to stay in the host region), or, as in the case of our family groups in the West Bank, taking care of a child with a disability [51].

To generate topics for core activities, a list of stressful aspects of living in a collective reception center was gathered, by asking the group members to write examples of stressful experiences on small notes, which were collected in a bucket. It was then explored how then explored how to cope with these stressors and shared ideas by creating a treasure box. Parental sources of support were examined by drawing a sociogram, while children painted a picture of their hometown memories. Parents and children drew a fantasy figure together on a large piece of paper, demonstrating their talents and strengths and making the figure into their own "code of arms" reflecting their families' pride and values. In another example on the theme of stressful aspects of living in an asylum seeker center, families wrote a script for a documentary about life in a refugee center. Activities and exercises can also be adapted to cultural traditions, such as coffee ceremonies in Eritrean culture (see also [52]).

Family Groups in Different Contexts

Multifamily groups can easily be adapted to different contexts and cultures. Besides implementing family groups in our Western therapeutic setting with refugees and veterans, the method has also been adopted for implementation in a conflict region. In cooperation with Birzeit University and a Community-Based Rehabilitation (CBR) program on the West Bank (occupied Palestinian territory), the approach has been adapted for use in groups of mothers/caretakers of children or other family members with a disability [34, 51]. CBR field workers working with mothers and caretakers of people with a physical or psychosocial disability had noticed that the women they work with found relief in seeing each other at social, educational, or cultural activities. Working together with two academic colleagues from the Institute of Community and Public Health of Birzeit University, CBR workers were next trained in using the multifamily group facilitation skills to organize support groups for these mothers. Over a 5-year period, the CBR program established about 30 'mothers groups' which are facilitated by CBR workers. They use basic techniques to facilitate listening and sharing stories and experiences about caring for the person with the disability or about more general family issues they find difficult to deal with. Together the group members develop ideas to help each other, and to laugh together. Nahreez, one of the CBR workers, says: "It was hard for us to learn to not always come up with solutions for the mothers, but to 'sit on our hands' (see Box 15.3) and to facilitate the group in such a way that the mothers themselves offer suggestions to each other." Maha, who has a child with autistic spectrum disorder, says: "I struggled to toilet train my son, but the ideas that I got from another mother in the group have really helped me. It is so special to be in this group and to feel that you are not alone. The members of my group all have autistic children and we can learn so much from each other. Especially because even the professionals, like doctors and psychologists, are often not able to help us!"

Effectiveness of Family Groups in Different Contexts

Although research has demonstrated that multifamily groups are effective for families dealing with depression [25, 29], eating disorders [23, 54], schizophrenia [30], and children's behavioral difficulties [32], few studies exist that have been conducted in war or conflict-stricken and migrated populations (see Box 15.4).

Box 15.3 Principles of Multifamily Groups
- Families supporting other families, based on acknowledgment and equality. All family members recognize the struggles in other members of other families and may learn from solutions that are brought forward.
- Building on resources and generating hope: "Yes, we can."
- Sharing experiences and eliciting the narration of stories creates acknowledgment and social cohesion, starting with natural curiosity.
- Participants of family groups are the experts, helping each other.
- Group facilitators "sit on their hands," maintain responsibility for participants' interactions, but refrain from intrusive interactions. They facilitate participants interacting.
- Power of pleasure: Fun activities are part of family groups in order to foster positive interactions.

Box 15.4 The Benefits of MFG (for Refugee Families)
- Overcome isolation and stigmatization
- Become more flexible when faced with possibilities of multiple perspectives
- Regain a sense of control by offering help to others, instead of feeling isolated and helpless
- Allow families to discover and practice new competencies
- Increase hope instead of hopelessness
- Help children and parents to understand each other and share pleasurable moments.

Weine et al. [52] organized family groups in the USA for refugees in the aftermath of the Balkan war. The preventive intervention was the Balkan custom of drinking coffee while sharing stories (CAFES). The results indicated that a multiple family group was effective in increasing access to mental health services and that depression and family comfort with discussing trauma mediated the intervention effect [52].

Concluding Remarks

In this chapter we advocated for a family approach in programming in response to violence, war, and migration. Family members are unique in their capacity to provide support to each other, in particular to children who are vulnerable due to cumulative stressors and discontinuity in their lives. When all family members suffer from distress, their capacities to support each other may be diminished. Families' resources can be depleted due to severe adversities and long-lasting cumulative stress. Dysfunctional family adaptation can become a source of additional stress and a risk for parent-child relational problems and child development. Preventive or early intervention programs that are focused on strengthening families as a source for natural support may be effective in helping families adapt to changed situations. We have described multifamily groups as a method to work with refugee families. The advantages of working with families within groups can increase acknowledgment and create a social support network, as well as improve the quality of parenting and interaction among family members.

References

1. Asen E, Scholz M. Multi-family therapy: concepts and techniques. London: Routledge; 2010.
2. Bala J, Kramer S. Intercultural dimensions in the treatment of traumatized refugee families. Traumatology. 2010;16(4):153–9.
3. Barnes M, Figley C. Family therapy: working with traumatised families. In: Lebov L, editor. Handbook of clinical family therapy. New Jersey: Willey; 2005. p. 309–29.
4. Bornstein MH, Bohr Y. Immigration, acculturation and parenting. Immigrat Acculturat Childhood. 2011;6:15.
5. Bryant RA, Edwards B, Creamer M, O'Donnell M, Forbes D, Felmingham KL, Silove D, Steel Z, Nickerson A, McFarlane AC, Van Hooff M, Hadzi-Pavlovic D. The effect of post-traumatic stress disorder on refugees' parenting and their children's mental health: a cohort study. Lancet Public Health. 2018;3:e249–58.
6. Bronfenbrenner U, Morris PA. The bioecological model of human development. In: Lerner RM (red.). Handbook of child psychology. Theoretical models of human development. vol 1. Hoboken: Wiley; 2006. p. 793–828.
7. Child Protection Working Group. 2019. Retrieved from https://www.unicef.org/iran/Minimum_standards_for_child_protection_in_humanitarian_action.pdf.
8. Cicchetti D. Resilience under conditions of extreme stress: a multilevel perspective. World Psychiatry. 2010;9(3):145–54.
9. Cowan PA, Cowan CP, Schulz MS. Thinking about risk and resilience in families. In: Hetherington EM, Blechman EA, editors. Family research consortium: advances in family research. Stress, coping, and resiliency in children and families. Hillsdale: Lawrence Erlbaum Associates, Inc.; 1996. p. 1–38.
10. Dalgaard NT, Montgomery E. Disclosure and silencing: a systematic review of the literature on patters of trauma communication in refugee families. Transcult Psychiatry. 2016;52:579–93.

11. Dalgaard NT, Montgomery E. The transgenerational transmission of refugee trauma: family functioning and children's psychosocial adjustment. Int J Migrat Health Soc Care. 2017;13(3):289–301.

13. El-Khani A, Ulph F, Peters S, Calam R. Syria: the challenges of parenting in refugee situations of immediate displacement. Intervention. 2016;14(2):99–113.

14. Ellis BH, Hulland ER, Miller AB, Barrett Bixby C, Lopes Cardozo B, Betancourt ThS. Mental health risks and resilience among Somali and Bhutanese refugee parents. https://www.migration.policy.org/research/… 2016.

15. Eruyar S, Maltby J, Vostanis P. Mental health problems of Syrian refugee children: the role of parental factors. Eur Child Adolesc Psychiatry. 2018;27:401–9.

16. Falicov CJ. Migration and the family life cycle. In: McGoldrick M, Garcia-Preto N, Carter B, editors. The expanded family life cycle: individual, family and social perspectives. Massachusetts: Allyn & Bacon; 2011. p. 336–47.

17. Fazel M, Reed RV, Panter-Brick C, Stein A. Mental health of displaced and refugee children resettled in high-income countries: risk and protective factors. Lancet. 2012;379:266–82.

18. Fazel M, Betancourt TS. Preventive mental health interventions for refugee children and adolescents in high-income settings. Lancet Child Adolesc Health. 2018;2(2):121–32.

19. Fazel M, Wheeler J, Danesh J. Prevalence of serious mental disorder in 7000 refugees resettled in western countries: a systematic review. Lancet. 2005;365(9467):1309–14.

20. Figley C. Helping traumatized families. San Francisco: Jossey-Bass; 1989.

22. Haan MD. The reconstruction of parenting after migration. A perspective from cultural translation. Hum Dev. 2011;54:376–99.

23. Hughes EK. Multifamily therapy may add to the effectiveness of single-family therapy for adolescents with anorexia nervosa. Evid Based Ment Health. 2018;21(1):e4.

24. Kagitcibasi C. Autonomy and relatedness in cultural context: implications for self and family. J Cross-Cult Psychol. 2005;36(4):403–22.

25. Katsuki F, Takeuchi H, Konishi M, Sasaki M, Murase Y, Naito A, et al. Pre-post changes in psychosocial functioning among relatives of patients with depressive disorders after brief multifamily psychoeducation: a pilot study. BMC Psychiatry. 2011;11(1):56.

26. Kerig PK. Refugee children and their parents. J Trauma Stress. 2018;. https://onlinelibrary.wiley.com/doi/toc/10.1002/(ISSN)1573-6598

27. Kia-Keating M, Capous D, Yuang L, Bacio G. Family factors: immigrant families and intergenerational considerations. In: Patel S, Reicherter D, (eds.) Psychotherapy for immigrant youth. Cham: Springer; 2016. p. 49-71.

28. Kien C, Sommer I, Faustmann A, Gibson L, Schneider M, Krczal E, et al. Prevalence of mental disorders in young refugees and asylum seekers in European countries: a systematic review. Eur Child Adolesc Psychiatry. 2018:1–16.

29. Lemmens GM, Eisler I, Buysse A, Heene E, Demyttenaere K. The effects on mood of adjunctive single-family and multi-family group therapy in the treatment of hospitalized patients with major depression. Psychother Psychosom. 2009;78(2):98–105.

30. McFarlane WR. Family intervention in schizophrenia: new approaches and outcomes in single- and multi-family group formats. In: Past, present and future of psychiatry. World Scientific Publishing Co. Salem, USA; 1994. p. 513–8.

31. McGoldrick M, Giordano J, Garcia-Preto N, editors. Ethnicity and family therapy. 3rd ed. New York: Guilford Press; 2005.

32. McKay MM, Gonzales J, Quintana E, Kim L, Abdul-Adil J. Multiple family groups: an alternative for reducing disruptive behavioral difficulties of urban children. Res Soc Work Pract. 1999;9(5):593–607.

33. Mooren T, Bala J. Goed ouderschap in moeilijke tijden [Good parenting in difficult times]. Utrecht: Pharos; 2016.

34. Mooren T, Reiffers R, Rabaia Y, Mitwalli S, Koenen S, de Man M. The multi-family approach to facilitate a family support network for Palestinian parents of children with a disability: a descriptive study. Lancet. 2018;391:S49.

35. Nadeau JW. Family construction of meaning. In: Neimeyer ER, editor. Meaning reconstruction and the experience of loss. Washington, D.C.: American Psychological Association; 2003. p. 95–113.
37. Olson DH. Multisystem assessment of stress and health (MACH) model. In: Catherall DR, editor. Handbook of stress, trauma, and the family. New York: Brunner-Routledge; 2004. p. 325–47.
38. Price SJ, Price CA, McKenry PC. Families & change: coping with stressful events and transitions. Los Angeles: SAGE; 2010.
39. Rutter M. Resilience as a dynamic concept. Dev Psychopathol. 2012;24(2):335–44.
40. Sim A, Fazel M, Bowers L, Gardner F. Pathways linking war and displacement to parenting and child adjustment: a qualitative study with Syrian refugees in Lebanon. Soc Sci Med. 2018;200:19–26.
41. Shonkoff JP, Garner AS, Siegel BS, Dobbins MI, Earls MF, McGuinn L, et al. The lifelong effects of early childhood adversity and toxic stress. Pediatrics. 2012;129(1):e232–46.
43. Tankink M. 'We are now married with the UNHCR': domestic violence in the context of refugee camps. In: Tankink M, Vysma M, editors. Roads and boundaries: travels in search of (re) connection. Amsterdam: AMB; 2011. p. 116–25.
44. Timshel I, Montgomery E, Dalgaard NT. A systematic review of risk and protective factors associated with family related violence in refugee families. Child Abuse Negl. 2017;70:315–30. https://doi.org/10.1016/j.chiabu.2017.06.023
45. Tol WA, Song S, Jordans MJ. Annual research review: resilience and mental health in children and adolescents living in areas of armed conflict–a systematic review of findings in low-and middle-income countries. J Child Psychol Psychiatry. 2013;54(4):445–60.
46. van Ee E, Kleber RJ, Mooren TT. War trauma lingers on: associations between maternal posttraumatic stress disorder, parent–child interaction, and child development. Infant Ment Health J. 2012;33(5):459–68.
48. Vindevogel S, Verelst A. Supporting mental health in young refugees: a resilience perspective. In: Song S, Ventevogel P, editors. Child, adolescent and family refugee mental health. Springer Nature. 2020. p. 53–66.
49. Walsh F. Strengthening family resilience. 2nd ed. New York: Guilford; 2006.
50. Walsh F. Family resilience: a developmental systems framework. Eur J Dev Psychol. 2016;13(3):313–24.
51. War Trauma Foundation. The multi-family approach in humanitarian settings. Diemen: WTF; 2015.
52. Weine S, Kulauzoviv Y, Klebic A, Besic S, Mujagic A, Muzurovic J, Spahovic D, Sclove S, Pavkovic I, Feetham S, Rolland J. Evaluating a multiple-family group access intervention for refugees with PTSD. J Marital Fam Ther. 2008;34(2):149–64.
53. Weine SM. Developing preventive mental health interventions for refugee families in resettlement. Fam Process. 2011;50:410–30.
54. Wierenga CE, Hill L, Knatz Peck S, McCray J, Greathouse L, Peterson D, et al. The acceptability, feasibility, and possible benefits of a neurobiologically-informed 5-day multifamily treatment for adults with anorexia nervosa. Int J Eat Disord. 2018;51(8):863–9.

Engaging Refugee Families in a Family-Strengthening Intervention to Promote Child Mental Health and Family Functioning

16

Rochelle L. Frounfelker, Tej Mishra, Bhuwan Gautam,
Jenna M. Berent, Abdirahman Abdi,
and Theresa S. Betancourt

Introduction

This chapter focuses on barriers refugee families and children face in engaging with mental health services and identifies practical recommendations and strategies for practitioners to overcome these barriers and encourage involvement of refugee families in programs that promote child and family functioning. We write from our own perspectives as community leaders, healthcare professionals, and researchers engaged in community-based refugee mental health work. Although our experiences are based within the context of refugee third country resettlement in the United States, we discuss issues that are equally relevant for mental health professionals who are looking to implement mental health programming in humanitarian settings that follow best practices around community-based protection, mobilization, and support [13, 33, 40]. Tej Mishra, Bhuwan Gautam, and Abdirahman Abdi write as individuals with Bhutanese and Somali Bantu refugee life experience who have dual roles as community leaders and members of a larger research team involved in the implementation of evidence-based prevention interventions in their

R. L. Frounfelker (✉)
Division of Social and Transcultural Psychiatry, Department of Psychiatry, McGill University, Montreal, QC, Canada
e-mail: rochelle.frounfelker@mail.mcgill.ca

T. Mishra · J. M. Berent · T. S. Betancourt
Research Program on Children and Adversity, Boston College School of Social Work, Chestnut Hill, MA, USA
e-mail: tmishra@bu.edu; berent@bc.edu; theresa.betancourt@bc.edu

B. Gautam
Bhutanese Society of Western Massachusetts, Inc., Springfield, MA, USA

A. Abdi
Shanbaro Community Association, Chelsea Collaborative, Chelsea, MA, USA

© Springer Nature Switzerland AG 2020
S. J. Song, P. Ventevogel (eds.), *Child, Adolescent and Family Refugee Mental Health*, https://doi.org/10.1007/978-3-030-45278-0_16

respective communities. They reflect on what they want outsiders to know about their communities and steps outsiders should take in order to develop successful relationships with refugees. Rochelle Frounfelker, Jenna Berent, and Theresa Betancourt write from their perspective as researchers, clinicians, and public health practitioners affiliated with academic institutions, reflecting on the successes and challenges they have experienced engaging in community-based research and family interventions with refugees.

The Family Strengthening Intervention for Refugees (FSI-R)

Our experience with community-based prevention interventions is based on work with Somali Bantu and Bhutanese refugee communities in the Greater Boston, larger Massachusetts, and Maine areas in the United States. The senior author (TSB) initiated partnerships with both refugee groups with the goals of understanding the challenges and strengths of refugee families and using this information to adapt an evidence-based family intervention to meet the needs of the populations [6]. The work is informed by a community-based participatory research approach (CBPR) [37] that aims to create equitable partnerships between researchers, service providers, and Bhutanese and Somali Bantu refugee communities. In CBPR, different stakeholders come together around shared goals and interests to build the capacity of community members and facilitate the successful development and implementation of community-based interventions [14, 20, 37]. Although our work is done within the context of a research partnership, it is aligned with UNHCR guidelines on using a community-based approach in humanitarian settings [31]. Such an approach emphasizes building partnerships between humanitarian workers and refugee populations, identifying and supporting capacities and skills of war-affected individuals, and has the goal of empowering and reinforcing the dignity and self-esteem of vulnerable communities [31].

The initial phase of our work consisted of using qualitative methods to conduct community needs assessments and identify mental health syndromes and cultural idioms of distress used in both refugee groups to discuss child mental health problems [6]. The second phase of work involved using this information to adapt an existing evidence-based intervention developed by Boston Children Hospital's Dr. William Beardslee [2–4]. This intervention, the family-based preventive intervention (FBPI), was designed to prevent depression in children of depressed caregivers and has been adapted for use in a diverse range of cultures, including HIV-affected families in Rwanda [7]. The relevance and utility of the intervention for families affected by the Rwandan genocide led the senior author (TSB) to see the potential of using the core components of the FBPI with other war-affected populations in the United States. The adapted Family Strengthening Intervention for Refugees (FSI-R) involves a series of separate and joint meetings (partitioned into modules) with children and parents to discuss the past challenges the family has faced, identify strengths that have helped the family get through difficult times, and build positive coping strategies to overcome current stressors for supportive family relationships. The intervention includes psychoeducation material on mental health, promoting resilience, and positive parenting (see Table 16.1). In the third phase, we conducted an FSI-R pilot randomized controlled trial of the intervention to assess its feasibility and acceptability in both Bhutanese and Somali Bantu communities [5]. Throughout these three phases, we encountered various challenges engaging Somali Bantu and Bhutanese refugees in the work.

Table 16.1 FSI-R Curriculum

Modules	Theme(s)	Content	Aims
1–2	Introduction	Introduction to the intervention's goals and structure. Creation and discussion of a "family narrative". Identification of family strengths and challenges. Identification of family goals.	Prepare caregivers for intervention. Begin to establish a trusting relationship with caregivers. Understand family's circumstances from caregiver point of view.
3	Children and family relationships	Creation and discussion of a "Family Narrative" from a child's point of view. Identification of family strengths and challenges.	Establish a trusting relationship with children. Understand family's circumstances from child's point of view.
4	Responsive parenting and caregiving	Identify ways to engage and respond to children, build and maintain positive parent-child relationships. Identify and model ways to discipline children and alternatives to harsh punishment. Explain importance of adults' active involvement and communication with children.	Introduce strategies to manage stress and reduce harsh punishments.
5	Engagement with the US education system	Importance of parental engagement in the US education system. Coaching on specific, age-appropriate structured activities families can incorporate into their daily routines to talk to their children about school.	Educate caregivers on the education system in the United States. Empower caregivers to engage with schools and their children's educational experience.
6	Supplemental module: Promoting health, Well-being, and safety	Discussion and demonstration of stress management. Guide for healthy eating and engaging in physical activity. Discussion of household hygiene. Effective strategies for prevention and wellness. Identification of the health risks of excessive alcohol consumption. Staying safe in the community and at home.	Help caregivers learn about good physical and mental health. Identify strategies that promote health, well-being and safety.

(continued)

Table 16.1 (continued)

Modules	Theme(s)	Content	Aims
7–8	Communicating with children and caregivers	Building communication skills. Identifying ways to respond well to hard questions. Preparing for family meeting.	Prepare caregivers and children for the family meeting. Build skills related for improved child-parent communication.
9	Uniting the family	Facilitate a family meeting. Create shared understanding of resettlement and focus on family strengths. Recognize each family member's experience and views.	Promote positive communication between children and caregivers.
10	Bringing it all together	Create a plan with the family for how they will apply what they have learned going forward. Discuss ways to involve all family members in these strategies, activities, and routines.	Empower the family to practice and implement new strategies and skills learned throughout the intervention.

Barriers to Care

There are numerous barriers that prevent refugee children and families from engaging in mental health services (see Table 16.2). In third country resettlement, structural barriers include issues such as transportation and time. Oftentimes, families have limited access to cars or public transportation, making traveling to a second location for services difficult [8]. There are multiple and complex challenges and priorities such as securing employment and housing, navigating welfare and healthcare systems, and adjusting to a new educational system that consume the time and energy of refugee families and children [15]. In humanitarian settings such as refugee camps, families must focus on securing the basics of food, clothing, and shelter in order to survive through a time of great uncertainty and upheaval [33]. Additionally, general healthcare services, let alone mental healthcare, may be extremely limited in scope. Thus, even if families are concerned about the well-being of their children, they may not be able to access services for very practical reasons.

Additionally, there are many salient cultural barriers. On a very concrete level, language barriers between refugees and providers are a significant concern [24, 41]. In both humanitarian settings and third country resettlement, refugee population knowledge of, and fluency in, the primary language spoken by humanitarian workers and healthcare providers varies greatly. Likewise, there may be very few clinicians who speak the language of certain refugee groups, and finding translators to bridge the provider-client communication gap can be challenging [8]. Our work

Table 16.2 Refugee child and family barriers to accessing mental healthcare

Category	Barriers
Structural	Transportation. Competing priorities – housing, food, employment, education. Time constraints. Limited availability of services.
Cultural	Language. Stigma. Poor alignment between Western/European conceptualizations of mental health and those of local communities.
Other	Focus on clinic-based, as opposed to community-based services. Providers fail to engage with and promote buy-in from refugee communities.

with the Somali Bantu community highlights these issues. Due to educational barriers in Somalia and limited educational opportunities in refugee camps in Africa, few Somali Bantu were fluent in English prior to resettlement in the United States; additionally, the Somali Bantu we work with speak *Maay Maay*, a little-known non-written language used by some of the Bantu ethnic-minority in Somalia. Although some providers rely on family members for translating with clients, this is inappropriate, as it not only violates confidentiality, but also means that clients may be less inclined to be open and honest with providers because others are present. In addition to language barriers, there may also be an overall lack of fit between Western treatment modalities and the beliefs, values, and norms of refugee populations. In some cases, this leads individuals to seek out traditional healers and non-Western forms of treatment used in their country of origin [41]. Based on our experience with Bhutanese and Somali Bantu communities, there is widespread use of religious and traditional healers for a range of health problems, including mental health. Refugee populations frequently do not disclose the use of complementary or alternative medicine out of fear of being judged by Western healthcare providers.

Other barriers include stigma around mental health problems [8, 25, 26, 35] and general distrust of providers [15, 18, 24, 30]. Beyond stigma, refugee groups may frame, conceptualize, and understand mental health issues and symptoms very differently from Western psychiatry. As one of our authors, a refugee community leader succinctly explains, "Who cares about mental health issues if you don't know what they are?" In the Bhutanese and Somali Bantu communities, it is common for individuals to not recognize that something they are feeling or experiencing may be a manifestation of a mental health condition (e.g., that feeling tired and lack of energy could be a symptom of depression). There is frequently limited prior experience or awareness of formal mental health treatment [8, 28]. In addition, practitioners may have a lack of understanding of local and nonthreatening terms for describing emotional and behavioral conditions. Learning local language, culture-bound mental health syndromes, and culturally relevant idioms of distress can help to demystify emotional and behavioral problems and increase community engagement [6].

Beyond the Clinical Encounter

There are strategies to overcome these barriers and increase engagement in services [9]. For instance, in the context of third country resettlement, some programs increase accessibility of clinical care for children by providing services in school settings [10, 11, 42]. Other strategies include using cultural brokers/refugee community health workers as part of the clinical team to address and overcome language barriers and other cultural issues [29]. Furthermore, mental health providers can provide psychoeducation to refugee communities around mental health, diagnoses, and therapy options [27, 34]. Another strategy is to reframe the components and critical ingredients of Western therapies, such as cognitive behavioral therapy, using terminology that is more aligned with the belief systems and worldviews of refugee groups [16].

There is a larger question about the appropriateness, both in terms of access and acceptability, of clinical services for refugee populations [19]. Is therapy and psychiatric medication adequate to address the underlying causes of mental health problems? While historically there has been a focus on clinic-based, individual-level mental health interventions for refugees, there is increasing interest in interventions that adopt a more ecological perspective in terms of being both more embedded in community settings and also working with larger systems, such as entire families, that impact child psychosocial well-being [21–23]. Indeed, IASC Guidelines on mental health and psychosocial support in emergency settings highlight that while clinical services delivered by mental health professionals are warranted, the vast majority of supports should focus on advocating for basic services and security, supporting community-based initiatives for children, and providing more focused psychosocial supports for individuals and families [33]. In addition, it is worthwhile to consider interventions aimed at preventing mental health problems among refugee children and promoting the functioning of the entire family, thereby decreasing the need for acute care services [12, 38, 39].

Engagement and Buy-In from Refugee Populations

Community-based mental health prevention programs will not be successful if outside practitioners attempt to come into a community and impose an intervention on the population, no matter how well-intentioned. There must be mutual understanding about, and interest in, interventions based on a partnership between healthcare providers and the community. To build good rapport and a positive relationship with a specific refugee community, it is important for practitioners to understand community dynamics more generally and how communities negotiate accepting and participating in new programs designed to help the community more specifically. Certain refugee communities have a history of communal living and decision-making, where there are covert leadership structures. The leaders can be educated individuals who are widely known and respected in the community, oftentimes people who have been community heads and leaders since their time in the country of origin. Leaders are also often individuals who either volunteer or work as case managers, healthcare navigators, pastors, *pandits*, and so on in the resettled country. It is important to realize that there can be multiple community "leaders" who sometimes have rivalries among themselves. This creates divisions and subgroups within the larger refugee group based on whom a designated leader most frequently serves and provides assistance to.

When securing buy-in for community-based interventions, it is imperative that these groups (i.e., their respective leaders) be brought together to illustrate how interventions can address a shared interest for the whole group. These community dynamics are typically formed based on culturally defined subgroups that are oftentimes "invisible" to outside practitioners and do not become apparent until project activities are initiated. Body language, indirect styles of communication, and other culturally specific expressions make it difficult for outsiders to understand the sentiments, demands, and expectations of the community. Thus, it is ideal to involve members of the community in initial discussions related to potential community-based interventions to conduct preliminary informal investigations to understand these dynamics and plan accordingly. Reaching out to refugee self-help organizations in the community is one way to establish relationships. For instance, in our experience, Bhutanese refugees are a very heterogeneous population with subgroups formed based on characteristics such as ethnicity, language, religion, and historical caste dynamics. We experienced setbacks in the initial phases of our work with the community because we were not aware of these hidden community dynamics and unknowingly excluded subgroups in initial project planning and staff hiring decisions. We temporarily stopped program activities to develop better relationships with community members, build trust with refugee project staff in order to facilitate more open discussions about community dynamics, and identify strategies to use moving forward, such as implementing more transparent hiring practices and engaging in more purposeful outreach activities to connect with subgroups in the community. The lessons we learned from our work are well articulated in a UNHCR community-based protection policy brief, which emphasizes that developing community relationships and selecting community partners by necessity take considerable time and sensitivity [32].

Community advisory boards (CAB) are an essential part of deepening engagement with community stakeholders. They are formed and maintained to act as a liaison between a refugee community and an intervention program. Advisory boards need to be representative and formed in close and transparent processes with community partners. Gender, age group, occupation, status as parents or nonparents, participation of children, and other sociodemographic factors should be considered when inviting members to join the group. Roles and expectations, including time commitment and frequency of meetings or other forms of involvement, should be outlined clearly with the group. Individuals with no or minimal exposure to higher education may find it hard to understand the concept of mental health prevention interventions, and it can be intimidating for them to provide their input and opinions. Although this may pose added challenges, it is critical that people of all education and economic backgrounds are included to garner diverse perspectives. In some cases, separate groups for men and women and for adults and children may be appropriate. It can also be important to set up policy and/or clinical advisory boards depending on the topic of focus. Thus, programs should have plans to invest resources and time to educate and involve members for the duration of the project, as well as to engage such partners in disseminating the findings of collaborative research.

It is not ideal, nor practical from a community member perspective, to reach out and invite individuals to meetings only when service providers deem their input "necessary." Due to project priorities, individuals outside the refugee community can easily forget this. We learned this the hard way and have had to rebuild CABs numerous times over the lifetime of the project. The most challenging aspect of this work is in retaining board membership. It should be acknowledged that CAB members are, in most cases, volunteering their time amidst competing priorities related to their own family and personal life. Benefits of CAB participation must be made explicit in order for individuals to continue participating and provide input. If the project cannot provide financial benefits, programs should consult with the same group and find ways that render motivation for them to participate. Some form of compensation for donating time and expertise is very important for reasons of fairness/social justice, as well as to reward individuals for continuous participation. Also, overcoming relevant barriers to participation, which in our case included meals, transportation, and childcare, should also be considered. Workers in humanitarian settings should collaborate with affected communities to identify relevant, context-specific barriers that need to be addressed.

Youth CABs are especially important if the intervention or program aims to engage or address the needs of children or families. Children often have unique perspectives, needs, and challenges from adults, and due to increased intergenerational divides between adults and children of refugee families, child involvement in refugee programming is even more critical. With trust and rapport, children can share their experiences and views on important issues such as school, bullying, family dynamics, drug and alcohol use, and other pertinent issues that program implementers might not be considering or addressing appropriately. Consequently, programs or interventions can be better adapted to foster their engagement and address their needs [17]. In community-based work, including public health research, outreach, and coalition-building, children are considered a vital resource for catalyzing community change [1]. Youth CAB involvement can also foster leadership skills, as well as professional, personal, and general life skills, and help empower children and youth to be active members of their communities [17]. Similar to the adult CABs, consideration of age, gender, background, and other cultural elements is critical when recruiting members for the board.

Design Interventions Using Community Knowledge

In order to develop and promote the successful implementation of community-based interventions, practitioners must value ideas and opinions of members in the refugee community. This requires ongoing communication between CABs and outside practitioners. There are multiple benefits to this communication. First, there is tremendous scope of knowledge sharing, including an understanding of the community culture to be shared with outside practitioners. In turn, there is an opportunity for members of the refugee community to learn about community interventions. This is one way to reach the goal of community empowerment by sharing knowledge capital on both sides. Second, building relationships between practitioners and community members makes collaboration between the two parties more desirable, as members of the community feel that their opinions are valued by outside practitioners and integrated into program designs and implementation activities. Finally, specific to interventions designed to promote child mental health, family member relationships, and how the dynamics of these relationships impact well-being, are contextually dependent. Community members understand cultural dynamics such as multiple marriages and tribal/caste systems that affect family functioning. As such, community members know more about what is best for families than any outside individual or group. It is almost unimaginable for a program to effectively address these issues without informed involvement of individuals who know the culture as well as the objectives, goals, and content of the intervention.

Engaging Families in Intervention Work

For interventions such as the Family Strengthening Intervention for Refugees (FSI-R), which is designed to address the strengths, challenges, and goals of all family members, family engagement is essential for success. If the family is too busy, not interested, does not recognize the value, or is preoccupied with other issues, then they likely will not benefit from the information, skill-building, and sharing of perspectives and feelings that the program elicits and depends on. Engagement can pose an even greater challenge when working with low-income, underserved, or transient populations [36]. From our own experiences, the engagement challenges can be further exacerbated among families who have undergone the refugee experience and are experiencing additional resettlement stressors.

Through implementation of the FSI-R, we have experienced several challenges to family engagement. A major challenge is helping families recognize the value of participating. The idea of a family coming together and discussing their history, while focusing on strengths and resilience, and learning techniques for positive parenting and communication may seem quite unfamiliar and strange to many families. Furthermore, the concepts and value are abstract, with uncertain direct benefits. The family may either not find it useful or not be able to realize the long-term value of the intervention on their family's well-being and functioning. For many refugee families, prevention programs are a completely foreign and Western concept. With no previous exposure to such concepts or wide societal endorsement, it takes both time and effort to get buy-in of the benefits and engagement of the family members.

Another major challenge includes navigating time constraints and competing priorities experienced by families, especially among underserved populations. Many of the caregivers in the families we work with have long work hours, overnight shifts, and long commutes. Consequently, both caregivers are rarely home at the same time. The children are also in school, sometimes work, and are often engaged with other activities and social lives. With competing priorities around work, childcare, and elderly care obligations, finding an appropriate time that family members are all home and available for each module is challenging.

Lastly, engagement is also dependent on managing family expectations. Unfortunately, given the nature of the FSI-R, we cannot address the needs of all families, and often times they are focused on resolving more pertinent issues rather than focusing on parenting skill-building or communication techniques. Many of the families we work with might be navigating challenging US systems, such as welfare, housing, taxes, healthcare, education, etc. It is often common for the families to want to focus on handling many of these more pressing, consequential issues, and they turn to the FSI interventionists for support with these challenges. It is understandably difficult to help the family handle these issues while also gaining their attention, engagement, and commitment to the FSI program. Competing priorities and challenges are equally relevant in humanitarian settings, and intervention components and delivery strategies need to be adapted to respond to local realities.

Despite these challenges, we have learned important lessons and, together with the team and consultation of both adult and youth CABs, have created effective approaches to improving engagement. For one, we emphasize flexibility with the interventionists and families. Our interventionists strive to keep a schedule that allows flexibility to meet the family's needs around scheduling sessions. Oftentimes, sessions are held on the evenings and weekends and rescheduled multiple times to allow for more family members to be present. Another approach to engagement is to tailor the intervention to the unique needs of the family and spend more time focusing on modules that are particularly important or relevant to them and less time on other modules. We also designate a certain amount of time prior to each session to help the family navigate more pressing issues. Some of these issues may be out of the scope of the intervention, but we strive to address them and/or link the family to other resources in the community before proceeding with the contents of the intervention modules. That way, the family will be more likely to feel relaxed and ready to focus on the other elements of the intervention. Furthermore, we train our interventionists to coach the families on how to best address these issues, with goals of enhancing capacity building and empowering the family, so that they might be able to handle them on their own in the future and decrease reliance on community health workers and case managers.

Interaction between the interventionist and the family is another important component to improving engagement. The FSI-R is designed to be conversational and includes role-plays, vignettes, art, poster boards, and other forms of interactive communication, rather than a one-way direction of information sharing.

Interventionists have separate sessions with children to help gain their trust, build rapport, and privilege their experiences and perspective on the family. Interventionists also bring crayons and small toys for the children to play with while participating in the FSI-R to help increase engagement. Lastly, our staff for the FSI-R are recruited and trained from the community, which is another key piece in facilitating family engagement. They are trusted, well-respected, and often considered leaders in the community, who, of course, speak the local languages. Equally important, they understand the culture and the needs of their community and serve as critical players in helping the FSI-R meet the needs of each family.

Conclusion

There are numerous challenges to engaging refugee family and children in mental health services. In order to overcome these challenges, it is important to move beyond clinic-based encounters and develop community-based prevention interventions developed in partnership with refugee communities. Developing and maintaining community partnerships are critical throughout all phases of work, ranging from identifying refugee community problems and strengths, designing interventions, to implementing programs. Navigating refugee community dynamics can be extremely challenging, and transparency and open communication via CABs are essential. When implementing interventions, there are additional practical and cultural challenges that must be overcome in order to successfully engage refugee families and children. Ultimately, putting in time and effort to develop and sustain refugee community-provider partnerships can lead to successful and effective interventions.

References

1. Adolescent Health Initiative. Creating and sustaining a thriving youth advisory council. 2nd ed. Ann Arbor: The Adolescent Health Initiative at Michigan Medicine; 2019.
2. Beardslee WR. Prevention and the clinical encounter. Am J Orthopsychiatry. 1998;68(4):521–33. https://doi.org/10.1037/h0080361.
3. Beardslee WR, Gladstone TR, Wright EJ, Cooper AB. A family-based approach to the prevention of depressive symptoms in children at risk: evidence of parental and child change. Pediatrics. 2003;112(2):e119–31.
4. Beardslee WR, Wright EJ, Gladstone TR, Forbes P. Long-term effects from a randomized trial of two public health preventive interventions for parental depression. J Fam Psychol. 2007;21(4):703–13. https://doi.org/10.1037/0893-3200.21.4.703.
5. Betancourt TS, Berent JM, Freeman J, Frounfelker RL, Brennan RT, Abdi S, Maalim A, Abdi A, Mishra T, Gautam B, Creswell JW, Beardslee W. Family-based mental health promotion for Somali bantu and Bhutanese refugees: feasibility and acceptability trial. J Adolesc Health. 2020;66:336.
6. Betancourt TS, Frounfelker RL, Mishra T, Hussein A, Falzarano R. Addressing health disparities in the mental health of refugee children and adolescents through community-based participatory research: a study in two communities. Am J Public Health. 2015;105(S3):S475–82. https://doi.org/10.2105/AJPH.2014.302504.

7. Betancourt TS, Ng LC, Kirk CM, Munyanah M, Mushashi C, Ingabire C, Teta S, Beardslee WR, Brennan RT, Zahn I, Stulac S, Cyamatare FR, Sezibera V. Family-based prevention of mental health problems in children affected by HIV and AIDS: an open trial. AIDS. 2014;28(3):S359–68. https://doi.org/10.1097/2FQAD.0000000000000336.

8. Colucci E, Minas H, Szwarc J, Guerra C, Paxton G. In or out ? Barriers and facilitators to refugee-background young people accessing mental health services. Transcult Psychiatry. 2015;52(6):766–90. https://doi.org/10.1177/1363461515571624.

9. Colucci E, Valibhoy M, Szwarc J, Kaplan I, Minas H. Improving access to and engagement with mental health services among young people from refugee backgrounds: service user and provider perspectives. Int J Cult Mental Health. 2017;10(2):185–96. https://doi.org/10.1080/17542863.2017.1279674.

10. Ellis HB, Miller AB, Baldwin H, Abdi S. New directions in refugee youth mental health services: overcoming barriers to engagement. J Child Adolesc Trauma. 2011;4(1):69–85. https://doi.org/10.1080/19361521.2011.545047.

11. Fazel M, Garcia J, Stein A. The right location? Experiences of refugee adolescents seen by school-based mental health services. Clin Child Psychol Psychiatry. 2016;21(3):368–80. https://doi.org/10.1177/1359104516631606.

12. Fazel M, Betancourt TS. Preventive mental health interventions for refugee children and adolescents in high-income settings. Lancet Child Adolesc Health. 2017;2(2):121–32. https://doi.org/10.1016/S2352-4642(17)30147-5.

13. Inter-Agency Standing Committee (IASC). IASC guidelines on mental health and psychosocial support in emergency settings. Geneva: IASC; 2007. Retrieved from: https://www.who.int/mental_health/emergencies/guidelines_iasc_mental_health_psychosocial_june_2007.pdf

14. Israel BA, Schulz AJ, Parker EA, Becker AB. Review of community-based research: assessing partnership approaches to improve public health. Annu Rev Public Health. 1998;19(1):173–202. https://doi.org/10.1146/annurev.publhealth.19.1.173.

15. Karageorge A, Rodes P, Gray R, Papadopoulos R. Refugee and staff experiences of psychotherapeutic services: a qualitative systematic review. Intervention. 2017;15(1):51–69. https://doi.org/10.1097/WTF.0000000000000137.

16. Kohrt BA, Maharjan SM, Timsina D, Griffith JL. Applying Nepali ethnopsychology to psychotherapy for the treatment of mental illness and prevention of suicide among Bhutanese refugees. Ann Anthropological Pract. 2012;36(1):88–112. https://doi.org/10.1111/j.2153-9588.2012.01094.x.

17. LoIacono Merves M, Rodgers CR, Silver EJ, Sclafane JH, Bauman LJ. Engaging and sustaining adolescents in community-based participatory research: structuring a youth-friendly community-based participatory research environment. Family Commun Health. 2015;38(1):22–32.

18. Majumder P, O'Reilly M, Khalid K, Vostanis P. 'This doctor, I do not trust him, I'm not safe': the perceptions of mental health and services by unaccompanied refugee adolescents. Int J Soc Psychiatry. 2015;61(2):129–36. https://doi.org/10.1177/0020764014537236.

19. Miller KE. Rethinking a familiar model: psychotherapy and the mental health of refugees. J Contemp Psychother. 1999;29(4):283–306. https://doi.org/10.1023/A:1022926721458.

20. Minkler M. Linking science and policy through community-based participatory research to study and address health disparities. Am J Public Health. 2010;100(S1):S81–7. https://doi.org/10.2105/AJPH.2009.165720.

21. Murray KE, Davidson GR, Schweitzer RD. Review of refugee mental health interventions following resettlement: best practices and recommendations. Am J Orthopsychiatry. 2010;80(4):576–85. https://doi.org/10.1111/j.1939-0025.2010.01062.x.

22. Pejic V, Alvarado AE, Hess RS, Groark S. Community-based interventions with refugee families using a family systems approach. Fam J. 2017;25(1):101–8. https://doi.org/10.1177/1066480716680189.

23. Pejic V, Hess RS, Miller GE, Wille A. Family first: community-based supports for refugees. Am J Orthopsychiatry. 2016;86(4):409–14. https://doi.org/10.10337/ort0000189.

24. Priebe S, Giacco D, El-Nagib R. Public health aspects of mental health among migrants and refugees: a review of the evidence on mental health care for refugees, asylum seekers and irregular migrants in the WHO European Region. Copenhagen: WHO Regional Office for Europe; 2016.

25. Saechao F, Sharrock S, Reicherter D, Livingston JD, Aylward A, Whisnant J, Koopman C, Kohli S. Stressors and barriers to using mental health services among diverse groups of first-generation immigrants to the United States. Community Ment Health J. 2012;48(1):98–106. https://doi.org/10.1007/s10597-011-9419-4.

26. Scuglik DL, Alacoon RD, Lapeyre AC, Williams MD, Logan KM. When the poetry no longer rhymes: mental health issues among Somali immigrants in the USA. Transcult Psychiatry. 2007;44(4):581–95. https://doi.org/10.1177/1363461507083899.

27. Shannon PJ. Refugees' advice to physicians: how to ask about mental health. Fam Pract. 2014;31(4):462–6. https://doi.org/10.1093/fampra/cmu017.

28. Shannon PJ, Wieling E, Simmelink-McCleary J, Becher E. Beyond stigma: barriers to discussing mental health in refugee populations. J Loss Trauma. 2015;20(3):281–96. https://doi.org/1 0.1080/15325024.2014.934629.

29. Singh NN, McKay JD, Singh AN. The need for cultural brokers in mental health services. J Child Fam Stud. 1999;8(1):1–10. https://doi.org/10.1023/A:1022949225965.

30. Svenberg K, Skott C, Lepp M. Ambiguous expectations and reduced confidence: experience of Somali refugees encountering Swedish health care. J Refug Stud. 2011;24(4):690–705. https://doi.org/10.1093/jrs/fer026.

31. UNHCR. A community-based approach in UNHCR operations. Geneva. 2008. Retrieved from: https://www.refworld.org/pdfid/47da54722.pdf.

32. UNHCR. Understanding community-based protection. Protection Policy Paper. Geneva. 2013. Retrieved from: https://www.refworld.org/pdfid/5209f0b64.pdf.

33. UNHCR. Community-based protection and mental health & psychosocial support. Geneva. 2017. Retrieved from: https://www.refworld.org/docid/593ab6add.html.

34. Valibhoy MC, Kaplan I, Szwarc J. "It comes down to just how human someone can be": a qualitative study with young people from refugee backgrounds about their experiences of Australian mental health services. Transcult Psychiatry. 2017;54(1):23–45. https://doi.org/10.1177/1363461516662810.

35. Valibhoy MC, Szwarc J, Kaplain I. Young services users from refugee backgrounds: their perspectives on barriers to access Australian mental health services. Int J Human Rights in Healthc. 2017;10(1):68–80. https://doi.org/10.1108/IJHRH-07-20160010.

36. Wallace NM, Berent JM, McCarthy TG, Senn TE, Carey M. Recruitment and retention of low-income, urban participants in a longitudinal study: recognizing and strengthening participants' motivations. Behav Ther. 2014;37(8):226–30.

37. Wallerstein NB, Duran B. Using community-based participatory research to address health disparities. Health Promot Pract. 2006;7(3):312–23. https://doi.org/10.1177/1524839906289376.

38. Weine SM. Family roles in refugee youth resettlement from a prevention perspective. Child Adolesc Psychiatr Clin N Am. 2008;17(3):515–32. https://doi.org/10.1016/j.chc.2008.02.006.

39. Weine SM. Developing preventive mental health interventions for refugee families in resettlement. Fam Process. 2011;50(3):410–30. https://doi.org/10.1111/j.1545-5300.2011.01366.x.

40. Weissbecker I, Hanna F, El Shazly M, Gao J, Ventevogel P. Integrative mental health and psychosocial support interventions for refugees in humanitarian crisis settings. In: Wenzel T, Drozdek B, editors. Uncertain safety: understanding and assisting the 21st century refugees. Cham: Springer; 2019. p. 117–53.

41. Wong EC, Marshall GN, Schell TL, Elliot MN, Hambarsoomians K, Chung CA, Berthold SM. Barriers to mental health care utilization for U.S. Cambodian refugees. J Consult Clin Psychol. 2006;74(6):1116–20. https://doi.org/10.1037/0022-006X.74.6.1116.

42. Young M, Chan KJ. School-based interventions for refugee children and youth: Canadian and international perspectives. In: Brewer CA, McCabe M, editors. Immigrant and refugee students in Canada. Edmonton: Brush Education; 2014. p. 31–53.

Index

© Springer Nature Switzerland AG 2020   271
S. J. Song, P. Ventevogel (eds.), *Child, Adolescent and Family Refugee Mental
Health*, https://doi.org/10.1007/978-3-030-45278-0